D0368688

HEALING MIRACLES

FROM MACROBIOTICS:

A Diet For All Diseases

JEAN CHARLES KOHLER
and
MARY ALICE KOHLER

PARKER PUBLISHING CO., Inc. ● WEST NYACK, N.Y.

This book is a reference work based on research by the authors. The opinions expressed herein are not necessarily those of, or endorsed by, the publisher. The directions stated in this book are in no way to be considered as a substitute for consultation with a duly licensed doctor.

Library of Congress Cataloging in Publication Data

Kohler, Jean Charles,
    Healing miracles from macrobiotics.

    Bibliography: p.
    Includes index.
    1. Macrobiotic diet. 2. Diet therapy.
I. Kohler, Mary Alice,   joint author.
II. Title. [DNLM: 1. Neoplasms--Diet therapy--
popular works. 2. Rice--Popular works. 3. Thera-
peutic cults--Popular works. QZ201 K79h]
RM235.K63   615'.854   78-23780
ISBN 0-13-384339-4

Printed in the United States of America

Comments by Physicians
Acquainted with Macrobiotics

This book is must reading for all cancer victims. Jean Charles Kohler, a musician-teacher, recovered from cancer of the pancreas, a death sentence in modern medicine. He and his wife, Mary Alice Kohler, have written a powerful challenge to modern medicine. And why not? There is nothing unreasonable about this duo presenting their well-documented theory, data, and experience; after all, medicine is too important to be left to doctors.

The Kohlers, followers of Michio Kushi, have made a major contribution by presenting his thought and his practical methods (even including "macrobiotic lunch boxes") in clear, understandable language. But they have also made an important contribution of their own by recounting their own amazing history and the detailed case reports of others close to them.

Scientifically trained doctors can be expected to reject these exciting case reports as "mere anecdotes." Perhaps more disappointing, the medical profession can be expected to ignore the urgings of the Kohlers that medical scientists collect the data and apply their statistical approach to determine the effect of macrobiotics.

The reason for this intransigence lies in the deep-rooted antipathy of modern medicine to applying nutritional approaches to the prevention and cure of disease. Only in the past few years, as the failures of the "miracle cures" of modern medicine are becoming increasingly obvious, has this attitude begun to change. Thus, this book, dealing with yin-yang, sugar, megavitamins, Laetrile and the rest of the nutritional spectrum, appears at a remarkably timely moment.

The healing miracles (and there is nothing inappropriate in that term) described by the Kohlers, occurring in people of all walks of life, provide a recipe that cannot be overlooked by any American who is ill today, from cancer or any other condition. Nor can this book be disregarded by anyone who is responsible for the care of others. The Kohlers themselves, aware of the urgency of their message, open their book with the statement, "If you or a member of your family are seriously ill, may we suggest that you begin reading this book with Chapter 11."

I would add — if you and your family are in good health, you must immediately begin reading this book with page one.

Robert S. Mendelsohn, M.D.

  Medical Director, American International Hospital, Zion, Illinois

  Associate Professor, Department of Preventive Medicine of the University of Illinois College of Medicine

  Former National Director of the Medical Consultation Service of Project Head Start

  Former Chairman of the Medical Licensure Board of the State of Illinois

  Author of the nationally syndicated column "The People's Doctor"

* * *

I have had personal experience with the macrobiotic diet, and feel that there are healthful benefits to be derived from it. At this stage of knowledge in nutrition, I do not believe much can be gained by "scientific" argument over its merits or demerits. The diet appears to be a wholesome vegetarian one with logical nutritional value. More than that, if pursued carefully, it will enable one to avoid the intake of a host of additives, preservatives, hormonal compounds, synthetics, extenders and pollutants and contaminants that certainly can, and do, harm our bodies, especially for those of us who have some weakness, tendency or already established health problem.

Over and above my searches through medical and scientific material I have sought the guidance of the Lord.

To those of you who seek health and healing, I can advocate that you do the same.

Richard A. Prindle, M.D.

  Director, Thomas Jefferson Health District, State of Virginia

  Member of the Teaching Staff of the Medical School of the University of Virginia

  1972-1977: Head of the Western Hemisphere Family Health Division of the World Health Organization

  1968-1971: Assistant Surgeon General of the United States

*   *   *

Macrobiotics began for me with the illusion of adequate health. Actually, I had become grossly insensitive to an ever worsening general condition in spite of my training as a physician and a keen interest in physical fitness. My history included long-time consumption of a diet of approximately 70% animal food, especially cheeseburgers, eggs, citrus fruits, french fries and other common foods.

As I began eating the strange, tasteless (then) macrobiotic foods whose names eluded me, the sense of a great adventure developed despite strong intellectual skepticism about such simplistic approaches. By day three, even waking up became a great joy, so many wonderful changes were coming. Over the ensuing months, changes continued, including an increased sense of body and mental lightness, increased endurance (running 6 miles a day without fatigue), and a new feeling to my skin.

I am convinced, by now, that countless others have also become entrapped within cycles of ill health and deterioration, and lack the experience and encouragement of a 9-day macrobiotic resurrecting experience.

Macrobiotics has become the fundamental discovery of my life, and I feel it has saved my life. However, it must be constantly emphasized that the unexpected healing of any serious disease is a multilevular process involving multiple unknown factors favorably interacting with natural diet, stress reduction, personal and family growth processes, and a widening philosophy of life."

Alan Kenney, M.D.
Moncton, New Brunswick, Canada

*   *   *

As a person who is firmly convinced that the balanced, vegetarian approach of Macrobiotics contributed substantially in my fight against cancer, I can only say that this is just the tip of the iceberg which will eventually have impact on the practice of medicine in the West.

We are slowly coming to realize that the incredible progress we have made through technology is not enough, and that dietary and lifestyle influences may in fact be considerably more important in the prevention and treatment of degenerative disease. Macrobiotics, when appropriately practiced, offers new approaches, from centuries of wisdom.

Anthony J. Sattilaro, M.D.

> Graduate of Health Systems Management Program, Harvard School of Public Health
>
> M.D. Degree Hahnemann Medical College, Philadelphia
>
> For 15 years by certification of American Board and College of Anesthesia, practiced and taught Anesthesia at Pennsylvania Hospital, Methodist Hospital, and University of Pennsylvania in Philadelphia, and was Attending Anesthesiologist at Hartford, Connecticut
>
> Now Associate Clinical Professor at Thomas Jefferson University, Philadelphia
>
> President, Methodist Hospital, Philadelphia

FOREWORD

by a world-renowned author and lecturer on macrobiotics

When I first met Professor and Mrs. Jean Kohler at my home in Brookline, Massachusetts, on September 26, 1973, I was immediately impressed by their sincere desire to find a solution to the severe health problems from which they had been suffering for several months. Whenever people come to me for advice, I ask whether normal medical treatments have been sufficiently tried, and if there is any possibility that such methods can help the problem, I will suggest that the individual continue to pursue that direction. However, as with many cases that are referred to me, theirs was apparently hopeless according to modern medical standards. Several minutes after we had begun our conversation, therefore, I suggested that they consider trying the macrobiotic approach.

In a short time, I knew that their situation was hopeful, both by observing their physical condition and through our conversation. Professor and Mrs. Kohler were extremely sincere, open, and humble, as well as persevering enough to understand what I was about to present to them. I noticed especially their compassion for other people. I felt I could present as fully as possible the wholistic, or macrobiotic, approach to changing their daily life from its previous pattern, since I could trust not only their power of comprehension, but also their love for each other. Any serious situation requires the understanding and support of a patient's spouse, relatives, and friends, who frequently share his or her daily life. In the case of Professor and Mrs. Kohler, it was apparent that they could offer each other mutual encouragement. Practicing the modifications in their daily life would require a certain amount of will, though the advice I gave them was very simple.

When we understand the Order of the Universe — the eternal law of God which functions without exception throughout the whole universe, including our human lives — the course of symptomatic illnesses, even if they appear critical, can be reversed. The universal Law of Change — or yin and yang, the antagonistic, complemental factors in all phenomena — is the basic principle of life, and therefore seemingly miraculous events result following its acceptance. Thousands of people throughout the world and many teachers throughout history have dedicated their efforts to the liberation of humanity from mental, physical, and social ills through the application of this basic principle.

The *biological* application of yin and yang, or macrobiotics, is not included within any particular field of medical science, as defined by modern concepts. It is, rather, a Way of Life to regain happiness, freedom, and health. It is not a special teaching or religion, but is part of the common knowledge which everyone originally has in the form of native or intuitive understanding. The dietary use of yin and yang, along with the corresponding change in an individual's way of thinking and living, is only one among countless applications of the Order of the Universe. However, it alone could release many people from needless physical and mental illness.

The happy outcome for Professor and Mrs. Kohler in solving their health problems is one of thousands of instances which I and many others have witnessed, recently and in the past. It is my hope that everyone can profit from the stories recounted in this book and can discover that such apparent miracles are possible, requiring only the simplest efforts, when we orient our habits of eating and way of life to agree with our natural intuition, insight, and judgment. It is my sincere wish that all people everywhere may have an opportunity to learn this wonderful Order of the Universe — the Way of Change — which is universal and endless.

Michio Kushi,
Founder and President,
East West Foundation

A Word from the Authors

Throughout this book, the word "cure" must be construed as *our* interpretation of the success my wife and I have observed from the use of macrobiotic principles in our lives and those of many of our friends. Michio Kushi, the remarkable man to whom this book is dedicated, is largely responsible for this success. But he is a philosopher and teacher rather than a licensed physician, and therefore makes no pretentions whatsoever of recommending "cures" or of making "medical" judgments.

Of course, even members of the medical profession, because of their meticulous training, are cautious about the use of the word "cure," especially in regard to diseases such as cancer, arthritis, multiple sclerosis, and others known to recur after remissions that can have the appearance of a cure. They would certainly not employ the term in speaking of the application of a macrobiotic food program, believing that it would not have the remotest chance of healing any illness. But for want of better terms, we use the words "cure" and "patient" simply to facilitate communication. In reality, those who visit Michio Kushi are like friends and visitors with whom he shares his knowledge, certainly not like patients.

However, no matter what medical people may say, or what our macrobiotic friends can legally say, I am convinced that I am, more than five years after major exploratory surgery, confidently and comfortably free of cancer of the pancreas, duodenum, and blood stream. My reasons for making such a statement are outlined in the Sequel to Chapter 9. Whether we use the term "cured," or "controlled," or "in a state of remission," those of us whose stories appear in this book are elated with the good health we are enjoying and expect and intend to enjoy throughout a very long life, now that we have found the way to align ourselves with the flow of the universe.

Many experts would declare that the proof we offer to promote our approach, far from being scientific, is nothing more than testimonials. But it happens that these "testimonials" are backed by medical records; and, additionally, the *number* of cases we describe is too great to be mere coincidence. This number seems impressive to us, at least, since we have limited ourselves to cases we know personally (as a result of an event that happened in September of 1973), with the addition of a few selected from those on file with

Michio Kushi's staff in Boston. And we feel that the chain of events presented in this book is so extraordinary that there has to be a basic truth in what macrobiotic philosophy expounds: namely, that *almost all illness is due to the patient's being out of balance with the laws of the universe and that the way to obtain relief from the illness is for the patient to get back into balance with these universal laws.* This applies mainly to food and to the patient's mental attitude. No drugs or surgery are required or desired in most cases; and generally what works for cancer will, with some modification, work also for a heart condition, for diabetes, multiple sclerosis, arthritis, allergies, cataracts, glaucoma, obesity, sickle cell anemia, and many other ailments.

Through this book we are hoping to help promulgate information about the amazing changes we have seen macrobiotics accomplish — changes which lead us to believe that *a solution for cancer is here now and has been all along, in addition to a solution for most other diseases.* It isn't, obviously, the cure-in-a-pill the public wants: there are many, many more people who would rather die than change their eating habits than there are people who are willing to give up the foods they will have to do without. A person with a serious illness will have to learn to live in accordance with universal laws, to continue to be very careful about what he or she eats, for an indefinite time, or the illness may return. But one learns to accept the laws willingly, gradually recognizing their derivation and their immeasurable benefits. For those whose desire to live gives them sufficient courage and self-discipline, or for those who are not ill, but who are strongly motivated to improve their health and to ward off future illness, we hope these pages will be convincing evidence that, as unbelievable as our claims seem, they are, nevertheless, actual examples typical of those that have worked for thousands of people.

Almost any doctor, nurse, medical technologist or scientist will be convinced that the miracles we claim for this food program are simply not possible: there could be no single diet that could bring obvious improvement in a wide diversity of illnesses. In the first place they may feel that, while there is increasing evidence that diet is a causal factor in many diseases, there certainly is no reason to believe that diet alone is going to save a terminal patient from death when he or she has only a very short time left. Yet we know of cases, my own among them, where that is exactly what happened. Second, if such a diet did exist, it would not be this strange and totally unfamiliar one called macrobiotic, which, we claim, saved all our lives. Since it bears little resemblance to currently accepted "balanced diets," most experts will regard this regimen as lacking in a number of basic requirements such as protein (because of no meat), calcium (no milk), Vitamin C (no citrus fruits or juices except the limited amount acceptable in their native areas), and so on. But just in our own brief experience my wife and I have seen many refugees from modern-day "food-group" diets who have recovered from major illnesses by adopting the wisdom of antiquity in eating simple grains, vegetables, beans, and seaweed. That these foods *do* contain all the essential nutrients is explained in Chapter 9, while the rationale for believing that modern nutritional reasoning is faulty is summarized in Chapter 7, page 95.

Our purpose in writing this book is two-fold: first, to give reassuring examples to people who are afraid of and bewildered by their illness, but are determined to recover; and second, to try to beg, coax, persuade, and finally challenge medical and research organizations to give respectful attention to the macrobiotic approach. We feel that the success of the people in this book is sufficient to warrant investigation by medical research groups. Even if the friends we tell you about here could look forward to no more than they have already had — months and months of unpredicted freedom from medication and from any serious discomfort or inconvenience — the record is remarkable enough to bear looking into.

As we describe later, we made many overtures to try to get medical authorities to check out our claims, to try to suggest that they incorporate macrobiotic ideas into their own practice. Perhaps at first they will be willing to offer this information only to terminal patients, who have nothing to lose and everything to gain by trying this approach. We are confident that doctors will find that macrobiotic principles, when correctly followed, will be consistently helpful in alleviating many illnesses. It is encouraging that a few medical people are beginning to listen with interest to the "new" but ancient concepts we try to set forth in this book, which was in the process of preparation, off and on, for about three years. For the first two years the theory of relating diet and cancer, believed in by only a very few people, was in a nearly static condition, and no matter what thrust we attempted we wound up in a blind alley. Then suddenly the situation began to change, and we have watched in wonderment as several of those blind alleys we had groped around in seemed to have opened up automatically. Chapter 6 has details of these breakthroughs. Yet we decided to record our trials and errors in the manner in which they unfolded for us, so that you might share in our appreciation of the significance of the prog-ress that we had feared would be years in coming about. Besides, we know from experience that there's a long, long way ahead to general acceptance. Only enough ice has been chipped off the 'berg to fill a small thimble. Too many times has Walt Whitman's familiar truism been applicable: "It is provided in the essence of things, that from any fruition of success, no matter what, shall come forth something to make greater struggle necessary."

What follows is not a documentation of hundreds of statistics, but rather a description by "confirmed" amateurs about adventures we hope will comfort and help many of you. We are jealous enough of our amateur standing that we would not want anyone to think that we are trying to resemble doctors, be doctor "substitutes," or prac-tice medicine. We simply share here a sincere and honest account of some absolutely incredible experiences which drastically altered our lives after the bottom fell out of our world! If *your* world has just been shattered by a diagnosis of serious illness for yourself or a member of your family, it is suggested that you begin reading this book with the first nine paragraphs of Chapter 10, and then move on to Chapter 11, so that you can get to the heart of the therapy early.

Jean Charles Kohler
with Mary Alice Kohler

This book is dedicated to

MICHIO KUSHI

with profound admiration and gratitude

by all of us

who participated in its creation

Contents

15

CHAPTER 1

Cancer? We've Been There — and Back!

Mary Alice Kohler (late summer 1973)

THE WAY THERE

When we landed at the Indianapolis airport the last day of September in 1973, my husband and I had mixed feelings of great hope and (for me, at least) submerged apprehension. Five days earlier, in Boston, we had been told by a Japanese philosopher who had a profound knowledge of Oriental medicine that we could solve my husband's cancer problem, which the doctors at the Indiana University Medical Center in Indianapolis had said after surgery on August 21 would take his life in one month to three years — with no chance for a reprieve. This was the word of Dr. John Jesseph, the chief surgeon. And Dr. Philip Christiansen, the other doctor on the case, had decreed, "I know of nothing coming out in research in the next ten years that could possibly help him." The grim sentence had been handed down.

Often we hear people say, in cases like this, "I couldn't believe anything of this kind could happen to *me*!" My husband, too, would have been voted by most people as one of the world's most unlikely candidates for a terminal cancer. Let me give you a little of the background.

Jean was 56 years old, a professor of piano at Ball State University in Muncie, Indiana. He had always believed strongly in keeping in good physical condition. Instead of taking the elevator to his studio on the fourth floor of the Ball State music building, he always climbed the stairs, often two at a time. His hobby was gardening, but a much more active gardening than most people do, for he had some 500 rose bushes in border planting around the outside edge of the yard and in foundation planting around the house. There also was a constantly increasing collection of evergreens of many rare varieties in all sizes, as well as a number of unusual Japanese maples.

Since he was continually replacing plants or moving them to get a better location, much of their care was strenuous work. He frequently sprayed the plants against fungus or other diseases — a task which required a lot of exercise. (Should he have been more wary of breathing the chemical sprays?)

In addition to the yard work, he practiced piano several hours every night, and then did a series of vigorous calisthenics such as push-ups, chin-ups, rope-jumping, and weight-lifting. It would seem that the exercise program was more than adequate.

He didn't smoke or drink — except perhaps a small glass of wine three or four times a year. He didn't care for strong, peppery foods. He drank milk and cocoa instead of tea or coffee. In a casual way, we tried to balance meals as well as we knew how from articles I swished through in cookbooks and magazines. Also, we dutifully ate six or seven almonds a day because clairvoyant Edgar Cayce in his readings declared that three almonds a day could ward off cancer. Not that we thought we'd ever have to be really concerned about having cancer — but just in case — and anyway almonds are quite tasty!* It would seem that we were eating properly.

Oh, but wait! Like most Americans, Jean had always eaten meat at least twice a day. We did use a lot of canned and packaged foods — "intelligently" selecting those advertised as being especially nutritious, of course. And all that exercise created quite a thirst, which had to be satisfied with quantities of soft drinks. (Jean always said he was a "Pepsiholic" rather than an alcoholic.) Then there was that sweet tooth, which required desserts, especially of the creamy variety, with plenty of whipping cream; and thick, tall milkshakes were pretty frequent. Some years ago an annual checkup revealed a threat of diabetes, so the soft drinks became "diet" drinks, and saccharin and sucaryl replaced sugar in desserts and cocoa. (Would sugar have been less harmful?) Almost every night he had a dessert-type midnight snack. Too late we found out that all these things are common to a large majority of cancer victims!

---

*In November of 1975 we received a thoughtful and helpful letter from Mr. G. Edward Griffin, president of American Media publishing firm and author of *World Without Cancer,* who had been kind enough to look over our manuscript. He commented that it was "interesting to note that you had tried to follow Edgar Cayce's recommendation of eating several almonds every day. Note, however, that when Edgar Cayce was giving his readings, the typical almond in the United States was of the bitter type. Since that time, they have been cross-bred to the point where the sweet almonds today have a much different flavor. The bitter almond was very rich in vitamin B_{17}. The sweet almond has none whatsoever. Therefore, if you had followed Edgar Cayce's advice in terms of the almonds available at the time he gave his readings, you would have been receiving a high dosage of vitamin B_{17}."

In the summer of 1973 Jean was eagerly involved in more concerts than usual, in addition to the regular teaching. This meant more hours of individual practice, more hours of rehearsing with other faculty members — and as a consequence fewer hours of work in the yard. Thus there was no activity to drain off the tension of a heavier work load. Earlier in the spring he had been gardening, however, so when in late May a rash developed around his ankles he assumed it was a gift from some sort of poison weed in the yard. Always before, such things had cleared up after a couple of weeks. But this time the itching kept spreading, although the rash was only on his ankles. Finally the itching became severe enough that he couldn't sleep at night, so it was time to check it out with our doctor. Antihistamine pills gave no relief, nor did changing our laundry detergent. So then a blood sample was analyzed — and our doctor was alarmed. He wanted Jean to get over to the I. U. Med Center immediately. We did talk the doctor into waiting a few days till the last recital was over, but finishing out the last several days of teaching for that term was forbidden.

On August 8 Jean entered the Medical Center for tests, and we still were expecting some easily corrected ailment to be found. However, days of intensive testing, including a painful liver biopsy, showed nothing. Exploratory surgery was indicated — for a guy who had had only a handful of sick days in his whole life! But the itching could be controlled only with drugs, and we knew he shouldn't continue that — so there seemed no choice.

The surgery was on the morning of August 21. About eleven o'clock, Dr. Jesseph came into the room where I was waiting and told me quietly that a large tumor — *malignant!* — had been found on the head of Jean's pancreas — that it had spread to the intestine — that it was loose in his system — that surgery to the pancreas would almost certainly be fatal — they were finding more and more of this type of cancer — they could keep him from suffering as the disease progressed — yes, we should tell Jean — always tell the patient, especially a man — plans he may want to make — travel perhaps — not much time — with the help of chemotherapy maybe a month, six months, maybe a year. A *month!* But this isn't just a character in a story, you know. This is a real person — this is *Jean!* And this isn't our usual luck. We've always counted on being lucky. I fought back fainting and could hear my voice saying, "I can tell you we'll try off-beat methods." I was thinking — I guess — of all the reading we'd done during the past few years on psychic and spiritual phenomena. I think I figured we'd try faith healing — or something — but I knew we'd try *something*.

"Well, we hope that whatever else you try, you'll stay with us on the chemotherapy."

"Oh, we will!"

"And I would hate to see you drag around everywhere and spend all your money trying one off-beat cure after another."

"We won't be foolish." I probably said something like that.

Dr. Jesseph explained that he had made a by-pass from the gall bladder into the intestine below the tumor, so that the bile would no longer back up into the liver and cause the relentless itching.

I don't know how long it was before they brought Jean back in — all pallid — and *gray*. Cancer color. Gray.

Sometime that day I phoned Jean's sister in Mount Vernon, Indiana. What a blow for her! Her mother — Jean's stepmother — had died a few years earlier with cancer that started in the breast. It took four years of surgery here, surgery there, radium treatments, and the final illness during which Elaine nursed her as tenderly as anyone has ever been cared for. I knew Elaine was thinking we'd have a repeat performance with Jean. Their 80-year-old Aunt Viola, who had taken care of Jean for several years after his mother died when he was four, lived with Elaine and her husband. How heartbreaking for her!

I phoned the head of the Ball State School of Music, hardly knowing what I was saying. Our good friend for 26 years, he said we should try many other things, and encouraged me by telling of recent successes in ostensibly conquering terminal cancer. But we both were thinking of friends we knew who had gone the radium route. ... And I phoned our close friend Mari, who with her seven-year-old son Ivan had become an extension of our family since her divorce a couple of years earlier. Actually, I phoned a mutual friend to tell Mari the crushing news because I knew she would become terribly upset — and that shouldn't happen if Ivan was around. I phoned another friend, a devotee of the Summit Lighthouse organization, who had frequently given us counsel from a wealth of knowledge in psychic and spiritual matters and Far Eastern philosophy. One of the most beautifully spiritual people we know, she was quietly confident that Jean could be cured in spite of the dire predictions.

I made rules: no matter what, we were going to be cheerful when we were with Jean — absolutely no tears when we were in his room. I told his sister, and I told Mari. Furthermore, when he came home, we would set up visiting on a rigid schedule, so that we could keep things as well-ordered as possible and not have Jean exhausted by long conversations.

Mari drove over to Indianapolis to see Jean and to take me home. (I had stayed in a motel near the hospital for a couple of nights.) When I got home the piano and I had a long, long cry. We knew the trials ahead would be slow and difficult. We knew how hard he would try to make things sound as they had before — how the motor control just wouldn't be there, how the memory would gradually become sluggish, how he'd be weak and gray and lose days of practice when the chemotherapy would make him sick and he'd have to build up the practice again. But we would keep encouraging him and telling him it would all come back — till the time came when it was too obvious that the skill would never return.

Elaine phoned and wanted to come up to see Jean right away. I argued that she should wait till he was stronger, and he had said that himself. But she insisted, and I was tense and angry about it. I reminded her that we'd have no weeping when we were with Jean. She came up by bus the next day, bringing special touches with her — a rosebud from her own garden (nurtured in water and aspirin all those hours!), a silly figurine, good cheer, assurance and comfort, and the latest copy of *Psychic* magazine. I hadn't had time to look at our copy, but she showed me an article in it that was to make quite a difference for us (more later about this account of Dr. Carl Simonton's use of psychic techniques in cancer cures).

Elaine stayed at Mari's, because I was too distraught to have anyone else around — even Elaine or Mari. In a couple of days Elaine's husband George drove up, bringing our blessed Aunt Viola, who made the trip without any obvious ill effects! Hospital rules allowed only three visitors at a time, so I went to the waiting room on that floor and George went downstairs for lunch. By the time an hour had gone by, I was explosive. What if I would have Jean for only month and they had kept me away from him for a whole hour of that precious time! I wasn't exactly rational, but George seemed to understand my distress. He had never yet failed — and he didn't fail this time — to come up with a perceptive remark at the precise moment to de-fuse the tension in family situations before any real confrontation developed.

We decided there might be some hope for Jean in psychic methods, which had been of interest to all of us for some time. Elaine and Viola were in a Spiritual Frontiers fellowship in Evansville and Mount Vernon, and we had all read many of the Edgar Cayce books, as well as many others on psychic phenomena. Here in Muncie at our Unitarian Church, we had had meetings of people who were interested in such matters. In early June we had taken the Silva Mind Control course in Indianapolis, where we learned techniques of relaxation and concentration which would help us attain a meditative state of mind. We learned that the mind is a powerful agent in making us well or sick — that we should vigorously avoid negative thoughts or statements, even in jest, because our "subconscious mind doesn't know when we're kidding." They told about many cases like that of Brian Piccolo, the famous football player, whose standard quip, when people commented on his strength and fine physique, was, "Sure, and I'll probably die of heart cancer!" Heart cancer is comparatively rare, but it got Brian Piccolo. His subconscious mind took him seriously.

We were supposed to make it part of our lives to meditate ten or fifteen minutes every morning and evening, relaxing the mind to be receptive to messages from within ourselves as well as from higher vibrations, pondering among other things the fact that we would never become ill from diabetes, cancer, or any other serious disease. We learned all this, and we were completely convinced of the power of the mind, but we were always extra busy. Since we weren't the type to have serious illness anyway, and since we stayed perpetually lucky, we didn't bother with the meditation routine. (Could we have prevented all we went through later that summer?)

Most of all, we had great faith in a clairvoyant in Muncie — a very calm, charming, no-nonsense lady who had given us a reading in July of 1971 and with whom we had periodic contact whenever we sent others to her for help. She can tell people so many things that *have* happened in their lives that it lends credence to what she says about the future. She had told Jean that he would have a long life, for she saw him as a very old man. "But," she said, "I see you in a hospital — something internal, I think — but it will turn out all right." (We had envisioned an illness in perhaps twenty years or so.)

Elaine thought I definitely should try to get in touch with our daughter Shirley, who, with husband Dick and their daughter Julie, was traveling on the west coast. I had thought about it many times, but had decided there was no use to spoil their trip when there was nothing they could do to help Jean. With Elaine's encouragement, I phoned various people they had planned to see, and found friends in Texas whose home they had not yet visited. I told them what had happened and suggested they have Dick phone me when they arrived. In a few days Shirley phoned, displaying the strength she always had in times of crisis, and they decided to come home without further stops.

A day or two after the surgery I saw Dr. Christiansen in the corridor and asked him for a sketch of the location of the tumor. Then I asked what the shortest life expectancy was for people who had Jean's condition. "Oh, three months." (Three months was a little better than one month.)

"And what's the longest time?"

A shrug. "Three years."

"Well, if we have three years, maybe something will be discovered that can cure it." That's when he made the pronouncement that there would be nothing to help.

"He will *seem* to be getting well, and will probably make a good recovery from surgery — but it won't last. He will start going downhill rapidly."

I could hardly talk, but I asked whether Jean should try to go back to work. "If he feels like it — probably part-time."

Elaine made it a point to ask Dr. Jesseph what the prospects were for Jean. He told her there was no hope whatsoever. A day or two later I asked one of the younger doctors for the sketch I wanted, and got a rough but adequate sketch this time. At least we would have an idea of where to beam our concentration if we could succeed in concentrating.

The family decided to ask all our psychic friends to work for us. We were home in the mornings, so I had a chance to see our mailman and ask him to help. He was studying to be a psychic healer and eagerly agreed to send healing to Jean during his meditations, and to ask his friends to do likewise. A very wonderful minister here in town, and a mutual friend who is a skilled chiropractor, agreed to work on it with their psychic group. We phoned to ask for similar help from an outstanding Methodist minister who was a good friend of the Mount Vernon family, but who had moved to Franklin, Indiana. (He had been the guiding light of Elaine's Spiritual Frontiers group.) Our psychic friends sustained us by telling us of miracle cures they had known, and of course we had read of dozens of such cases. Later we were to learn that son-in-law Dick phoned from Texas to his parents in Traverse City, Michigan, and his father volunteered to ask the order of Carmelite nuns there to say masses for Jean.

All the friends who called at the hospital or who heard about our trouble said we would be in their thoughts, although I imagine most of them had thoughts of despair. I wondered whether such a clamor had ever been set up for one person, from so many different types of people! We had little doubt that all this got us started on the road to recovery. (Those who are inclined to scoff at such beliefs should hold their fire until they have read a great deal about these subjects.)

One nurse at the Medical Center was very much "into" psychic knowledge, and with her we had shared brief but insightful exchanges. By contrast, none of the doctors had displayed the slightest interest in our psychic explorations — not even in the article about Dr. Simonton. During the days of preliminary examinations Jean was telling a couple of them about our clairvoyant's hospital prediction and one came up with a spark of humor in the remark, "It's a shame she didn't tell you exactly *what* the trouble would be!" (We were quite surprised some months later, when we had occasion to request copies of Jean's medical records, to find that one intern had written into his rough-draft report the comment that "[the patient's] clairvoyant told him he would live to a ripe old age but would have a rocky summer hospitalization in his future. Another clairvoyant friend suggested he have a blood and urine test when she found out about the itching." This friend was Mari, who in mid-July had had a dream that Jean was surrounded by doctors in surgical gowns!

On August 26 the chemotherapy was started intravenously. It was pathetic to see Jean take his daily "walks" in the corridors. He was very thin and weak, but most of the time he forced himself to take two walks a day, using the trolley carrying the chemotherapy bottle as a support, with Mari or Elaine on one side and me on the other. He did seem to gain strength, but the long incision made it painful to get in or out of bed, or when he had to cough; and the veins in his arms kept collapsing from the strain of the intravenous injections. I was worried about real damage to his arms and hands, which sometimes became badly swollen. Several times he had terrifying chills. It seemed as if not just the bed, but the whole room was shaking. Then he'd have a high fever. In spite of all this, by the time the Mount Vernon family had to leave on Sunday we were beginning to think there might be a glimmer of hope that we could keep Jean around for a while.

Jean himself had a great deal of hope by now. At first, when he was just barely conscious after surgery, he had believed the doctors and had figured he had very little time to live. He was too groggy to have much feeling about it, and anyway we had grown to believe strongly in reincarnation, which holds that we have more learning experiences on another level, with eventual return for further development here. So dying didn't alarm him. However, once the anesthetic wore off enough for him to regain real awareness, he knew that he couldn't let our clairvoyant be wrong, nor could he miss the chance to see all those rare evergreens grow up, nor could he abandon Ivan, to whom he had become a kind of guardian "Uncle Jean," who frequently jerked the energetic youngster back into line, taught him to play piano, and saw to it that his attitudes changed enough so that he began to learn quite well in school. (Ivan had been in desperate need of such strength, for his parents' divorce had been a shattering experience for him at an age when he was particularly sensitive and impressionable.) When finally the five days of chemotherapy were over and Jean could go home the next day, he told Dr. Jesseph that he had decided to live to be an old man. "It's very if-fy," was the reply.

We signed out of the Medical Center on August 30, after making an appointment for another five days of chemotherapy starting September 26.

On the gentle drive home, I was thinking back over the twenty or so times Mari and I had made the trip since August 8. It was during those trips that I reflected on what had happened and what might now happen. One of the main things that sustained me was the statement of our lady of clairvoyance: "I see you as a very old man." (Or was she only seeing him as an old man because his serious illness would make him look that way in the next few months?! Still, she had been right about a hospital siege, and something internal. On the other hand, "It will turn out all right" could be interpreted more than one way! But I tried to suppress those ideas in order not to give power to negative influences.) Even more strength came from the ancient philosophy that there is a purpose in everything. There had to be some reason for all this.

Another source of help came from the article in the *Psychic* magazine Elaine had brought. Titled "Meditation and Psychotherapy in the Treatment of Cancer," it was written about a Dr. O. Carl Simonton, chief of radiation therapy at Travis Air Force Base.[1] It told of the outstanding success he had been having in treating cancer patients by using a combination of group therapy, meditation, instilling the will to live, and continuing cobalt radiation treatments. In regard to the meditation, three times a day, for a fifteen-minute session, the patient was to relax by imagining a peaceful scene or incident, then concentrate on the cancer location and imagine white blood cells swarming around the infection to carry away the cancer cells killed by the radiation treatments. At the end of the meditation the patient was to imagine himself well. Dr. Simonton had long noticed that those patients who had some definite goal

("I can't die yet — I have to get my son through college!") had a
much better recovery percentage than those who expressed no such
desires. These were techniques we had studied in the Silva course!

I had started trying to get in touch with the extraordinary Dr.
Simonton by phone while Jean's family were still here. On the Mon-
day morning after they left I was told that he was in a meeting and
would call me back when it was over. In less than an hour he phoned.
He listened with understanding kindness to my story. Then he said
he would send me the name of a book to order and the address of a
place where I could order a tape of one of his lectures. "Cancer
works slowly," he reassured me, and said there was time to wait for
the material to arrive. When I asked him about other cancer cures
we'd heard about, he said we should stay with any method as long as
it seemed to be working. "He can tell if he's getting well," he remarked. (Underscore that statement!) I asked him whether it would
be possible for Jean to recover and he said yes! So maybe there was
hope after all. I kept thinking of this as we drove back and forth to
Indianapolis.

Dr. Simonton said he was leaving the Air Force soon to open
his own clinic (see Appendix), but that Travis AFB would know how
to reach him if we wanted to contact him after reading the book and
hearing the tape. Although I offered to send a check for the telephone interview, he said not to bother, since the Air Force paid his
salary. I felt sure we'd go to Dr. Simonton's clinic as soon as Jean
was able to travel.

Note for Chapter 1

[1]Jean Shinoda Bolen, M.D., "Meditation and Psychotherapy in the Treatment of Cancer,"
Psychic, July/August, 1973, pp. 19-22.

CHAPTER 2

The Way Back

Mary Alice Kohler

My husband didn't behave too much like an invalid when we got home, and my plans for limiting visiting time became obsolete. He took sunbaths and ate well and walked rather strongly. In a day or two he began practicing a little. There was almost none of the fumbling I had dreaded! (But I remembered, "He will *seem* to be getting well," and I dared not hope too much.)

For a couple of months a remarkable young woman, a Ball State student, had been helping us with yard work. Pattye left for California just a day or two after Jean came home, but she gave us some books she didn't want to take along. One she had urged us to check was the Jethro Kloss *Back to Eden*. In this we read statements such as, "No disease can exist in a pure blood stream."[1] And, "Man does not go astray from nature because he lacks intelligence, but because he wishes to gratify his own desires."[2] Kloss gave us our first insight into the fact that any disease can be cured by proper diet, exercise, and mental attitude: his approach to food was definitely spiritual. In the many cases he described, the miracles were effected in terminal illnesses by the use of herbs, massage, compresses, and enemas as preludes to proper diet and exercise. We were impressed by his long discussion on cancer, analyzed the whole book carefully and worked out an elaborate "Kloss system" for Jean. We could use a wide variety of foods, potatoes being especially good, as were tomatoes (but not at the same meal). Vegetable juices, fruit juices, and fruit were recommended. But no meat or dairy products — make a note of that. We still think the Kloss book has great value, in spite of being very disorganized. Anyone who wants to use his ideas should study the entire book carefully to work out the contradictions.

In a couple of weeks another friend brought us a pamphlet from the Kelley Research Foundation in Grapevine, Texas (now located in Winthrop, Washington). Their booklet, "One Answer to Cancer" (see our Bibliography), told of foods which had been typical of the diet of cancer victims — exactly the things Jean used to eat.

Their recommendations, resulting from Dr. Kelley's own remarkable recovery from the last stages of pancreatic, metastasized cancer, were so similar to those of Kloss (again, no meat or dairy products) that we phoned to ask about going there for an examination. They told us that they had to have their patients referred to them by an M.D., and they hoped we could work that out. (We had heard that the referral was made necessary by pressure from the medical profession.) After considerable searching, we found a doctor who was about to retire who agreed to sign the referral which the Kelley Foundation had mailed to us — and we made flight reservations to Dallas for September 25. The examination would take one day and $300 and would result in a diet tailored to Jean's individual needs, plus food supplements, plus enemas, plus faith, all of which could be practiced at home. We could fly back to Indianapolis in time to keep our chemotherapy appointment at the Medical Center.

However, a few days before the 25th we drove down to Mount Vernon to visit Jean's family. A friend here in Muncie who had a habit of helping us had told us of a nutritionist in Evansville — Mrs. Judith Viehe (see Appendix: INDIANA) — who knew about an Oriental diet which was supposed to cure cancer, so we made an appointment to see her while we were down there. Well, she knew her field so well that we were willing to listen to her theories. She persuaded us that with Jean's type of cancer fruit juices (and chemotherapy!) were likely to spread the toxins throughout the body, and she told us of the total benefits of the "macrobiotic" diet. She stated a basic principle of this ancient philosophy — one we were to hear many times afterwards — that all illness is simply a matter of being out of balance with the laws of the universe, and that proper food can bring us back into balance. "Yin" and "yang" (the expansive and the contractive, light and dark, hot and cold, sweet and bitter, and all other opposites) need to be taken into consideration in building our lives. Judith told us about her study in Boston with Michio Kushi, the foremost authority anywhere on macrobiotic diet, and when Jean asked whether we should get an appointment with him she thought it would be an excellent idea. However, she avoided giving us too much encouragement, since, as she said, cancer in the pancreas is a very "deep" cancer. After much deliberation, and a phone discussion with Mr. Kushi, we cancelled the flight to Dallas — and the chemotherapy — and made reservations to Boston instead.

By phone we had been given instructions to stay at "Newton House," one of several mansions which were rented in the Boston area for the purpose of teaching people about macrobiotic methods. Bill and Andrea Kaufman managed Newton House, and Andrea cooked dinner every evening for those who stayed there for varying periods of time to learn how to recover from whatever illness they had. Usually there were about twenty people around. As she cooked, she gave quiet and inspiring instructions to anyone who wanted to absorb this philosophy. I learned that brown rice is sacred — not even one grain should be wasted — and that the atmosphere must be kept serene in the kitchen while this food is being prepared. I learned how to prepare vegetables in the macrobiotic way and in what order to sauté them, how to make miso soup and put seaweed in it, how to make bancha tea (the only beverage Jean would be allowed to have) and how to vary the diet while using these simple but royal foods.

At Newton House we heard much talk about the fabulous "Michio": he had a phenomenal ability to analyze ailments at a glance, and his extensive knowledge was respected by all who came into contact with him. Through arrangements made by widely scattered macrobiotic centers, he constantly lectures at well-attended seminars in many cities in this country and abroad. (On a recent tour of his native Japan, he gave 36 lectures in 30 days.) There is a broad range of lecture topics — philosophy, world religions, anthropology, world history, social problems, and health, for example, including special sessions for medical doctors. Mrs. Kushi almost always accompanies him on his travels, giving classes in macrobiotic cooking and other phases of Oriental culture.

As glowing as the praise had been for the astounding Michio, we were not disappointed. At eleven o'clock on the night of the 25th we kept our appointment at Mr. Kushi's home, after his return from his evening lecture. As at Newton House, we took off our shoes at the front door, and sat on cushions on the floor. We had a lengthy discussion with Mr. Kushi, during which he showed me a small blister on Jean's right eye, explaining that that indicated the trouble was in the pancreas. (In Oriental medicine the exploratory surgery, in most cases, would not have been necessary!) He also said that the blue-gray color of the whites of Jean's eyes indicated cancer.

Then came the instructions: "These things — *out:* all meat, all dairy products." (Again!) "All sweets — no sugar, no honey, no syrup. All chemicalized foods. All canned foods, for at least two years. All fruits, including bananas. All fruit juices. Potato, tomato," (Sorry, Mr. Kloss!), "eggplant, asparagus, avocado, spinach, beets, mushrooms, sweet potato. All refined foods. All soft drinks. All nuts — temporarily. All spices, yeast, alcohol." Well, at least the last one wouldn't be difficult — and Jean didn't like avocado or mushrooms or any of the vegetables except potato and tomato.

"Now, these he *can* eat: 50 percent of food should be grain, especially brown rice. Also millet, corn, buckwheat, rye, barley, oatmeal, wheat flours, whole-wheat and buckwheat spaghetti. 25 percent should be cooked vegetables." (He gave a long list of many vegetables not forbidden above.) "Pumpkin or squash may frequently replace half the cooked vegetables. 10 percent beans, especially garbanzo or azuki, 5 percent seaweed, 5 percent miso soup, 5 percent raw vegetables. Chew each mouthful at least 100 times. Two or three meals a day, eating as much as desired but not overeating. At the end of the meal, the beverage may be bancha tea, which may be taken during the day if thirsty; but in general drink as little as possible. No other beverage. No snacks — and never eat for three hours before the night's rest. No nap for one hour after meals. A hot ginger compress to the abdomen every evening. All activities are fine. Do not feel you need a lot of bed rest because you have been ill."

About a half hour after midnight we were asking the final questions. How long did he think it would take to be free of the cancer? A moment's silence. Then, "Three to six months." What an exciting birthday gift just a half-hour after Jean's birthday had begun! Six months, or less, to *life* instead of six months to live! And to think that we first planned to start chemotherapy that day! We were welcome to phone Mr. Kushi at any time we had questions. Then it was back to our shoes and back to our motel.

We stayed in Boston three more days, sightseeing a little, being lost a lot, learning how to cook all that strange food, and eating meals at Newton House. We bought many books about the macrobiotic way of life, and packed boxes of food to bring back on the plane, to last until our natural foods store in Muncie could order what we needed. Jean had done a lot of traveling for a man just a month away from surgery.

If we could believe our macrobiotic friends, we had the rudiments of a knowledge that could solve most health problems, or keep well people healthy. Moreover, their eventual goal is the establishment of "one peaceful world" — a large order, it seemed to us! In an over-simplified form, one ramification of the philosophy is that if we are in good health we can better turn our attention to the building of a peaceful world, and better contemplate the purpose of human beings in the universe.

We were to become more and more convinced that we could believe them. One of the most amazing, and totally unexpected, benefits for us personally was that after only five days of macrobiotic food, Jean's hands were suddenly much more flexible. He could reach farther on the keyboard than ever before! This condition has remained to the present time.

While he was enjoying this new-found flexibility, my own hands were staying warm from wringing them over what to do with all that food. I had acquired a lot of respect for it in Andrea's kitchen, but to be faced with it all alone so far from Boston was a frightening prospect. But gradually we got all other food moved out and grains and beans, whole-wheat spaghetti and noodles, flours, seaweed, tea, and seeds squirreled away. Never very capable in the kitchen, I had many a struggle and spent many an hour studying macrobiotic cookbooks and keeping us fed, and we ate many an experiment that had fizzled.

Mari, too, although a skillful gourmet cook, studied the new cookbooks — and in a short time was brightening our lives by adding gourmet touches to this ancient food. She began to remember much of all this from her childhood in Japan, although the Japanese people for years had been digressing more and more into Western ways (and more illness). We took some of the food down to Mari's almost every evening and she cooked the rest of the meal, with many innovative touches. All her Japanese friends here in Muncie added enthusiastic ideas and help. We were also lucky in that our faithful little Mazda natural foods store stocked everything we needed, and we had one meal a week at the Harvest Moon natural foods restaurant near the campus. The people in both businesses took a helpful interest in Jean's recovery.

In the fall term (just two and a half weeks after surgery) Jean had begun teaching a half-load, armed with a key to the elevator. But on the second day he was half-way up the stairs before he remembered he had the key, and that was the last it was needed. At first I drove him to school, letting him out to walk the last block, the last two blocks, the last three blocks, still chewing the unleavened bread I was learning to make. Before long he was walking the near-mile both ways twice a day — and had time to chew a whole piece of bread on the way in. He bought a survival (!) jacket and boots — and no matter what the weather was dealing out, he walked. He began a gradual program of calisthenics each night.

Now there were a few times when he got too cocky. One night

he practiced till about 2:00 a.m., taught and had meetings the next morning, and was supposed to go back to hear student exams in the afternoon. But at noon he had one of those awful chills, followed by the high fever. I was heartsick. (Our first warning from the cancer enemy, I thought, but of course I only fussed at Jean and told him it was the result of getting over-tired. Later I learned that it didn't occur to him that it could be anything *else* but over-fatigue resulting from post-surgery weakness.) A few weeks later the same thing happened after our first heavy snow, when he insisted on shoveling the whole driveway. And there was one other time like that. But that was all — and it's now been more than eleven months. For a long time he looked gray when he got even a little tired, and that was scary, but eventually even that symptom disappeared.

One distressing feature was that there was a continual weight loss. He felt better and stronger all the time, but his weight continued to go down. Our macrobiotic friends would say only that "there is some weight loss at first." (But 45 pounds?!) Of course, the inactivity in the hospital and the weakening effects of the surgery would cause some loss. Still, knowing that weight loss is symptomatic of cancer would have made me very uneasy except that I was losing steadily, too. (I had decided to follow the same diet, so that we'd have some sort of check.) My eventual loss was 22-23 pounds — down to 83! Since I didn't have cancer, it had to be because of the diet, although we ate large amounts of food and didn't count a single calorie.

About mid-November we developed a constant "dark-brown" taste in our mouths which was so persistent that we finally decided to phone Mr. Kushi about it. He said we had become too "yang" and could now add a little fruit to our diet — and a small, thin portion of baked or broiled fish once a week. We had been promoted! He was completely placid about our weight, and said that when the proper time came we would gain. Two days after we began putting boiled raisins and dried apples in our rice for breakfast the dark taste disappeared. (Check the breakfast menus in Chapter 13.)

Every morning and evening after the first of October Jean did some breathing exercises recommended by our lovely Summit Lighthouse friend. Then he would meditate on getting rid of the cancer and on being completely well, using Silva and Simonton techniques. Also, during his walks, he did a lot of "psyching out" of things he wanted to improve.

Soon after Jean's surgery, Elaine had phoned Gordon Melton in Chicago, one of the national leaders of the Spiritual Frontiers groups. He phoned us one evening and we asked him whether he would either give us an appointment or suggest someone else who had had success in psychic healing. We thought if the distance wasn't too great we would make the trip to confer with such a person. Mr. Melton said he didn't know why we'd want to travel when two of the best people anywhere — a man and wife team — lived right here in Muncie! He gave us their name and we hit it lucky — they were home and would come over that very evening. They generously gave the entire evening to discussing their ideas and giving Jean a relaxation session. In time we got a few people together and took a course of six lessons from the psychic couple. Some of it was similar to the Silva Mind Control course, but Jean was given a lot of specific attention. He and Mari seemed to derive considerable benefit from these sessions.

All the psychic methods we had any association with had religious or spiritual emphasis, mostly in a universal sense, but with frequent references to Christianity, Buddhism, and other orthodoxies.

Every few days after Boston I would check the little blister in Jean's right eye. After a couple of months it suddenly became almost invisible, and soon I couldn't find it even with a magnifying glass! The whites of his eyes gradually became clearer. (Could I possibly now begin to have *real* hope?)

During the winter quarter Jean began teaching a full load, and on January 7 he gave one of the best recitals he'd ever played, using a program that would have taxed the strength of one who had never been ill. It was a miracle that he was even alive, and yet he was doing more than he ever had before. The wonderment of it was great. Shirley, Dick, and Julie had spent frequent weekends with us since September and they came down from Kalamazoo for the recital. Elaine came from Mount Vernon. Mari had a gala party for everybody. It was a high point in the lives of all of us!

As early spring began to emerge on an occasional day, Jean started more arduous work in the yard than ever before. More plants were moved, more new ones added, and better care given to all of them. No matter how much work he did he felt rested after less sleep than he used to need. In late February, in a blizzard, he found that his legs would run again, even up hill! The calisthenics were getting back to pre-surgery level, and on April 19, he was able to take the four flights of stairs to his studio two at a time. The last barrier to recovery was overcome.

When we went back to Boston on April 7 to confirm what we knew was true (Remember Dr. Simonton's saying, "He can tell if he's getting well?"), it still was exciting and comforting to have Mr. Kushi say, again after a careful examination, that all signs of cancer had disappeared. There still was a small tumor, he said, but only about the size of a walnut, and it was no longer malignant. Also, there was some hardness in the abdomen which might in time cause trouble. Therefore, to finish dissolving these potential trouble spots, we were to continue the diet as it was for another six months (although by July we could add a little pure maple syrup!). After six months we would be able to relax the diet quite a lot. Mr. Kushi said we would soon begin to gain weight, a prediction which is now slowly coming about. Mari was with us on this trip and we celebrated by sight-seeing in Boston and Washington, D.C., then driving in a rented car to some rare-plant nurseries in Pennsylvania and New Jersey before flying home again from Washington.

Actually, we'll always keep basically to the macrobiotic diet. Many unpleasant complaints we had come to accept in pre-cancer days have disappeared — the bad taste in the mouth in the morning, the need for deodorants, the chronic pains in the joints here and there, "common colds." There's no mucus in our systems for a "cold" to hang on to. But it will be fun to digress once in a while, and add a few more foods that we will enjoy. We plan to stay young till we're at least 90 or 95, and of course we'll never have to worry about overweight, no matter how much we eat!

The more we studied about the macrobiotic way the more we felt the need to let others know about it. [Chapters 3 and 4 detail our various attempts, carried to the point of being obnoxious. Books with macrobiotic information and other data helpful for starting and continuing a macrobiotic life are listed in the Appendix and Bibliography.]

The macrobiotic philosophy was rescued from oblivion a number of years ago by George Ohsawa, Michio Kushi's teacher. To a life style that had been part of certain civilizations of 3,000 years ago or more, Ohsawa gave the name *macro* (comprehensive) *biotic* (way of life). Followers of Shintoism, of Lao Tsu and his Taoism, of Buddha, and of Confucius, as well as people of ancient Western countries, had generally embraced a macrobiotic type of life as a natural part of their culture. They enjoyed the ensuing benefits of sturdy health, longevity, and peace until corrupted by outside influences of wider travel and communication. Ohsawa dedicated his own life to bringing the ancient philosophy to the attention of all those who would listen in European countries, particularly France and Belgium, while Michio, after a time, came to this country. One of Ohsawa's favorite philosophies was, "Nothing is so curable as an incurable disease, but nothing is so incurable as the patient himself"—for people as a rule are reluctant to change their habits, especially in regard to their food.

Our fervent hope is that more people who need help will learn about the macrobiotic methods. It should be emphasized that to follow this particular "diet" ("food program" or "way of eating" would be more accurate) is not a deprivation but a privilege. We believe it is an open gateway to curing almost any illness, or to avoiding illness throughout life.

These may seem like fantastic statements we make, but we feel that being given a way to cure a malignant tumor in the pancreas — definitely a terminal cancer by medical standards — is a fantastic experience. Far from being kept alive only by drugs and medication, Jean hasn't needed even an aspirin tablet in all these months. We know his continuing good health to be a permanent condition even though no physician would verify the fact.

Doctors will not be likely to admit publicly that he is cured until an autopsy 35 or 40 years from now proves that he has no more cancer cells than normally healthy people always have. But even if the cancer is only in a state which the medical profession would call "controlled," it has been so completely subdued for so many months that we do not feel we should wait for the autopsy to try to convince others that cancer need no longer be a dread disease, or that other serious illnesses can be partially or wholly conquered. In time, a dietary cure for cancer may be accepted, just as acupuncture, long scorned by the medical profession, is now becoming respectable.

We are extremely fortunate, of course, and if you think back over the way things happened it seems as if everything fell into place for us like pieces in a large puzzle. A part of the puzzle, too, is being able to recognize the good luck in situations that do occur. Jean says, for instance, that having an "incurable" cancer is one of the best things that ever happened to him. It gives him a chance to improve his health even beyond the good constitution he originally had, and it gives him the opportunity to share good health with many others. Very few people have the strength of optimism and the self-discipline that he has — but these qualities can be developed. Perhaps his special ability to interest others in this way to a good life is the purpose I was looking for behind his illness.

Notes for Chapter 2

[1]Jethro Kloss, *Back to Eden* (New York, N.Y.: Benedict Lust Publications, Beneficial Books, 1971), p. 160.

[2]*Ibid.,* p. 114.

CHAPTER 3

Where Do We Go from Here?

Jean Kohler

AN INCREDIBLE DISCOVERY — A DIET FOR ALL DISEASES!

The adventure of curing my absolutely terminal cancer of the pancreas and small intestine was an exciting experience, as my wife described it in the preceding chapters. The most exciting part of all was the realization, on our second visit to Michio, that the diet that had saved me from a fast-approaching death would indeed work for almost any illness. We had often read the macrobiotic belief, of course, that illness is caused by being out of balance with universal laws, but to have Michio's affirmative answer to my question as to whether the diet would relieve heart trouble, arthritis, and a host of other ailments seemed like an incredible discovery. Words can hardly express the vastness and importance of it.

However, this astounding discovery was soon followed by another one almost as unbelievable but not at all wonderful — namely, that it seemed impossible to let the world at large know that there was help for thousands (even millions) who needed it. Skepticism we expected as only natural. I was a bit incredulous myself when I first heard that there was a way of healing terminal cancer through diet.

Many people with conventional opinions are also suspicious of our interest in psychic phenomena and the power of the mind in healing ourselves, although I hope that few are as adamant as the chief of one cancer center who said to a respected psychotherapist, Dr. Lawrence LeShan, when discussing a theory of mental attitude in relationship to cancer, "Even if you *prove* your theory, I still won't believe it!"[1] To such people our searching into psychic matters makes us suspect in other areas as well, including our belief in macrobiotics as a way of relieving illness.

Skepticism also leads many people to question whether certain of the cases included in this book were really terminal or incurable by medical standards. The answer is definitely yes. The prognosis for me, for example, was in a way a "double terminal" one, and therefore the increasingly vigorous health I am enjoying in my sixth year after surgery should be all the more proof that the macrobiotic program can bring about a real cure, rather than some kind of inexplicable remission. The reason I use the "double" label is that in addition to the large malignant tumor on the pancreas, which the doctors regarded as incurable and fast acting, there was the matter of the cancer of the small intestine. Intestinal cancer is not by any means incurable but Western doctors generally consider it as such if it is not treated by surgery followed usually by radium, cobalt, or chemotherapy. In my case, since the tumor on the pancreas was inoperable and fatal anyway, the surgeon wisely decided not to undertake the usual approach of removing part of my intestines (thank God!). Moreover the doctors were certain that the cancer cells were loose in my system and were sure to form malignant tumors any place at any time.

As regards the effectiveness of the macrobiotic diet versus the finality of my illness, since I didn't die from the pancreatic cancer, and the intestinal cancer was not treated by surgery, and neither of these organs was treated by chemotherapy, it seems obvious that the change was brought about by the diet, plus a positive belief in it. For all that malfunction to clear itself up with no relationship to the diet would be practically an impossibility. As we have pointed out, medication could have had no bearing on my recovery, for I have had none at all since the end of August, 1973. This reasoning seems to us to be satisfactorily convincing. (I did spoil my record by taking two aspirins for a 1977 toothache!)

The "credentials" for the other people whose stories are in this book are equally verifiable. Without macrobiotics, some of us would be dead or severely invalided and under the threat of a slow death. Instead, we are all well and active and are all planning to continue to improve in health and strength for years and years to come.

The potentiality as well as the validity of the macrobiotic way in helping sick people seemed so obvious to me, and yet so many people, both sick and well, remained unimpressed, that it became an obsession with me to look for ways to spread the news. Knowing from the beginning that I was going to get well, and then watching the recovery come about, meant so much to me that I could hardly understand why other people didn't feel the same way about themselves — why most of them didn't want to take my experience and use it in their own lives.

The depth of my feeling about this knowledge was manifested in a very personal reaction which began happening before I left the hospital and continued at irregular intervals for about two years. It was a very private thing and even Mary Alice did not know about it until I mentioned it to her in July of 1976. By that time it had stopped. I refer to the fact that I had spells of crying, always when alone, and not for the reasons one might expect. The tears were shed not because of pain or discomfort, or fear, or self-pity, or anxiety. Rather they were the result of moments of exhilaration, happiness, and wonder that I, among the thousands who had died of cancer of the pancreas, was going to survive and be in better health than ever. I was absolutely convinced that I was going to conquer the malignancy, and the wonder of it overwhelmed me.

The only other tears during my convalescence occurred when my eighty-year-old Aunt Viola came into the hospital room to visit me, having traveled some two hundred miles (in spite of somewhat delicate health after a number of illnesses and several surgeries) to get there very soon after my own operation. Far from being an expression of grief, those tears, also, overflowed because of a feeling of joy and deep gratitude that she would make a trip so difficult for her in order to encourage me. Since I never did feel fear or despair, I wanted very much to help other people avoid these emotions.

Gradually I began to be less frustrated by the reluctance of many people to part with their fears. Many seemed *more* afraid of the type of hope I felt I could offer! Since the patients who accepted macrobiotic ways made great strides toward getting well, I very much wanted to figure out how to reach a larger audience so that the small percentage who *were* receptive would comprise more people. I know there must be thousands upon thousands who, like me, *are* willing to learn to heal themselves, who *are* looking for a reprieve from the apparent death sentence, and who want a lifetime reprieve rather than a temporary one. I don't intend to keep quiet, because if our friend had kept quiet when I first learned I had cancer, I could not be making this much noise now.

Of course I realize that the lack of acceptance of new concepts is woven into the story of the human race. Actually macrobiotic and psychic beliefs are simply renewals of age-old concepts, many of which were gradually discarded as superstitions because people lost the ability to get in touch with their original universal psychic nature. (Macrobiotic philosophy holds that this loss was the result of eating wrong foods.)

There is a double-barreled reason why most people resist ideas that are contrary to their current beliefs: (1) The "new" concept seems incredible by their standards and (2) their disbelief is reinforced by their confidence that if the concept were valid the majority of experts in the particular field would promote it or at least not oppose it.

A quick look at some historical facts shows the fallacy of placing too much credence in the experts and in the commonly accepted beliefs of any era. For centuries people had the notion that "royal blood" was different from that of the commoner. Not only the laymen but apparently even the scholars of the time were convinced of this. And probably the most difficult truth of all unbelievable truths for people to accept was that the earth is round and that only gravity keeps us all from flying through space as astral bodies! The story of Galileo is an even better illustration. If only his critics had *looked* through his telescope at Jupiter's moons!

Hearing that French peasants insisted rocks had fallen from the sky, the French Academy of Science announced publicly that of course rocks could not fall from the sky. And when Thomas Jefferson learned that two scientists had agreed with the French peasants he said that he could much sooner believe that the scientists lied for some personal reason than he could believe that rocks did indeed fall from the sky. Of course today we know that the French peasants were right and the Academy of Science absurdly wrong. We call these rocks meteorites.

The French Academy did no better when some of its members heard one of Edison's first phonographs. They threw out the man who brought it to them and said that no cheap ventriloquist was going to fool them. It apparently didn't take much to fool that august body of learned men!

In another instance some scientists working in the Arctic were befriended by the Eskimos of the region. Wishing to show their appreciation they selected one man from the tribe and brought him back to civilization so he could return and tell the tribe about the home of the scientists. They thought this was a kindness to the tribe, but it proved to be the cruelest thing they could have done as far as the man they selected was concerned. When he returned home and told his tribe what he had seen, his name was changed to mean "the man who always lies," and he was forever branded a consummate fabricator. The Eskimos first of all could not grasp the facts of the entire nature of the planet Earth: they could not conceive of a place where there was not constant ice and cold, with no whale meat to eat. Nor could they comprehend the crowded population, or the highly advanced technology.

Their derision reminds me of the story of the old farmer when he saw his first train. This happened back in the days when locomotives were a new thing. He surveyed the mass of tons of steel and iron sitting on the track, hopelessly immobile. When someone asked him what he thought of it he said, "They'll never start 'er." After the train was roaring down the tracks the same someone asked again, "What do you think now?" "They'll never stop 'er," was the reply.

The idea of television was incomprehensible to most of us fifty years ago, yet today it is commonplace. And just six months before Sputnik one of the leading British astronomers said that there could *never* be space travel!

My Dad felt, as did most people, that man could never land on the moon. When the first serious discussions about space travel began he thought it was all nonsense. Later on he happened to be visiting us during the time of the second moon walk. When he realized that the TV coverage of that event had pre-empted his beloved St. Louis Cardinals he was unhappy, to put it very mildly. After watching the moon walk for a few minutes he shuffled disgustedly out of the room snorting, "When you've seen one moon walk you've seen them all." I think he felt that replacing *his* baseball team on TV for this lesser event was a Cardinal sin.

For centuries acupuncture has been practiced in most parts of the world. Almost any place where Orientals have lived in any numbers they have had some of their members practicing acupuncture, acupressure, and moxabustion.* In addition many Occidentals have received benefits, both in their own country and in the Orient, from acupuncture treatments. However, the Western medical profession chose to scoff at the idea that "sticking needles in your toes will cure a headache." The *only* reason that today acupuncture is *beginning* to be accepted in medical circles in this country is the fact that when former President Nixon went to China he took along a couple of distinguished doctors. During the tour a *New York Times* reporter traveling with the party needed an emergency appendectomy. The doctors, as well as a number of reporters, watched the operation, for which acupuncture was used as an anesthetic. They could hardly disregard what they saw, and the reporters sent back

---

*A process of easing tension at acupuncture points to allow ki energy to flow more freely, effected by bringing heat, as from a lighted cigarette, to within about ¼ -inch of the ki points (which are explained in the DeLangre books listed in our Bibliography).

stories about the use of acupuncture. That was the beginning of the slow acceptance by medical organizations of something they had very successfully ignored for so long.

A similar situation exists in regard to chiropractors. Most doctors regard practically all chiropractors as ineffective, at best; and probably for the most part they regard them as downright quacks.* Yet I know of dozens of people who have received tremendous relief from chiropractors after the doctors had been totally ineffective. One dramatic case that I know of personally concerns a European musician who was involved in a car accident in his country before coming to the U.S. to live. After he had been here a couple of years he began to lose all feeling in his right arm — an anxious condition for anyone, but for a pianist it becomes nothing short of agonizing. He went to a prominent neurosurgeon who did everything he knew to do and finally told the pianist that he was going to have to face the fact that he would be paralyzed in his right arm for life! It happened that the pianist had as a social acquaintance another doctor, and he asked this friend whether he knew of a good chiropractor. The response was, "Why do you want to have anything to do with those quacks?" The pianist pursued his questioning because in his country doctors respect chiropractors. Grudgingly his doctor friend admitted, "Well, there is one who gets lucky sometimes." The pianist felt that he definitely could use some luck so he went to that chiropractor. After only five treatments he was completely cured! In fact, after the fifth treatment he had an appointment with his neurosurgeon just one hour later, and the feeling began to come back in his arm as he was driving to the doctor's office. The doctor examined him and couldn't believe what he found. Finally he said, "Well, it either is a miracle or it was psychosomatic!" Our friend didn't bother to tell the doctor that it was neither — it was a chiropractor. Nothing would have been accomplished by making the doctor angry.

Later our friend went back to his country to settle a lawsuit involving his accident, taking along a statement from the neurosurgeon regarding the cause of his trouble and a corresponding statement from the chiropractor. They did not agree. The doctor said the trouble was in the "C-6" vertebra, while the chiropractor said it was in the "C-5" vertebra. The court appointed a committee of three doctors to decide the truth of the matter and they found the chiropractor's report to be the accurate one.

*However, I was surprised to learn that Indiana law requires that the state medical board be comprised of one chiropractor and one osteopath, in addition to five medical doctors!

You will notice that except for the tabloids, articles about the successful practice of chiropractics almost never appear in newspapers and periodicals. From the lack of material in the major news media one would think chiropractors did not exist in this country. Incidentally, a macrobiotic tenet is that much of the need for a chiropractor is the result of poor diet (although obviously not in the case of an accident), and that one reason chiropractic treatments are not necessarily long-lasting in their effectiveness is that poor diet soon recreates the same problem.

In spite of our awareness of these and other examples of disdain for new ideas, I was nonetheless eager to share our discovery about macrobiotics and healing. I felt that my case, at least, was so well documented with medical reports that surely some major magazine would be interested in publishing our experiences just for the human interest side if no other. Chapters 1 and 2 were written with that in mind about a year after surgery. We submitted them as a separate article to the *Reader's Digest,* hoping that publication would, if nothing else, have their medical reporters inquire into our story and the macrobiotic program. It was rejected — not because it was not interesting, or was untrue, but because it did not have the backing of the medical profession. The *Digest* was not one whit interested in evaluating macrobiotic successes.

An agent for a professional news service read our story in our University newspaper and asked to try to sell it to some nationally known magazines. After many months he gave up, mainly because the story was too controversial. A *National Enquirer* reporter phoned from Florida, but lost interest when I told him that I attributed my good health more to Oriental nutrition than to psychic phenomena.

The managing editor of one of our local newspapers was going to run the entire first two chapters in a series of installments and spent quite a lot of time planning it, but was finally overruled by the general manager. We did get cooperative press and radio coverage locally when we needed it for workshops which we sponsored on macrobiotics. Likewise, in the same newspaper there were two lengthy feature articles, several months apart, giving details of my cancer cure.

We felt even more frustrated when we began to realize that the only material on macrobiotics in national publications was unjustly detrimental, as we shall see later.

The lackadaisical attitude of the general public was revealed in one more way when measured against two area television programs — a 15-minute interview on an Anderson station (twenty miles from Muncie), and a comprehensive feature story by Guy Johnson of Channel 13 in Indianapolis. Mr. Johnson's show was a popular one watched by thousands of people. Many local friends (none of them ill) commented that they saw the show and were impressed by the editor's work. But although our segment of it appeared two or three times at different hours of the day and evening, we had only a handful of responses from sick people wanting help.

So far as national TV is concerned, a feeling of futility that has frequently distressed me occurs when I chance onto certain programs — whether they are soap operas, guest appearances on talk shows, or documentaries — dramatizing or describing the frustrations and uncertainties of doctors and patients in dealing with one major illness or another. It gives me an altogether different perspective, having been cured of the incurable, to listen and watch the action. It all seems misdirected and unreal.

One of the most disturbing times I had resulted from a Dick Cavett show with columnist Stewart Alsop as a guest. Mr. Alsop was dying of leukemia. The program was devoted to a discussion of how he felt to be dying, and of a book he had written about his feelings and experiences. What I was watching was a re-run which had been taped a couple of months earlier. By the time I saw the show Mr. Alsop was dead! It was a strange sensation to be sitting alone in my study watching the adventures of a dying man, feeling all the while that I knew — and many others knew much better than I — of an easy and inexpensive way to cure his leukemia. Oddly enough, here I was healthy and happy after macrobiotics had conquered a really tough cancer for me, but Mr. Alsop was no longer with us. Although he had had the best medical care available, no doubt at great expense, all those involved with his care thought that little could be done for him. What is even more discouraging is the knowledge that if he were still alive we would probably find it just as useless to try to help him now as it would have been then! If we wrote him of our success and beliefs, he probably would regard the letter as the hallucinations of some kind of nut and throw it in the wastebasket. If he was mildly hopeful about the diet and showed it to his doctors, then they probably would throw it in the wastebasket. If they compromised on the diet *and* chemotherapy, it would be likely to have poor results because of the toxic effect of the chemicals.

The television commercials also seem unnecessary and sometimes even vicious, as viewed from my own present lack of need for medication. The vast number of ads for aspirin, DiGel, Bufferin, Excedrin, Alka Seltzer, ad infinitum (no pun intended) — as well as the ads for food — indicate how most Americans live and what most of them want. I also find the ads for vitamins and food supplements obsolete, not having taken any of them since September of 1973!

Along with our naivete in thinking it would be easy to get our story into print, as we described earlier, we felt sure we could persuade some well-known individuals and organizations to investigate the work of Michio Kushi in Boston. Considering the millions spent on cancer research it would seem that it would be a simple matter to have qualified doctors and research organizations check out Michio's work in an objective manner.

However, such was not the case. Just as with Dr. Max Gerson, who apparently had surprising success in curing many illnesses through diet (in some ways similar but in some ways quite different from the macrobiotic diet), it seemed it was going to be impossible to secure any significant attention from the field of medicine or medical research. At least Michio has had a pleasant relationship with most of the doctors he has known (mainly because of his awesome knowledge coupled with his unassuming and modest manner), contrasted to the attempts by organized medicine to discredit Dr. Gerson. Dr. Gerson is now deceased but his work was never fairly evaluated by the medical profession, who were not swayed even by the prestige of a glowing testimonial from Dr. Albert Schweitzer, whose wife was cured of tuberculosis of the lungs by Dr. Gerson and his diet. Schweitzer referred to Gerson as "the greatest medical genius of the century."[2] As related by Dr. Gerson's daughter, Mrs. Johnna Oberlander, Mrs. Schweitzer "was just over 50 when she came to Dr. Gerson. The climate of Africa had given her the lung condition. Dr. Schweitzer was extremely grateful for what my father did. He said, 'My wife wouldn't be here today if it hadn't been for Dr. Gerson!' Mrs. Schweitzer died this January at the age of 79."[3] To author S.J. Haught, Schweitzer wrote, "I agree with you that Dr. Gerson's cancer therapy had great merits and know with which difficulties Dr. Gerson had to struggle. I would be grateful to you if you try to tell the people of America about Dr. Gerson's merits and about the results he obtained with his therapy...I wish you the best in your difficult task."[4] In spite of Schweitzer's praise, and the renown earned by Dr. Gerson (or perhaps *because* of it?), no major research organization, so far as I know, ever made any study of his findings.

As we stated indirectly in our Introduction, we have found that the research and medical professions tend to be so "locked in" to their traditional way of doing things that they have trouble noticing that there could be any other way. Public service groups sponsoring various fund drives for major illnesses have the same characteristic. I suppose that if they *should* happen to take a good look at the macrobiotic philosophy and perchance become somewhat curious about it, the moment they came across the affirmation that almost *all* illness can be avoided, or in many instances relieved for those who are already ill, they would be likely to toss out the whole thing as ridiculous. It is admittedly a premise that is hard to believe!

To me, the public service appeals for the cancer fund, the multiple sclerosis fund, the arthritis fund, and all others seem terribly misguided. I hear and read their statements saying, "There is no cure for arthritis but help us with research to find one." Many other similar statements are made about other major illnesses. Yet there *is* an answer for arthritis! There *is* an answer for multiple sclerosis! And we believe it is a cure which is all-beneficial with no possibility of the future damage likely to result from the popular chemical-drug-surgery syndrome.

In January of 1974, nearly five months after I left the hospital, we mailed a newsletter to many of our friends detailing our cancer cure, and also gave it to others who were interested in health problems. We sent a copy, including the comment that we believed the macrobiotic diet would cure most types of cancer (as well as most other illnesses), to a national honorary president of the American Cancer Society, whose main purpose is research. We received a pleasant letter in return saying that she was glad I was feeling better! There was no response at all to our suggestion that the organization contact the East West Foundation in Boston.

As another example relating to the efforts of public service groups, among all the frustrating and upsetting experiences we have had in attempting to let others know of our message of freedom from illness, the most vivid and maddening came just a year after surgery. In August of 1974 we took the vacation trip that we had planned for 1973. (In '73 it had been abruptly canceled by the hospital tests and the bomb following surgery.) This year we planned to really enjoy ourselves and celebrate our victory over those dark days of the previous summer. Our plans called for a trip to the East Coast and then down the coast line to Florida. We arrived in the Miami area rather late at night, picking up a newspaper in the motel lobby as we checked in.

Just before going to bed I glanced at the paper and was stunned to see an account of a group of children and teenagers in the Miami area, all suffering from leukemia, who had formed an organization to help each other accept their tragic suffering and eventual death. I glanced at the date on the paper and it was August 20th, 1974; but I was reading it at 12:30 a.m. on the 21st!! *Exactly one year from the date of my surgery!*

We were determined to try to help them although we knew it was doubtful that anything could be accomplished by our meddling. The next day Mary Alice tracked down the adult sponsor for the group. She learned that this indomitable lady and only six or seven other volunteers raised about a hundred-thousand dollars every year to help children and teen-agers with their terminal illnesses! The lady described the suffering the kids endured following such treatments as radium, cobalt, chemotherapy, and other ordeals. She told how they were a consolation to each other in all that they went through until their final moments. We felt a strong sympathy for these unfortunate youngsters, but were powerless to do anything. After talking to the lady on the phone, Mary Alice didn't even have the heart to mention what she had planned to say about the macrobiotic diet program. Being worlds removed from the organization's purpose and history, we would only have disturbed a compassionate and dedicated woman. As in the case of other groups we had tried to interest in our ideas, this organization of children was so tied up with the conventional way of thinking that nothing we could have said would have made the slightest difference. Mary Alice mumbled something about our hoping to learn more about their work, and hung up, limp and defeated.

No matter how persistent a person may be, there finally comes a point when he or she wonders where to turn next to look for a way to accomplish a goal. We were asking ourselves, "Where do we go from here?" And we were beginning to think the answer was, "Nowhere."

Notes for Chapter 3

[1]Eda LeShan, "Can Your Emotions Help You Resist Cancer?," *Woman's Day,* March, 1975, p. 101.

[2]Flyer advertising *The Solution to the Cancer Problem* (Dr. C. Moerman). (Flyer printed by the International Association of Cancer Victims and Friends, Inc., Playa del Rey, Cal., 1976).

[3]S. J. Haught, *Has Dr. Max Gerson a True Cancer Cure?* (North Hollywood, Cal.: London Press, 1962; 12th printing, 1975), pp. 24-25.

[4]*Ibid.,* Foreword.

CHAPTER 4

"Prove It!"
Jean Kohler

As hard as it seemed to be to sell our enthusiasm for macrobiotics to wide-scope media and national public service organizations, it was even stranger that we found it difficult to win over those who most needed our discovery: wishing that sick people would try the macrobiotic way has been one of our sad frustrations. Even when doctors could provide no hope, the patients shied away from what macrobiotics had to offer.

Many times relatives and friends of sick people come to ask about our experiences, and become caught up in our zeal. "This is wonderful — just the thing for Cousin Mehitabel!" But when Mehitabel is confronted with the idea she will have none of it. Many people find all kinds of excuses to cover up the fact that they *need* their illness, that they are in fact afraid to try methods that might rid them of it — and then what would they do without it?! As Dr. Arnold Hutschnecker points out in his book *The Will to Live,*[1] people often have *decided* to be sick, or even to die, without consciously realizing it. He sets forth the proposition that even the cause of death is frequently chosen. These people may be very much afraid to die, but nevertheless they are unhappy and want to get away from it all — permanently!!

This theory ties in with the one we constantly come across to the effect that people are responsible for the development of their own disease. If this is so, then after working months or years to ripen the illness, it's no wonder they have trouble releasing it. They hang on to it with, literally, a death-like grip. They are "out of balance with universal laws," it's true, but until some new insight shocks them out of it, that's the way they *want* it.

Whenever we think of *The Will to Live* we think of Dr. Carl Simonton, who first told us about this book (see page 26). In an address given in June of 1974 Dr. Simonton declared that "most patients see themselves as victims of the disease and not as having participated in the development of it."[2] And, among the philosophical conclusions agreed upon in a list of principles drawn up by

47

his staff at Oncology Associates in Fort Worth is the one that "serious illness may be a form of passive suicide." His "shock treatment" is to ask patients point-blank, "Why do you want to die?"

Oriental medicine, of course, affirms that improper eating is the main cause of disease, and insists that we are responsible for learning *how* to eat properly. One of Ohsawa's favorite themes is *"mea culpa"* — "my own guilt." In discussing cancer, he declares that if it is "the most 'incurable' disease, it is also the most 'curable,' the easiest to conquer if you seek its cause, which lies within you. Introspection will tell you how you produced it. If you discover the mechanism, you can then change the orientation of your ever-darkening civilization. In this sense cancer can serve as your savior!"[3]

Having been raised in an environment of atrocious eating habits, however, many people find that the sensual or pathological pleasure they derive from food is just too hard for them to forgo. While we personally have not found our way of eating overly strict or confining, it does mean abstaining from many favorite and delectable dishes. It is not a diet for the gourmand or the person of very weak character. However, if properly approached, it can develop into a transfer to a much greater appreciation of a different type of food, so that in addition to deriving pleasure from meals, one has the knowledge that there is a noble purpose in building those meals from proper food. It is very challenging to get this idea across to most people, for it seems to be a fact that they would rather not live if they have to give up their favorite foods. Food is their haven — certainly an understandable human trait in view of the eating habits that have been becoming more and more prevalent during the last sixty years or so.

I fear that we cancer patients (characteristically unhappy people that we are) are likely to be especially stubborn in this regard. In the lecture mentioned above, Dr. Simonton and his wife, apparently in a mean and ornery mood, painted the following very unflattering picture of us cancer people. We have: "(1) a great tendency to hold resentment and a marked inability to forgive; (2) a tendency towards self-pity; (3) a poor ability to develop and maintain meaningful, long-term relationships; (4) a very poor self-image." Then, to top off these overly candid remarks, they state, "The heart disease personality is basically a much more socially acceptable personality than the cancer personality."

I had already known about and had been smoldering under another body blow delivered by Ohsawa, of all people, to the effect that cancer is the product of arrogance! Ohsawa — the foster father of macrobiotics! Even he pokes holes in our ego!

One man we knew of who had cancer of the throat typifies the mental aspect of malignancy. The doctors insisted that he have his vocal chords removed to save his life and they said it had to be taken care of without delay, since his chances of surviving grew less and less the longer he waited. He was determined not to have surgery, for the removal of his vocal chords was doubly disastrous in his case: his voice was an essential asset in his particular profession. However, his first (and last) reaction to trying the macrobiotic diet was, "I can't give up meat!" Since talking to us, he heard of the curative properties of distilled sea water, so he took a tablespoonful of sea water every day, hoping this would save his voice and his life. *That* much he was willing to do. Meanwhile his voice became more and more husky — and soon was silenced by surgery.

Through mutual acquaintances we sent a copy of our newsletter and a personal letter about curing cancer to a famous, brilliantly talented young musician who is dying of some type of cancer. We didn't receive so much as an acknowledgement, although there is little doubt the letter was received, for her friends had been most eager for her to have the information.

While we were in Boston the second time (April, 1974), we met a young man and his wife, both of whom, along with their small child, had been eating macrobiotically for several years and were firm believers in the benefits of the diet. His mother in St. Louis had developed cancer of the brain and by the time our friend learned of it and returned home to see her, she was practically dead. The doctors had administered chemotherapy treatments but at length they had given up and were just waiting for time to run out. Our friend insisted that the family call Michio to see what could be done. They were stubbornly opposed to the idea, but at last (since there was no other hope) they allowed him to place the phone call. Michio, because of his crowded schedule, can not travel to see patients, but fortunately he had as a guest a Japanese doctor of Oriental medicine who believed in the macrobiotic approach. This man was prevailed upon to fly out to see the patient. When he went into her room she was extremely weak, listless, and ashen. Our young friend went into the room with the Japanese doctor. He reported that within five minutes his mother was feeling much better, and he watched the color coming back into her face. The Oriental approach in this instance was to use acupuncture to help revitalize the patient and gain time, which it did most successfully. Then the Japanese man recommended certain herb teas as medicines in addition to the macrobiotic diet. He stated that if his instructions were carefully followed the patient would be able to walk in ten days. To the surprise of all, especially of the relatives who had opposed this approach, she began walking in only six days. Her color was much better and she was obviously making excellent progress. Then an unexpected thing happened. To the sorrow and puzzlement of our young friend his mother decided to go back to the chemotherapy treatments and drop the diet, without having any valid reason at all for doing so except that her deceased father (a doctor) would not have used the macrobiotic method! Our friend wanted me to talk to her by phone; I did so without success. The chemotherapy treatments didn't work any better this time than they had before, and the last I heard, she was dying again.

There are those who seem to use trial and error as an excuse for not getting well. Rather often we are contacted by people who are thrashing about trying page 10 of one system, page 75-a of another system, and other instructions from several other systems, for a total program of chaos and bewilderment. They are furiously busy making an unconscious pretense of trying to cure their illness. But this frantic grasping at small sections of a number of different programs is a disorganized jig-saw puzzle piecing together a picture of failure.

An attitude we find all too frequently is one where the patient says, in effect, "Prove it!" We naturally feel that the proof in my own case, and those of other Muncie-influenced cures, should be a strong enough platform to win over someone who has been told there are only a few months left on this plane. We are coming to the conclusion that these people want the iron-clad proof of acceptance by the medical profession — and this may be a long time in evolving. While such people are waiting and looking for proof, the noose is tightening. Since this book was started, a number of people we spent hours with, explaining the macrobiotic benefits that many others had enjoyed, have hesitated — and hesitated — right up to time for the funeral.

The need for proof is one thing that keeps driving us to try to convince some doctor to offer macrobiotic information to terminal patients, for the timid ones need the assurance that they have come to depend on from doctors. Also, it has occurred to us that perhaps many of those who seem to want to die would change their attitude if they could be presented with a more positive argument that life is still possible.

The national office of the East West Foundation in Boston is now collecting case histories to correct this situation. Records in the past have been non-existent, and the Foundation has lost track of people who have come to them for advice in fighting cancer. This casualness was, of course, a serious flaw; but Michio, in his philosophical overview of the entire history of the entire universe, knew that when the time was right, acceptance would come!

At best, however, any records Boston can compile at the present time would be only a collection of testimonials, some with medical documentation, rather than a controlled, experimental setup that would be required for approval by the medical profession. Yet a "control-group" experiment is likely to be inaccurate in the case of a dietary program, partly because of the typical human inability to avoid breaking rules where food is concerned, and partly because of the danger of misinterpreting instructions or forgetting them through careless study. I make these assertions even knowing about the Harvard blood pressure and cholesterol experiments that will be mentioned in Chapter 8. While their research was extremely valuable, involving dedicated macrobiotic people who would be unlikely to do any deliberate cheating, the individual interpretations of macrobiotics would of necessity keep the results from being meticulously accurate. Even so the medical profession apparently looked with favor upon the results of the project.

A couple of examples will help explain my modest opinions in the direction of dietary-control experiments. One zealous young doctor with whom I talked said that my experience did not prove a thing. One case history of any type meant absolutely nothing, according to him. He said, "Now if you take three hundred patients and have them eat macrobiotically without their knowing what they are eating and compare that group with another one of three-hundred patients who are eating conventional food without knowing what they are eating, then you would have a valid basis for comparison." Then he said, "But you're not going to experiment on *my* patients." I presume he included in this statement even his terminal patients whom he could not help. When we pointed out that it is impossible to have *any* patients follow *any* diet without their knowing what they are eating, the young doctor remained silent.

His remarks, however, show that it is an obvious fact that experiments involving diet can be controlled only with exceeding difficulty, if at all, the reason being that there is no way to check scrupulously on a rigid diet. If patients are not ill enough to need to be in bed, they will not stay confined to a hospital just for an experiment which should take at least three months. If they are at home, there is *no* check-up researchers could devise to show whether the participants are honoring their diet or are consistently cheating.

Even if the patients are in the hospital in a special ward, there is no way to prevent some deception through the help of sympathetic, although misguided, friends, relatives, and even nurses. To illustrate this point, the book about Dr. Max Gerson tells of "controlled" experiments in a German hospital treating lupus, a horribly disfiguring and fatal disease which is a tuberculosis of the skin. In one wing of the hospital a large number of male patients were being fed a special diet of salt-free food. The results were utterly disappointing. The doctor in charge had mailed Dr. Gerson a letter telling him that they were going to discontinue the experiments, when he happened to see the fattest nurse on the staff going into the experimental ward carrying an enormous tray of beer and many foods strictly forbidden to the men. When he asked her what she was doing, she blurted out that she couldn't stand to see the men eat only that terrible food so she brought them every afternoon a huge treat of everything they weren't supposed to have.[4] The disturbing fact is that neither she nor any of the men who were going to die of this awful disease had sense enough (or will power enough) to realize that by cheating that much they were destroying their only hope. All, apparently, reassured themselves that that little bit of cheating wouldn't make any difference! The time it took to eat these forbidden foods couldn't have lasted more than ten or fifteen minutes. And for that short amount of pleasure these men were willing to throw away their only hope of survival.

It would be rare for a group of patients to be penned up in one place as these men were and, therefore, control would ordinarily be even less manageable. We do have the ability to control laboratory experiments with mice, however, and such an experiment is being conducted in the biology department here at Ball State University. Dr. Peter Nash received in 1975 a government grant to study the differences between tumor cells and non-tumor cells in the A mouse strain. The study also compares the light microscope to the electron microscope in examining tumor cells versus normal cells. Begun in early February of 1976, the experiment, involving 72 mice, will require many months to complete; but we hope you will eventually hear good results from it.

In January of 1976, Michio Kushi and his wife visited Ball State for three days of lectures. At that time we got the idea of trying the macrobiotic food program on one group of cancer-prone mice. Michio and Peter mapped the whole thing out, and since February our natural foods restaurant has been delivering macrobiotic food weekly to "our" mice in the biology department at Ball State. Dr. Nash cooks the vegetables and makes miso soup for our mice, none of whom reject any of the food. The one thing that can't be controlled, apparently, is their fondness for turnips, which they always eat first. (Of course, the amount *is* controlled.) Dr. Nash reports that they are exhibiting a human tendency to postpone the most difficult work till last, in that they don't eat the beans, still rather hard after having been cracked and soaked overnight, till all the other food is gone.

If the score comes out in our favor in the mouse tests, we hope the medical profession may be persuaded to try further such experiments using macrobiotic methods, which may be convincing to themselves and hence to their patients. See Chapter 15.

As for my own cure, early in the game I learned that many doctors were going to be hard to impress. But there was a turn of events which made it seem as if I might have found a break-through.

To begin with, I had had a difficult time opening up a line of communication with the four doctors involved in my case. Ten months after surgery, I had written them telling about what we thought was a cure of my incurable cancer. We realized that they would naturally want to wait much longer to form any kind of firm judgment. However, we thought sufficient time had elapsed and the results were impressive enough for them to want to examine me again. Then, of course, we were hoping that they might offer macrobiotic information to some terminal patients. We knew a doctor could not guarantee any kind of results or even recommend the diet himself, but it would give some chance and hope to patients who otherwise had none. What could a terminal patient lose by this?! Many of them, as we keep saying, would not be interested, but some would grasp at the chance. Medical students have told me that doctors cannot make such suggestions because of possible malpractice lawsuits resulting from trying an approach not approved by traditional medicine. However, this obstacle could surely be overcome, it seems to us, by having the doctor explain the situation and by having the patient and his family sign a legal document absolving the doctor of any blame if the diet was unsuccessful.

At any rate, after sending our message to the four doctors, we were puzzled and surprised that not one of them bothered to even answer our letter. As we learned from a friend, our family physician of twenty-seven years became angry about the letter. He felt that I, a musician, was trying to tell him, a doctor, how to cure disease. Perhaps I did not write a sufficiently diplomatic letter, but I certainly had tried to avoid being presumptuous.

A few weeks before the second anniversary I again wrote my doctors long detailed letters reminding them of our program and the success with it. There were a number of important enclosures, including brief summaries of the amazing recovery of two other terminal cancer patients we knew.

Likewise, I mentioned that Michio was coming to our University in October for three days of lectures, including, we hoped, one for doctors in this area. I invited the Indiana University doctors to attend this lecture if it did materialize and suggested that they invite Michio to the Indiana University Medical Center for a lecture. Then ten days later I again wrote them saying that the date had been changed to January or February. A copy of this correspondence went to a doctor in the Pathology Department whom I had happened to meet and chat with after a recital at Ball State. For some time I received not a word in reply to this long-winded, one-sided correspondence, except from the doctor in pathology.

Then finally on August 21st, *the second anniversary of my surgery,* came wonderful news. I received a cordial letter from a doctor who had been in charge of my chemotherapy treatments two years previously, asking me to visit the Medical Center at my convenience for tests to try to learn the reason for my apparent recovery. I felt like a celebrity! Going back to the Indiana University Medical Center for the tests on August 26 made me feel as if I was going back for some kind of honorary degree.

We took along Mari and Ivan (whom you met in Chapters 1 and 2) and planned a gala day of it — a "vacation trip" fifty-five miles from home. Besides the tests, we had lunch at a Japanese restaurant, visited our favorite Japanese-maple nursery, and I even splurged on a new coat and house slippers! I felt I had "arrived." Quite a difference from the emotions we had in Miami on my *first* anniversary!

I was so elated about this happy opportunity that as I marched up the steps to the doctor's office I could even hear an imaginary brass band playing! I felt very fortunate and honored to find myself seated in the doctor's office after all the months of not getting any kind of reply to my detailed letters. He was exceedingly friendly and proceeded to tell me his reaction to my case. (The two other doctors involved at the Medical Center were the ones who had said that I had *no* chance for survival. While there was no reason to think that this doctor felt any differently, he had never had occasion to say so.) He expressed what I had rather assumed he believed all along — that even with the chemotherapy he hadn't expected me to be alive at the end of a year. For me to be not only alive, but functioning normally after one year seemed to him amazing. Then to be alive and functioning normally after *two* years he thought was a *miracle*! (I remember well his use of the word because of having already decided on the title for our book.) In fact, he said, they considered my good health so unique that they had checked back to be sure there wasn't some mistake in my medical records!

The doctor went on to say that he couldn't actually believe the diet brought about these remarkable results, but *something* obviously had and he was interested in finding out what it was. Then he came to the part that I found to be truly exciting. He asked if I would be interested in helping some of his terminal patients try this diet and even arrange for them to see Michio! Wow! This was what we had been hoping for ever since we realized the fantastic results we were getting after our first trip to Boston. I explained to him that the patients would need to have a strong will to live, be determined to stick to the diet, be able to go to Boston to consult Michio, and have a means of getting this food. That meant that someone in the family, in most cases, had to be willing to spend the time and acquire the skills necessary for macrobiotic cooking. This kind of cooking at first is a different world and the person attempting it needs much help.

Our doctor friend was certainly not long in getting started. The very next morning I had a call from him about a young man with lung cancer, which had spread to the testicles, who had taken all the medication his body would tolerate. The young man, too, responded quickly, phoning us within half an hour after the doctor's call. Now the macrobiotic approach *had* to work! If we could get results now the world would soon know that there is a cure for cancer!

But then — but then…Days went by, and weeks went by, and we heard nothing more from the young man or from the doctor. Finally we phoned his office and learned that the patient had had marital problems and had been preoccupied with them and with his illness to the extent that he had not done anything about trying the diet. Moreover, our fond hopes of having some other terminal patients try macrobiotics were gradually dissipated as we began to realize that nothing further was going to develop. We heard nothing more; so obviously that possible avenue of proof was not going to materialize.

However, after receiving the results of my August 26 tests, this doctor had done one very great favor for us by writing, on October 13, 1975, a "To Whom It May Concern" report stating that 26 months earlier I "was unfortunately found to have inoperable carcinoma of the pancreas," that I had been religiously following a macrobiotic diet (I fear I avoided admitting to him that I had done a little sneaking!), and that my surprising, happy, incredible response and freedom from symptoms of malignancy could not in any way be ascribed to the single course of 5-FU I had had before being released from the Medical Center in September of 1973. He was concerned, however, that my CEA (August, '75) was "elevated at 15 nanograms" and my alkaline phosphatase was above 700 "although the rest of his liver function studies and blood studies were completely normal." Details of my being able to control such tests by being carefully macrobiotic for a while appear in the Sequel to Chapter 9, as well as in a letter I wrote after receiving the doctor's report. Here is a part of my letter:

> Thanks so much for sending the report. We do appreciate it.
>
> I have some results of medical tests that I think will interest you. They seem to us to prove further the validity of our belief in the diet and Mr. Kushi's knowledge. Last May 7th I finally went to a local doctor for tests to see if I seemed as healthy to the medical profession as I felt. The tests he had run by a lab were normal *except for the very elevated alkaline phosphatase reading which was 1460. Also the SGOT test ran 225.* The doctor was puzzled by these results and thought perhaps the diet itself could be causing these elevated readings.
>
> We phoned Michio in Boston and he said immediately that *the trouble was that I was not following my diet strictly enough, that the high readings must be caused by spices and possibly too much salt.* He sounded correct in his diagnosis because I *had* been departing from my original strict diet. The deviation would have seemed minor to most people and I thought that since I felt cured of cancer I could safely take some freedom. Also, I was getting some spices, kind of by accident, because I was eating at least one meal a day at our natural foods restaurant and the cooks often did not set aside *our* portions of casseroles, soups, etc., before adding herbs and spices. I felt it was O.K. to eat those things, too. (Salt was not a prob-

lem for me.) However, *after he said still* **no** *spices I im-mediately eliminated all of them again. Seventeen days later I again had a blood test and this time the A.P. test was down to 985 and the SGOT down to 139. The reading on your test of August 26th showed 700 for the A.P. test. Last Saturday (October 11th) I had another test analyzed by the lab here and the A.P. was now 205 and the SGOT 42.* It is unfortunate that I didn't have a CEA at this time to see if this, too, would have improved. Since receiving your letter we again called Michio about *this* test and he said that cancer cells in the blood in my case are simply a matter of discharge.* He wasn't alarmed by it at all and, of course, neither am I.

The above excerpt seems to me to be exceedingly convincing proof that the macrobiotic diet truly does what we believe it is capable of doing. *For Michio to know instantly that spices could cause the abnormal alkaline phosphatase test (which relates to the condition of the liver) and for that reading to drop to nearly normal from May to October by eliminating them is amazing. That surely cannot be a coincidence!*

To return to my obstinate campaign, I have contacted many doctors in my search for one who might consider giving my ideas a try. As I would read in national news about doctors who had carried out innovative programs, I would phone them and then send a packet of information if they showed the slightest interest.

One prominent surgeon, who is also a writer, was very polite and asked to have our information. But he said I must include a laboratory report of the biopsy to prove the tumor was malignant or otherwise he would assume that it was benign. I mailed him our material and had the hospital send the biopsy report. No further word was received from him.

I phoned and then wrote to the president of a medical college, many of whose graduates might be working in disadvantaged areas. I thought he might be especially interested in this diet approach because it was comparatively inexpensive, especially suited for the poor. The president was quite cordial, and agreed to refer my information to his faculty. After studying the material, he sent a courteous letter stating in essence that if I did not claim so much for macrobiotics I might have a better chance of impressing those in the medical profession. However, I did not consider these claims — the same ones presented in this book — to be exaggerated. He

---

*For a discussion of "discharging," a typically macrobiotic experience, see Chapter 5.

also said that doctors would not give up the therapies they now use and "the only hope for a new one is integration." This is exactly what we would wish for! He made one statement that should be quoted: "I believe that attention to what we consume will help greatly in the fight against what consumes us." But none of his people "concerned with the care of critically ill patients," to whom he gave our material, ever responded.

I phoned one well-known physician who has been written up in some of our most popular magazines. He was a man of unusual humanitarian dedication toward helping the poor with their medical problems. I thought that since he was obviously a unique person and was active in helping the poor, he might be receptive to giving macrobiotic hope to some otherwise hopeless patients. However, he proved to be the most difficult man that I had ever approached. He was positive from his long years of medical practice that (1) no diet could possibly control cancer and (2) anyone who said that any diet could achieve the results we were suggesting was obviously a quack. He went on to say that he simply considered my case to be a mistake on the part of my doctors — that I, like most of the public, forgot that doctors were human and made mistakes the same as the rest of us. I asked about the biopsy report and again he said it must have been a mistake on the part of the technicians in the laboratory. I mentioned a macrobiotic friend of ours who was well along on the way to conquering rheumatoid arthritis. His rebuttal was that ever since the days of Mesmer (the French doctor who rediscovered hypnosis) it had been known that arthritis patients *seemed* to get better as a result of a kind of hypnosis or self-delusionment!

It soon became apparent that nothing I could say or do would have any effect on his entrenched beliefs, so I terminated the conversation, having lost one more round in my battle to try to inform the public.

I phoned the doctor in charge of cancer treatment at the Mayo Clinic and asked whether he would be interested in hearing about my good fortune in curing cancer, as well as learning about the success of some of our friends in this book. His reply was that he was not interested in "testimonials," no matter how impressive they were or how many of them we had to show him. (A friend of mine said later when I told him about this, "The legal profession accepts the validity of testimonials — they hang a person on the evidence of testimonials!")

Another source I tried was the Menninger Foundation in Topeka, Kansas, because I had heard of their fine reputation and had reason to believe that their thinking was more progressive than most. Perhaps *here* I would find a doctor who would present our kind of hope to terminal patients. At the time, I did not realize that the Menninger Foundation was primarily a psychiatric institution, so I was expecting the same type of hospital as the Mayo Clinic. The doctor with whom I spoke by phone was very cordial, requesting that I submit my medical record and any other evidence of the effectiveness of the macrobiotic program. I did so and had encouraging follow-up correspondence.

A couple of months later Dr. Stephen Appelbaum of the Menninger Foundation visited Boston and met with EWF associates Stephen Uprichard, Edward Esko, and Rod House. (Michio was in Europe at that time.) This exchange resulted in a reciprocal visit by Michio to the Menninger Foundation in December, 1976, to begin the implementation of a preliminary project to test the results of macrobiotics on a small number of patients. Hopefully this project will lead to more comprehensive tests, with cancer patients and perhaps with mental patients. Some of the experienced people from EWF would go to Topeka to assist with this latter phase of the work.

My next attempt was a very prominent surgeon with a national reputation. I was surprised and gratified by his very cordial reaction to what I had to tell him. Buoyed by more than ordinary hope, I submitted my usual packet of what I thought was impressive evidence. However, there was no response from the doctor, so it was another strike-out.

There was the usual luck (or lack of it) with an executive of the American Cancer Society. A reporter from a national magazine in New York phoned me in connection with an article she was writing about unorthodox approaches to the treatment of cancer. She had just talked to the Assistant Vice President for Professional Education of the American Cancer Society, who told her that he had never seen a single cure of cancer by an unorthodox approach. I suggested she tell him about my very well-documented case. After waiting a number of days to hear from him, I finally phoned his office. He returned the call, seemed interested, and said he would like to see my medical records. I mailed them, along with other case histories — and then heard nothing. It never ceased to amaze me that I usually received not even an acknowledgement that my messages ever arrived.

About a year after our macrobiotic life began, our continuing obsession to promote wider acceptance of proper food had led us into a local venture which turned out to be a mixed blessing. You may have noticed a couple of non-specific references to "our" restaurant; to be specific, it *is* ours. In September of 1974, Mary Alice and I purchased the Harvest Moon, the small natural foods restaurant where we had eaten about once a week since our first trip to Boston. It had been started two years earlier by two young couples interested in good nutrition of the vegetarian type.

When we bought it, it was being run by one man from the original four people. He was going to have to close it, since he was unable to make a living with it. We most certainly did not want a restaurant but we did feel strongly that there was a definite need for such a place; so we ended up buying it. We didn't expect to make much money, if any, but we certainly did not expect it to be the financial disaster which it unfortunately became. The loss ran into thousands of dollars, although we tried every practical frugality and every promotion we could afford. The reason for the financial loss is that even near a college campus the number of customers for this kind of restaurant is limited, although loyal, and the labor bill is staggering. (When only natural foods are used, of course, the preparation is unavoidably time-consuming.) We have a devoted and capable group of young people doing the work, with Mary Alice handling the general supervision, promotions, doing much of the buying, and keeping books. Our staff are willing to work very hard for extremely low wages, but even so, our labor bill must look like that of McDonald's and our income the first two years must have been less than any one of their restaurants takes in for a fraction of its french fries alone.

Many times we came close to giving up in despair, but somehow we would hang on, partly because we couldn't find time to close it out, mostly because it meant so much to our staff and our customers, and partly because it had become so intrinsically woven into our daily lives that parting with it would have been like losing a child. Well, one of the macrobiotic philosophies is that it's all right to make plenty of money as long as you don't hang on to it. The expense of maintaining the "Moon" did a neat job of "purifying" us in that respect!

Fortunately, the main benefit that we were counting on from our restaurant did come about. We planned to use the Moon as a source of information and a propaganda center for the macrobiotic diet and way of life. Here people know that, in addition to eating delicious, healthful food, they can read in our "mini-library" material such as Michio Kushi's lectures in a variety of publications, and the *East West Journal* (a monthly newspaper published by several of Mr. Kushi's students), the Muramoto *Healing Ourselves,* which is becoming quite well known, and macrobiotic cookbooks. Here, also, people with or without health problems can meet us for long discussions to help decide whether they want to try the macrobiotic system.

Largely because of our efforts at the Harvest Moon the East West Foundation invited us to become one of their Mid-west Centers, and thus we felt that our contacts, both local and distant, were radiating to some extent from the Moon.

After the Kushi visit to Muncie, many of the members of our staff became ardent macrobiotic supporters and eliminated the frequent use of some things that were "off limits." Those who left Muncie for better jobs with larger natural foods restaurants took with them the enthusiasm they had absorbed for the macrobiotic "flavor." And one young couple even started a restaurant of their own — "Our Daily Bread," in Atlanta, Indiana — which was imbued with macrobiotic characteristics. The Moon has a satellite!

Still we were dissatisfied with the number of people we were, or were not, reaching, and we began to think of another plan to bring our story and those of our friends to a larger audience. We still needed a more effective way to "Prove It."

Notes for Chapter 4

[1]Arnold A. Hutschnecker, M.D., *The Will to Live* (Englewood Cliffs, N.J.: Prentice-Hall, Inc., 1951; Fourth printing, 1961), pp. 48-68.

[2]"Management of the Emotional Aspects of Malignancy," lecture delivered by Dr. O. Carl Simonton, M.D., D.A.B.R., and Stephanie Simonton at the University of Florida, Gainesville, symposium on "New Dimensions of Habilitation for the Handicapped," June, 1974. Published in the *Journal of Transpersonal Psychology,* 7, no. 2 (June, 1975), 29-47.

[3]Georges Ohsawa, *Cancer and the Philosophy of the Far East* (Paris, 1963), ed. Herman Aihara, trans. Armand la Belle and Ralph Baccash (Binghamton, N.Y.: Swan House Publishing Co., 1971), p. 110.

[4]S. J. Haught, *Has Dr. Max Gerson a True Cancer Cure?* (North Hollywood, Cal.: London Press, 1962; 12th printing, 1975), pp. 34-35.

CHAPTER 5

Second Thoughts

Jean Kohler

Having probed all the impasses described in the previous chapters, we finally came to the conclusion that the only way to disseminate our information on a large scale would be to write a book, although judging from our attempts to find an outlet for a magazine article, we didn't have much hope of being accepted by a publisher. But after a couple of rejections, we decided to try one of the major companies and contacted Prentice-Hall, thus beginning an amiable working relationship with Parker Publishing Company, which handles their books on health.

However, now that our dream was suddenly real and tangible, we must admit that we began to have certain reservations about our big opportunity. First of all, we felt that we should have years of study about the macrobiotic or Order-of-the-Universe philosophy, so that we'd have a profound vantage point from which to make easily understood statements giving just essential information without any excess baggage. And we needed to know a lot more about food before trying to tell other people what they should eat and *why*.

What's more, no matter how we handle this thing, we're going to cause problems. As much as we want the information to be generally available, we have misgivings such as the possibility that people will try to do too much with it on their own, without having read our suggestions carefully enough or checked into other sources than this book (see Bibliography), or without having contacted Mr. Kushi or a closer East West Center (Appendix).

And doctors, although they may understand that this book is an accurate account of events, presented with a genuine desire to be helpful, may feel that it could exert a detrimental influence because many people might start disregarding their doctors' advice. Occasionally, of course, such disregard could have disastrous results, as when patients must depend on drugs to maintain life. We asked Michio about diabetes, for instance, in conjunction with macrobiotic food. He said that if patients are on insulin they should reduce the insulin as they feel the need for it decline, and that they can usually tell how much they need. But they certainly don't just stop taking it because of having started the diet. If they feel hyperactive, they will need less insulin; if sluggish, they will need more.

Much more common hazards, not serious if on a small scale, could result in not deriving necessary benefits from the diet. Such pitfalls would be: habitual cheating (as with any diet, "this little bit or that little bit" of cheating *can* be damaging), or even over-zealousness. One of our friends, for example, liked miso soup and felt that if a small daily serving was beneficial, larger amounts would do *more* good. She ended up with too much salt and a noticeable swelling in her face from taking too much liquid to satisfy the thirst. A phone call to Michio soon had matters straightened out. Another friend became rather seriously dehydrated because she was trying too hard to remain on a low-liquid level which in general is part of our program. A knowledgeable macrobiotic person tattled to Michio, and the girl was persuaded to be more easy-going about it and drink moderate amounts of bancha tea or water whenever she was thirsty. Consistent irregularities can, of course, be fatal!

Among other problems, would our approach add one more wild wind to buffet our weather-vane friends who try everything they read about? (Chapter 4) We wish instead that they would settle on one method. Please recall Dr. Simonton's admonition (Chapter 1) to stay with any method as long as it seems to be working. He didn't say to stay with a whole *bunch* of methods.

Even a single-minded effort to follow the road to recovery through macrobiotics will bring about various symptoms for its various converts. My wife and I, for example, frequently had the same annoyances, either concurrently or a few days apart. In Chapter 2 she mentions the weight loss and the "yang" taste in our mouths. Sometimes it was a small sore on the tip of the tongue or in the nose. Sometimes the fingernails grew fast for a while and sometimes slowly. The half-moon in the fingernails is supposed to disappear as a sign of good health. Ours disappeared and then reappeared for a while. Sometimes we would have soreness in the neck or a sore spot in the chest for a few days. My wife had problems with vision for several months.

A book which you would find valuable to have on hand is *Healing Ourselves,* a guidebook meticulously culled by admiring students from lectures of Naboru Muramoto, a scholar of Oriental medicine (see our Bibliography). We consider the book helpful and practical except for the chapter on teas and herbs. To use any of these you should certainly have the guidance of a macrobiotic friend. Michio always advises against the use of herbs, and the only teas we have known him to recommend are bancha (almost exclusively) and mu tea, which latter is suggested only rarely. (Be sure to check the food list for cancer from yin or yang causes, Chapter 13.) Having so many teas and herbs listed as all kinds of remedies puts one in the same sort of quandary as trying to follow several different systems for maintaining health. You need to know what you're doing in order to use teas as remedies. (In the Orient, the concept of using herbs as medicine is compared to *Den-ka-no-ho-to:* a family-treasure sword used only under extreme circumstances!)

However, among other very useful information, the Muramoto book outlines the progress of common symptoms as the body gradually rids itself of the poisons stored in every tissue from years of wrong foods. "Discharging," they call it — and it's a big part of the macrobiotic experience. But those who have worked their way through a few discharges and have reaped the benefits wouldn't give up macrobiotics for anything.

One problem we hope *not* to bring about by writing this book would be to cause some people to start this program without understanding that they should not give up the first minute things seem not to be going right, for on an individual basis discharging may work in strange ways. Often the "mb" diet seems to eradicate the major illness first and then continues at a slower pace to work on clearing out the stored-up debris in body tissues. This characteristic will be noted in some of the case histories in Chapters 14 and 15.

During my second summer I seemed to be going through this sort of process. I lost weight again, needed somewhat more rest, had a number of mild attacks of chills and fever, necessitating a few hours of extra rest in addition to a long night's sound sleep. These sessions, without exception, resulted from over-fatigue, as when too many events at once interfered with adequate rest, if I would happen also to become chilled during long meetings or rehearsals in cold air-conditioned rooms. Often, if I felt extraordinarily tired, my complexion would be slightly yellow or slightly dirty-looking. (In one of his lectures, Michio explained that "simply speaking, cancer is the result of excess carbon in the body, and this darker shade of skin is caused by the discharge of this excess."[1]) Edward Esko, executive secretary of Mr. Kushi's non-profit East West Foundation, said once during a phone call concerning plans for compiling this book that the "plateau" of symptoms I was experiencing in my progress was due partly to the summer season and partly to a discharge as my liver continued to rid itself of toxins.

Reading from a number of sources and information gleaned from macrobiotic friends confirm the idea that fever is usually an indication of trouble in the lungs or liver. And it is a common belief of ancient Oriental medicine that fever results from the intake of excess animal protein, which of course would cause too heavy a load on the liver and cause its storehouse to bulge to the point of suffocation. In this state, fever becomes a type of discharge. So there went some more of the meat and eggs I had burdened my liver with for 56 years; and my subsequent freedom from symptoms proved Mr. Esko to be accurate. My cancer had been subdued months earlier, but now I was following the route that a comparatively healthy person might travel after starting macrobiotics. (Experiences of this type are up-dated in the Sequel to Chapter 9.) Incidentally, it happens that fever can also be caused by an excessive intake of sugar and other foods of that type which oxidize immediately in the blood stream.

Many people seem to have one "cold winter." With Mary Alice it was the second one (1975), when to her the cold temperatures felt more penetrating and disagreeable than usual. She even had a couple of mild colds, although she was determined not to admit it until she had sniffled for three or four days. The third winter was my winter. After the several sessions of chills and fever during the previous summer, I had a few more during the winter, and found the cold weather so unpleasant and my stamina so lacking that I stopped jogging and doing calisthenics. For everything else — practice, teaching, and all other non-strenuous activities — I had adequate energy. When Mr. Kushi was here in January, he suggested a return to the very strict diet for three months. By spring my endurance began returning, jogging and calisthenics gradually became possible and finally easier than they used to be, and once more I needed considerably less sleep. And — I gained ten pounds during the summer! The best bonus of all was that my piano technique became better than it had ever been in my life. I was able to cover much more material in less practice time than ever before.

In July the Muncie doctor who had authorized the lab tests sent word through a patient (who happened to be our manager at the Harvest Moon) that he would be interested in my having another blood test. He gave no reason, and I assume it was simply out of curiosity. When he got the results he was amazed at my good condition, and so, I understand from our manager, was another doctor he showed them to. I'm sure I'm in the clear now on "discharging," and I feel great.

We'll list a few pointers on discharging that we've picked up from our studies here and there. They will give you a better idea of the commonly accepted theories until you can build your own reserve of basic knowledge:

(1) Warnings against overeating, from many sources, are frequent and consistent. From antiquity, moderation has been inherent in this Universal-Order way of eating. Out of respect for our sensitive, dutiful digestive system, we should not, as sick people have usually done, "work it to death." (Excesses as a factor in *serious* diseases are mentioned in Chapter 8.) Obviously, everything that should not have been stored in the body has to be rejected through some kind of a "discharge." As we said before, you can avoid both hunger and weight-gain on a macrobiotic diet, as long as you observe the recommended general percentages, and don't actually *stuff* yourself. Before long you become comfortable with the idea that eating all you want is certainly not the same as *over*-eating. (Mr. Kushi warns if you consistently eat too much of even macrobiotic food you could give yourself cancer.)

(1a) While overeating is abhorred, the opposite practice of fasting is considered by macrobiotic people only as a short-term curative tool. It is not necessary to prolong it or make it a regular habit. Our Chapter 9 mentions a few details about fasting.

(2) Relief from symptoms of a serious illness is often felt within twelve to fifteen days of proper eating. Absence of chemicals, of excess food and liquid, and of excess protein and mucus, allows the blood stream to begin to release toxins. In about three or four months, the body completely replaces all of its red blood cells, so that you begin to have a clean blood stream working for you. Muscle fibers and some internal organs are reconstructed, for many people, in about three years. In seven years the entire body constitution can be changed! (This can take as long as 12 years if you're one who insists on taking detours away from the basic macrobiotic food for periods of time, or on doing a lot of "bingeing." So do try to stay put as much as possible!) The length of time varies for different individuals, of course. And children, who have a faster metabolism, can make quicker repairs. Often one may feel worse during some of these times of change. But avoid the temptation to take medication to relieve the symptoms, for they are symptoms only, and inter-

ference from medicines serves merely to slow up the process of discharge and eventual relief.

So don't be scared off by having some discomforts or even by not feeling well part of the time — or even by the seven-year (or longer!) prediction. Most of the time you'll be unaware of the changes going on; and even during times when you recognize signs of "reconstruction," it beats being terribly sick from chemicals or having all your hair fall out or worrying that the effects of your treatment are no longer active and your reprieve is expiring.

(3) The weight loss that upsets patients and their families and friends is not at all worrisome, although it may be a bit of a strain on the vanity. The loss occurs because it takes the body a while to re-establish its original ability to change plant nourishment into blood. (One of our most interesting sources — Ohsawa's *Cancer and the Philosophy of the Far East* — emphasizes this process (his page 63): "If, in accordance with modern nutritional theories, we consume large amounts of animal protein, we lose the ability to produce for ourselves our own special proteins.") Actually the weight loss during the readjustment reduces the strain on the liver and gives it a chance to discharge old waste from the digestive system. The liver, being the organ that suffers the most damage from our overeating of wrong foods, eventually becomes so exhausted that it cannot carry out its intended function of filtering toxins from the blood. Thus, please don't succumb to the urge to try to gain weight by overeating!

(4) Skin discharges may also occur. During the macrobiotic process of healing, hands and/or feet may sometimes become very red, indicating that unclean blood is being filtered and discharged by the kidneys. If the palms of the hands become yellow, discharge is likely occurring through the gall bladder, pancreas, spleen, or possibly the liver.

Psoriasis, eczema, and acne stem from kidney problems, the waste going to the skin in an attempt to escape. The remedy is to ease the strain on the kidneys by proper eating, including limited salt and liquid, instead of trying ineffective salves and lotions. Pimples are caused by bad fermentation in the intestines, again showing up on the skin. And again the origin is in too much food, too much waste in the body, or in wrong food. Oh, ye red?-blooded Americans and other people who eat dairy food, saturated fats, sugar — ye pizza and soft-drink addicts! You're ingesting foods that clog the intestines so that you have a blood stream full of fatty acid and mucus, popping out into pimples! (Why did we have to find out how good all those things can taste?!) Sugar may *trigger* the discharge via the skin even though other foods are causing the basic problem. So when someone says that sweets make his or her face "break out," sugar isn't the only item that should be avoided!

"Surface" annoyances that bother a large percentage of people are dandruff and hair loss, often considered to be related to liver trouble. For years, I had had a severe dandruff condition, for which I had tried many of the popular nostrums. Now, without any medication, it has finally all but disappeared. It seems strange, though, that the cancer was cured long before the dandruff: I tell friends that cancer is easy, but dandruff is a tougher adversary! Being always on the lookout for slats for the macrobiotic soapbox, I am taking the improvement in my scalp and hair as one more index that the liver is getting stronger. And I'm viewing the absence of other skin irritations as a somewhat minor piece of evidence that the other organs mentioned in this discussion are approaching an above-average degree of good health.

In the cancer-and-philosophy book quoted above, Ohsawa asserts that the following skin troubles appear as an excess of protein: warts, rapidly growing nails, and foot calluses and corns, especially on the soles. He defines warts and corns as excrescences "non-existent in vegetarians" (page 64). I haven't discussed this with any other vegetarians, but my wife tells me that for several months she hasn't had "seed corns" on the soles of her feet, although they used to be a chronic symptom for her, as was a sloughing off of the skin on the soles of her feet. Likewise, she used to have a chronic condition in which her hands felt sticky for a day or two and subsequently would slough off skin in erasure-like crumbles. These symptoms did not, however, vanish in a few days of "total suppression of animal protein from the diet," as promised by Ohsawa. It was more like two years. He cites excess Vitamin C, sugar, potassium, phosphorus, and other factors which dilate our skin as other causes of falling hair, since the skin "loses its capacity to hold hair follicles" (page 67) if these substances are ingested.

One of the most common forms of discharge is diarrhea, which may last for months for some people who have many toxins to discharge. However, it is not accompanied by the feeling of weakness usually associated with this condition. Edward Esko told us that those people who experienced this annoyance, who were middle-aged or older, usually passed through this phase more quickly than people born after World War II, because the older people did not grow up in the age of artificial and chemicalized food. There's *one* benefit of "maturity"!

A good friend of ours, Ingrid Russell, whose case history is in Chapter 15, reminded us that in discharging we rid ourselves of toxins in the reverse order in which we acquired them. This is a principle which assists in our insight as we learn to cooperate with discharges; and as a matter of fact it could be an explanation for the phenomenon noted at the beginning of our description of discharging, that of attacking the serious illness first, for of course it would have been most recently in our minds as the one which brought us face to face with the need for drastic action. Ingrid is a past master at dealing with these things because of having "outlived" and conquered a number of them proportionate to the seriousness of her illness. She offered the helpful imagery that she thought of one stage after another as being like peeling back the pages of a book from back to front.

In one of his seminar lectures, Michio had some interesting descriptions of more or less short-range discharge resulting from specific foods:

> If someone becomes very angry, someone very happy, someone very depressed, what is the cause for the difference? It is what he or she is eating. Today I eat fish. Tomorrow I think more aggressively. But we forget to relate what we ate to the way we feel. If we are aggressive, or depressed, or sad, we may forget this is what we ate yesterday.
>
> *Student:* Does most food affect you so quickly, in just twenty-four hours?
>
> *Michio:* Some food can affect you that quickly. Some food takes 3, 4, 5 days. Suppose you "binge." You may eat cheesecake and plenty of fish and still you are thinking very clearly and feeling normal. At that time you think, "I must be getting very good." Then, a few days later, you feel the effect. By that time you have forgotten what you ate.
>
> *Student:* What if you ate lobster with a lot of butter?
>
> *Michio:* The effect would already begin that evening. But the peak comes about three days later. Then it diminishes in another three to four days. If you ate ice cream, the influence continues about three to four weeks. The peak comes about four days after eating it. At that time, some people become sick physically, or mentally depressed,

pessimistic. Then it gradually diminishes, taking about four weeks.

Student: Could it also make you sleep more?

Michio: Yes. Sleeping long means your brain nerves become paralyzed, like when you have a cramp in your leg and can't walk. When that condition appears in your brain, you become sleepy.

Later in the same lecture, Michio commented that brown rice can counteract some ill effects of other foods: "If you eat something in a restaurant, then go home and eat brown rice, your toxification will disappear. If your main food is day-to-day whole grain then you are safe."

In answer to a question as to how long it takes to discharge drugs, he said, "Drugs are very yin. (See Chapter 9.) Marijuana is 400-500 times more yin than sugar. ...LSD is again a few thousand times more yin than marijuana. It takes a long time to discharge. When you take marijuana for six months to one year it takes about one year to discharge after you stop. LSD takes about four years."

Thus, discharging can be a force to be reckoned with for a while for some friends of the macrobiotic way. But however it may be that some problems will occur — and some few people who do not exercise good judgment may even have serious trouble from going off on an extreme tangent — it is more significant that many thousands can be helped by having the material we have compiled here. It grieves us to think of the thousands who have died when the macrobiotic method could have saved them, if they had only had some way to know about that method.

My own stepmother is one example. She went to her local physician with a small lump on her breast and he said not to worry about it because he could tell by looking that it was not malignant. About a year later she returned for a checkup. Again he said not to worry about it, but he told her that if she wanted to ease her concerns he would send her to a specialist. She did and he did, so she found herself in the office of a specialist. This doctor told my Dad that his first reaction when he saw the tumor was that it was malignant. However, he said he had learned that he could not make an accurate diagnosis by just looking. Tests confirmed his fears, so a mastectomy was performed. Chemotherapy treatments were called for later, after which the doctors were so pleased with the results that my Dad made one of the few long-distance phone calls he ever made in his life to tell us that Wilma was responding very well to the medication. The doctors told him that the drug they were using seemed more effective for her cancer than for that of most patients. However, as so often happens with chemotherapy, the time was not long coming when it didn't work. Then another mastectomy was required, followed by her complete loss of vision in, and removal of, one eye. After that it was simply a matter of waiting for her time to run out. The only fortunate part of it was that she didn't suffer. For some reason, the malignancy seemed to strike part of her brain so that she didn't remember that she had cancer and she didn't feel any pain. She only knew that she had been sick for some time. The end came four and a half years from the time of the first mastectomy.

If we had known then what we know now, she could have been saved, for we believe she would have been one who would have adopted macrobiotics. And this kind of situation can be multiplied by many, many thousands every year who suffer from all kinds of illnesses.

We also feel obligated to find a means of disseminating favorable information about macrobiotics to counteract the detrimental, although infrequent, statements that have been printed in major publications. The practices of drug-oriented groups have warranted some of this criticism. Using brown rice as a cheap and easy food which can feed the "commune" type of household, such people may claim they are eating macrobiotically when actually they may have only a furry knowledge of what the total variety should be. Or, even if they should happen to have the food part of it worked out accurately, the benefits would be more than canceled out by their drugs.

Among publications of national circulation (prior to 1977), the only article we know of dealing *entirely* and *directly* with macrobiotics appeared in 1971. Dr. Frederick Stare, Chairman of the Department of Nutrition at Harvard, wrote "The Diet That's Killing Our Kids," a misleading accusation, which was later cleared up in a feature article in the Boston *Globe* of December 4, 1977.[2] Dr. Stare blamed macrobiotics for the death of one young woman (who, we learned, was using strong medication and yet unwisely went to the extreme of eating nothing but brown rice for nine months!). Macrobiotics or any other self-improvement regimen can be twisted into a fad by those who are emotionally unbalanced. Ohsawa lists the all-brown-rice diet as a temporary cleansing device, and macrobiotic leaders consider it as only a short-term fast, at least for Occidentals. They recommend it as a substitute for *total* fasting, for three to five days, or for seven to ten days at the most, and suggest accompanying it with small amounts of other grains and miso soup. In "Killing Our Kids" Stare also declared that the limited liquid of the "most dangerous fad diet around" is a "restriction almost bound to cause critical kidney malfunction." But macrobiotic followers have long known, and case histories being collected by the East West Foundation are bearing out the fact, that those who eat in this Universal manner have an absolute minimum of kidney complaints, if any. Among much other misinformation, Dr. Stare dismissed Michio's extensive work as "weekly lectures on the macrobiotic system delivered by a 'guru' at a Boston Unitarian church"!

Occasionally we have heard and read a few other brief antagonistic public statements against macrobiotics. One night as we were driving home from Michigan we heard on the radio a public service announcement warning against using reducing diets without medical guidance. It went something like this: "Don't take up some silly diet like an all-sweets diet or the macrobiotic diet." (!)

The *Reader's Digest* carried two articles on vegetarian diets, one in February and one in March of 1975, both including brusque references indicating that the macrobiotic diet is a foolish, even dangerous, quackery. The first, "Do We Eat Too Much Meat?", contained the warning that "a macrobiotic diet (based largely on brown rice) can induce scurvy, anemia, hypocalcemia, emaciation and loss of kidney function."[3] And again we say we believe that the *complete* program will clear up such ailments rather than cause them.

The article in the March *Digest,* "What's Your Food I.Q.?", was written by Elizabeth M. Whelan, co-author with Dr. Stare of a book about food additives. (As we have pointed out, macrobiotic knowledge excludes *all* additives.) This latter article, speaking of the way food fads come and go, noted that "Advocates of brown rice claim that it is a perfect food." (Well, it *is,* almost!) And: "Some of these fads may prove harmless. Others — particularly the macrobiotic diet's recommendation of the exclusive use of brown rice — can prove (and have proven) fatal."[4]

I'm sure all this criticism was committed with good intent, but unfortunately the macrobiotic facts are not presented accurately.

Incidentally, the shoe is sometimes on the other foot. Some university nutrition departments came in for their share of criticism in a United Press International news item of August 15, 1976, which told of a study released jointly by Rep. Benjamin S. Rosenthal (D., N.Y.) and Dr. Michael Jacobson, co-director of the Center for Science in the Public Interest. We need to be aware of this sort of background when we read advice from nutrition "authorities." This study revealed that "nutritionists often serve as food company directors, act as consultants and testify for the industry at Congressional hearings," thus leaving the consumer without unbiased advice. Dr. Jacobson said that "industry grants, consulting fees and directorships are muzzling, if not prostituting, nutrition and food science professors."

The article declared further:

> The Jacobson study was particularly critical of Harvard's Department of Nutrition. It said a prominent faculty member is on Continental Can Co.'s board of directors and has testified on behalf of Kellogg, Nabisco, Carnation, the Cereal Institute and the Sugar Association.
>
> The report said Kellogg sponsored a study by Harvard's School of Dental Medicine on the impact of sugar coated cereals on tooth decay.
>
> The cereal industry touted the results without revealing who paid for the research, the report said, and the study later was criticized in letters to the Journal of the American Dental Association where it appeared.

The report was also critical of the University of Wisconsin Food Research Institute, which "received more than $600,000 from such companies as Kellogg, Nestle, Campbell, Kraftco and General Mills." The director of the Wisconsin institute hotly denied that the money was used for any purpose other than research to keep food safe.

Another news story was ostensibly unaware of pointing accusations at macrobiotics. In the *U.S. News and World Report* of June 21, 1976, the article "What the Health Quacks Are Peddling Now" (pp. 45-46) estimated that two billion dollars are spent annually by Americans for all manner of "useless" treatments outside the realm of the medical profession. Commenting on new "quackeries," the article said, "In contrast to the standard treatment for cancer — surgery, radiation and chemotherapy — which may be painful and disfiguring, the quack remedy is simple and painless." It offers hope, which in itself may bring about an apparent remission. The American Cancer Society has a list of more than fifty "unproven methods of cancer management. ... Many of the cancer 'cures' rely heavily on special diets." People who may have heard vaguely of the macrobiotic diet may relate it to the latter statement, even though the *News* writer may know nothing about macrobiotics and therefore may have had no such relationship in mind.

We rack up a losing score, too, on a little test the *News* devised to protect you against quackery. But we hope you won't *really* consider us quacks because the test includes mention of services that are "supposed to cure a wide variety of unrelated ailments," or because our claims "seem to be too good to be true."

Since there is some discussion about arthritis later on in our book (especially in Chapter 10), we'd like to summarize here what the *News* article says about this disease. Although various types of arthritis afflict more than twenty-two million Americans, "medical science has no cure for the disease, and even control of arthritis is complicated and not always effective." Four-hundred million dollars a year are spent on quack remedies, according to the Arthritis Foundation in New York, as compared to twenty-million for "reputable" research. Because we believe in dietary help for relieving the agony of arthritis, we would be classed with the quack remedies, although precious little of that $400 million is spent on macrobiotics!

We did finally decide to get our material together to write this book, having come to the conclusion that any problems we may cause by doing so will be outweighed by the help it may give to people who are desperately looking for help; and it can perhaps set the record straight regarding attacks against macrobiotics. If we tacitly let things go by, we couldn't live with our conscience in the face of the forceful statement by President Joseph Kosarek of the International Association of Cancer Victims and Friends in his Message in the Vol. 11, No. 2, issue of the *Cancer News Journal.*

> It is disappointing that I had not learned the truth just two years sooner. The truth of cancer control was known in the time of my need, but was not made available to me. Among my fellow Americans there are people who had the knowledge to give this information and they did not. They are guilty of homicide. It is our humanitarian duty to help others learn the truth, to help others learn to lead healthy, productive, happy lives. Not to do so would be negligence of duty and guilt of negligent homicide. …As ministers of health, we have the moral obligation and duty to make available the opportunity of learning to our fellow man.

Notes for Chapter 5

[1]Quotations from Michio Kushi throughout the remainder of the book are taken from transcriptions from his frequent lectures in Boston and from seminars in this country and abroad. These lectures are reprinted, with occasional minor changes in wording, in various publications of the East West Foundation (359 Boylston Street, Boston 02116) and in Mr.

Kushi's books, specifically in *Order of the Universe* magazines, *East West Journals,* two volumes of the *Teachings of Michio Kushi,* and his latest books: *The Book of Macrobiotics* (1977) and *The Macrobiotic Way of Natural Healing* (1978). A complete list is in our Bibliography.

[2]Charles Radin, "The Message of Michio Kushi," *Boston Sunday Globe, New England* magazine section, December 4, 1977, pp. 67-84. (Available in many public libraries.)

[3]Daniel Grotta-Kurska, "Do We Eat Too Much Meat?," *The Reader's Digest,* February, 1975, pp. 195-200. Condensed from *Today's Health,* October, 1974, a publication of the American Medical Association.

[4]Elizabeth M. Whelan, "What's Your Food I.Q.?," *The Reader's Digest,* March, 1975, pp. 97-100. Condensed from *Glamour,* June, 1974.

CHAPTER 6

Hopeful Harbingers

Jean Kohler

As we promised in our Introduction, we'll tell you briefly about the windfalls that came about after all our frustrations had almost caused us to give up on trying to carry out our obsession.

The first sign of change we learned about was mailed to us by Edward Esko of the East West Foundation. It showed that, during all the time we were fuming, experiments and investigations were going on in the very areas we would have wished for, culminating in a government report which, if followed up as it should be, can be a boon to all humanity. On July 28, 1976, Gio B. Gori, deputy director of the Division of Cancer Cause and Prevention of the Department of Health, Education, and Welfare, presented a paper to the Select Committee on Nutrition and Human Needs of the U.S. Congress. From a Diet, Nutrition, and Cancer Program developed by the National Cancer Institute, the report was the result of the work of two hundred scientists, who came up with answers that made our eyes bug out — because much of it sounds quite macrobiotic! We thought it so remarkable that we wish it were practical to include the entire report here. However, you can order it from the Department of Health, Education, and Welfare. Subsequently (February, 1977) the staff of the Senate Select Committee on Nutrition and Human Needs (Senator George McGovern, S.D., chairman) prepared a booklet — *Dietary Goals for the United States* — which was equally significant. It is for sale for 95¢ (1977) from the U.S. Superintendent of Documents. If you think government documents are dull, these will change your opinion, for they're fascinating! We wrote "Wow!" in the margin many times in our copy. We made skeleton summaries of these two reports, lifting representative sentences and paragraphs, with significant (in our opinion!) passages underlined, and with our own comments enclosed in brackets. These summaries are available from the East West Foundation at a nominal fee to cover their costs in the matter. All we can do in this chapter is to toss you a few bones from the skeletons. We italicize the "choicest" ones.

We certainly hope the dust will not be allowed to collect on this type of research. One reservation we have is the fact that in the 1940's and '50's there was a similar surge of interest in diet-cancer relationship; but it died down when the virus, heredity, and other experimentations became popular. So until such time as diet theories become general and firmly established, perhaps our book will help you. Just remember that this scientific research *was* done and was given enough credence to be reported to the U.S. Congress; and if you're one of our friendly skeptics, please use the government reports to give yourself the confidence to depend on macrobiotics. If you have a serious illness, fate may not give you the time to wait for the information to become widespread.

The Gori report contains such statements as these:

> Until a few years ago, the role of nutrition in disease was recognized only for certain specific deficiency syndromes, such as beri-beri, scurvy and rickets. ...*Until recently many eyebrows would have been raised by suggesting that an imbalance of normal dietary components could lead to cancer and cardiovascular diseases.*
>
> Today the accumulation of epidemiologic and laboratory evidence in man and animals makes this notion not only possible but certain. ...It is possible to think of a coordinated effort of research and action to accelerate the application of this understanding in the maintenance of human health and in the prevention and cure of disease.
>
> *Epidemiologic and laboratory data suggest that diet is an important factor in the causation of various forms of cancer...*

Many, many cases have been investigated from migrant populations and from ethnic groups. Evidence is cited to show that even where other factors are different but diet is similar, disease patterns (not just for cancer but for others, such as cardiovascular diseases) are similar. By contrast, if diet is different, types of disease are different, even if other factors are the same.

Obesity, one of the most serious present-day afflictions, has here one more warning to face: "Of all dietary modifications, caloric restriction has had the most regular influence on tumor formation, ...generally inhibiting tumor formation. ...Furthermore, even within a group of animals being fed identical diets, the incidence of tumors tends to be consistently greater in heavier rats than in lean rats." And listen to *this:* animals fed the now much revered polyunsaturated fat, compared to a group eating saturated fat, had more colonic tumors!

One important observation was that in cases where long-term environmental hazards of various kinds, plus wrong diet, contribute to the final development of certain types of cancer, *the correction of diet alone may stop that development.* Therefore the conclusion was that in the investigation of carcinogenic factors "the study of nutritional influences should receive priority."

The report insists that the eventual definition of desirable dietary intake should not be generalized, but should be "formulated in such terms as to be applicable to the greatly varying requirements of individuals." Then the statement is made that at present it is not scientifically possible to "assess individual nutritional status." But those who are highly skilled in Oriental medicine can make this type of assessment by observation! (Chapter 7) (Or, if one must have some sort of Western medical evidence, one could examine the elaborate computer system Dr. William Kelley uses to determine that status. However, since he is a fallen angel with the "establishment" because of his unorthodox methods, it is not likely that he would be consulted to help remedy this need!) The report continues by saying that when such information does becomes possible, it may be used by "those in charge of global food policies, to make intelligent nutritional decisions that may affect the individual patient, the nutrition awareness of a given population, and the regulatory, manufacturing, and distribution policies of food resources." A lofty, commendable goal!

Research revealed that "dramatic results" had been obtained in initial work in intragastric and intravenous feeding of extremely weak patients, or those with cancer damage to the upper alimentary tract. (Compare this with our mention in Chapter 13 of feeding critically ill patients macrobiotically.) Also, *recent experiments "have suggested the intriguing possibility of using nutrition as a direct form of cancer therapy." (Recent* experiments — to "discover" age-old wisdom!) Speaking of research efforts in the future, "It is clear that, although the majority of these activities will be directed at the solution of the cancer problem, they will have considerable spinoffs for other nutrition dependent diseases, both in terms of prevention and in the *use of nutrition as therapeutic support."* What a significant statement! No wonder we're excited about this report.

They say that "nutritional support to the cancer patient could become a reality in the next few years," but that five to ten years would be required to determine desirable dietary intakes. (Meanwhile, if you've been told your time is limited, we'd suggest a macrobiotic parachute.)

The capital-letter enthusiasm is ours in this final paragraph of the report: "THE ROLE OF NUTRITION IN HUMAN DISEASE IS OBVIOUS, AND NO OTHER FIELD OF RESEARCH SEEMS TO HOLD BETTER PROMISE FOR THE PREVENTION AND CONTROL OF CANCER AND OTHER ILLNESS, AND FOR SECURING AND MAINTAINING HUMAN HEALTH."

Growing out of this report, the *Dietary Goals for the United States* begins with this Foreword by Senator McGovern:

> The purpose of this report is to point out that the eating patterns of this century represent as critical a public health concern as any now before us.
>
> We must acknowledge and recognize that the public is confused about what to eat to maximize health. If we as a Government want to reduce health costs and maximize the quality of life for all Americans, we have an obligation to provide practical guides to the individual consumer as well as set national dietary goals for the country as a whole. ...

Charles H. Percy (Illinois), ranking minority member of the committee, made these key remarks: "Without Government and industry commitment to good nutrition, the American people will continue to eat themselves to poor health. ... *Our national health depends on how well and how quickly Government and industry respond.*"

At a press conference to release the study of the Senate Nutrition Committee, Dr. D. Mark Hegsted, professor of nutrition at the Harvard School of Public Health, pointed out that degenerative diseases such as heart disease, some cancers, diabetes, hypertension, and obesity are now spotlighted more because infectious diseases are relatively controlled. Concerning the degenerative diseases, he declares that...

> an inappropriate diet contributes to their causation. ... The diet we eat today was not planned or developed for any particular purpose. It is a happenstance related to our affluence, the productivity of our farmers and the activities of our food industry. ... What are the risks associated with eating less meat, less fat, less saturated fat, less cholesterol, less sugar, less salt, and more fruits [we disagree!],

vegetables, unsaturated fat and cereal products — especially whole grain cereals? There are none that can be
identified and important benefits can be expected. ... *We
cannot afford to temporize.*

(Dr. Hegsted apparently had not looked too closely at the comments about saturated and unsaturated fats in the earlier report
presented by Dr. Gori.)

Other committee members spoke of easy access (as through
food machines and quick-lunch restaurants) to fats and sugars
versus difficult access to foods likely to improve health. There were
statements to the effect that the public has an over-confidence that
medical science can cure degenerative diseases. But, they said,
medicine does not have workable solutions (compare with the Ivan
Illich discussion in Chapter 8), *and therefore prevention (as through
proper food) is all the more important.*

As for other sections of the *Dietary Goals* booklet, since we
are strongly urging you to order your own copy, we'll give only a
minimum number of excerpts which we hope will emphasize its
value. They recommend accurate labeling of processed foods,
saying that at present labeling is voluntary and therefore such
information as percentage of sugar and presence of additives is
easily "hidden." E.L. Buckner (see later in this chapter) tells us that
unless the label specifically states that there are no preservatives or
other chemicals added, they could be among the ingredients. The
booklet mentions what many people now know — that additives
(especially by combination with other chemicals in the food or in the
body) are suspect as a cancer agent, and may also be contributing
factors to hyperactivity, especially in children, who, incidentally,
ingest a staggering amount of artificial coloring in beverages alone.

One reason children — and adults! — drink such harmful
amounts of harmful beverages, and eat so many junk foods is the
constant bombardment from television advertising. According to
one respectable source quoted by the Committee, more than 50
percent of the cost of television food advertising may be negatively
related to health.

This leads to a principal recommendation of the Committee:
government funding for public education in nutrition, including
extensive use of television, as well as instruction in school class-
rooms and cafeterias; funding for government study of new techniques in food processing to reduce risk factors; and funding for
the study of nutritional health concerns in agricultural policy.

Some of the goals are as follows (the numbering is ours): (1)

Increase carbohydrate consumption (although they do not know that it should be mostly *grain* carbohydrates); (2) Reduce fat consumption (There's almost *none* in the macrobiotic diet.); (3) Reduce butterfat, eggs, and other high cholesterol sources; use non-fat milk (Macrobiotics says *no* dairy products.); (4) Reduce meats (We say none at all.), and increase fish and poultry (still using only moderate amounts); (5) Increase fruits (ill-advised, we believe); vegetables, and whole grains (excellent!); (6) Reduce sugar (98 percent of American children are reported to have some tooth decay, and by age 55 about half of the American people have no teeth.) (We say that's not the *only* reason for eliminating sugar completely!); (7) Reduce salt. They quote studies showing that the desire for salt is acquired rather than being a "physiological necessity." We were pleased to read that these studies find evidence that "there is an important balance between sodium and potassium, required for the proper flow of fluids among and through cells," and the ratio they think best is downright macrobiotic! We consider it unfortunate, though, that they do not suggest replacing commercial salt, deficient in minerals and other essential elements, with sea salt or solar salt.

For related material, order the "Food Policy Recommendations" listed in the East West Foundation Special Publications in our Bibliography. This is an account of a September, 1977, meeting at the White House, a two-hour discussion by Michio Kushi and other macrobiotic leaders with government representatives in agriculture, public liaison, food policy, and other health issues.

Besides the government reports, we had another happy development. We had given up on generating interest from any organization, not knowing that the National Cancer Institute had sponsored the mammoth research program leading to the Gori report to Congress. (Because the contacts to the American Cancer Society had been futile we figured there would be no use to try NCI.) But suddenly an avenue did open up with an important organization: the International Association of Cancer Victims and Friends, based in California, which has as its purpose the study of new methods of cancer treatment. Founded in 1963 by Cecile Hoffman, when she was thwarted in her attempts to obtain Laetrile to help combat her cancer, the organization supports freedom of choice in cancer treatment. Legalization of Laetrile is one of their goals, now being realized as state after state follows the trend started by Alaska in September of 1976. They are also open-minded about other recently introduced non-toxic therapies. As a public service, they have taken on some legal battles to defend some of the doctors who have been harassed for using Laetrile, and to defend their own rights to privacy of their files.

Before their 1974 convention, we had written to several of the prominent speakers telling them about macrobiotics and suggesting that they contact Michio about the particular kind of cancer they were interested in. Not one answered.

Some time later we were contacted by Mr. and Mrs. E.L. Buckner of Chula Vista, California, who were hoping to compare the macrobiotic approach with their own dietary cancer cure, which had been worked out on a scientific basis by Mr. Buckner, a research biologist. (Some information about his method is given in Chapter 10.) The Buckners were members of the IACVF, and suggested that I get in touch with the executive director in regard to having Michio as one of the guest speakers for the 1976 convention. It was thereupon arranged for Michio to speak at one of the evening sessions. I had the honor of playing part of a recital during the evening's entertainment, and of introducing Michio before his lecture.

The speakers at the convention were excellent and the attendance was large. One thing we especially appreciate about the organization is the fact that they give every plausible system a chance to be heard from. (A few of these are discussed in Chapter 10, on "Alternatives.") Most of the cancer people there seem to have cured or arrested their ailment by means of the Laetrile method, the Kelley method, or some other Gerson-related method, sometimes accompanied by Dr. Simonton-type mental practices. But there were exhibits of other treatments, as well as a great variety of high quality exhibits on related subjects. People were very cordial, and showed interest in our field by asking many questions of Michio, and of us, and of Roy and Marijke Steevensz, sponsors of the East West Center in Los Angeles.

Another delightful benefit for us was to have some story-book acquaintances come to life. We had a long interesting talk with Dr. Max Gerson's daughter, Charlotte Gerson Straus, who had a booth there (see Chapter 3, and also her address in the Appendix). And, although we didn't get a chance to talk to him, we saw Dr. Ernest Krebs, Jr., who worked closely with his father and brother in the development of Laetrile (Chapter 10). Then we had quite a bit of time with Ida Honorof, who had an exhibit of her writings, as well as being one of the speakers. We haven't introduced her to you before, but she is a person to be reckoned with. We often say we hope she is always on our side. She publishes a hard-hitting, carefully researched newsletter called "A Report to the Consumer" (see Bibliography), and really comes out swinging. We doubt that anyone who read or heard her information on swine vaccine would have subjected him-her-self to that atrocity; and she has been equally outspoken on cancer misinformation, funeral "ripoffs," health hazards such as asbestos dust and pesticides, and many other varied topics.

Ida and the Buckners were the reasons we ended up at the IACVF convention, because Ida had picked up our story and had written an article about it for the *Cancer News Journal* published by IACVF. Sandra (Mrs. Ed Gooch), the lovely daughter of the Buckners, was telling the man who delivers vegetables to her home that her father had cancer. The delivery man showed her the Honorof article, and the Buckners tossed the ball to us. Then because Michio was "featured" at the convention, Gloria Swanson and William Dufty both came as major speakers, and both (of course) did a thoroughly professional job of it. Dufty is the author of (among other things) *Sugar Blues,* discussed in our Chapter 9. He said in his speech that as a former newspaper man he thought he could recognize history in the making, and that was exactly what was going on at the convention that evening, as East and West met on common ground to conquer one of the main threats of the human condition. He and Gloria Swanson were married in 1976, and they now carry on such endeavors as cooperating closely with the East West Foundation, frequently lecturing at their seminars, as well as traveling world-wide to promote *Sugar Blues.*

We are extremely grateful to the Cancer Victims and Friends for adding macrobiotics as one of their paths to restored health. President Joseph Kosarek (see end of Chapter 5) and Michio Kushi now compare notes from time to time. This organization can be a positive force in shaping the future for victims of cancer. For a time it was hurt by some internal wrangling (birth pangs?), but those problems seem to be solved now so that it can move ahead without further strife. Unfortunately, the only funding it has is that raised from its membership, for the government agencies related to health have done more harassing than helping. Those who might wish to aid IACVF endeavors could begin by subscribing to their informative and attractive *Cancer News Journal* (see our Bibliography).

In the matter of gaining the interest of the medical profession, the East West Foundation seems to have found the right buttons to push. In March of 1977 they sponsored a week-long seminar on the relationship of diet to cancer and other major illnesses. One day of the seminar was turned over to a conference with people in the medical field. The response of these guests was very gratifying, and during the conference, titled "A Nutritional Approach to Cancer," the atmosphere was one of friendly cooperation, resulting in a final agreement to keep in touch and try to find scientific ways to research the effect of the macrobiotic diet on cancer and other major illness. A very interesting diary recording this entire conference may be ordered from the East West Foundation.

As of June, 1977, ways of cooperating on research projects were beginning to be worked out with groups of doctors in various cities where Michio lectured. "Meanwhile, back at the Foundation," EWF is working with the Harvard Medical School, and particularly with Dr. Edward H. Kass of that school, pursuing the possibilities of controlled clinical research on the macrobiotic approach to cancer cases in Boston. Dr. Kass is one of three researchers who made the studies on blood pressure and cholesterol levels referred to in our Chapter 8. (See EWF Special Publications in our Bibliography.)

Monumental in its significance could be the association between the EWF and Dr. Richard Prindle, an influential figure in World Health. Do you remember that the paper we mentioned earlier in this chapter — the one read by Dr. Gori to the Nutrition Committee — stated that research on individual nutrition needs could make available to those "in charge of global food policies" information to help make decisions on such matters as "distribution policies of food resources"? Dr. Prindle would have the know-how to aid in the implementation of objectives of that sort, being uniquely qualified because of having been for some years head of the Western Hemisphere Family Health Division of the World Health Organization.

He became acquainted with Michio at the March 9 Conference and later had some further contacts with him. Jean also met Dr. Prindle that day, and was impressed with his pertinent comments during the meetings and at an informal session in the evening. During the following months we were in touch with Dr. Prindle by phone a few times to be sure of our accuracy in reporting the statement he generously supplied as a foreword for our book. We were especially happy in our understanding that he felt he could give support to the worldwide use of macrobiotics, particularly in the developing nations.

Dr. Prindle is at home with large-scale viewpoints, for even before his work in World Health he was from 1968 to 1971 the Assistant Surgeon General of the United States! A few months ago, in order to get away from the pressure of overseeing the work of some 500 people in the World Health Organization, he changed to a less (?) complicated position as Director of the Thomas Jefferson Health District of the State of Virginia (comprising the city of Charlottesville and an area of five counties — 10,000 square miles, staffed by 120 people, including some 50 nurses, 5 or 6 dentists, and several engineers). Besides that, he instructs young doctors at the University of Virginia Medical School.

Already warm supporters of macrobiotics were the other physicians whose statements appear at the beginning of our book. Outstanding in their field, they have given outstanding strength to the goals of the EWF, and they combine the knowledge of the East and West in their medical practice. Dr. Mendelsohn was honorary chairman of the 1978 Medical Conference, held this time during a week-long Summer Program sponsored by the Foundation at Amherst (Massachusetts) College.

As you well know by now, we had been ardently wishing that *something* would happen to make the advantages of macrobiotics convincing to doctors and hence to their patients. Many things that developed out of that day in Boston on March 9, 1977, began to point the way toward credibility.

On an infinitesimal scale by comparison, the day had far-reaching personal consequences for me. These consequences by chance went hand in hand with another surprising breakthrough — that of having two doctors suddenly become interested in my medical history. We describe these developments in the Chapter 9 Sequel.

As a related break-through, it was a kind of oblique benefit for macrobiotics that the Laetrile "revolution" got under way, with Alaska legalizing its use in September, 1976, followed by our own Indiana, and soon by one state after another. Acceptance of one unorthodox approach can smooth the way for another.

But even if things move in the smoothest possible manner, there is a long way to go to bring back good health — and its resultant peace — to this planet. We believe that your acquaintance with the macrobiotic way will be your personal contribution to this goal.

CHAPTER 7

Michio Kushi!

(MAK)

From the country of East, you have come
From the country of West, I have come
The day we two meet here
Is the day true happiness begins.
To make two into one
Is the way of eternity, the way of God.

With the endless life, we are living
In the endless dream, we are living
The day we all meet here
Is the day we are born in a true country.
To make all into one
Is the way of eternity, the way of God.

This poem of Michio Kushi's seems to us to express the inner purpose in all that he does. Of course, no one goes around analyzing Michio Kushi; but from his acts when we were privileged to be with him, and from his many essays, books, and seminar reports, it seems that everything he does leads toward the profundity revealed in this poem. The little song is the ultimate in simplicity — you can memorize it in a few seconds. Yet it is a pattern for saving planet Earth. If all people and all nations could meet each other, touch hands, and share the joy and trust and mutual appreciation that run deep in these few words, then a common energy could be used to solve the world's troubles.

We have never seen Michio refuse to answer anyone's questions, no matter how many hours of questioning he has been put through previously. Our time with him has been limited to our two private consultations in Boston, a number of midnight telephone conversations when we, or someone we knew, had problems, and his three-day visit to our University in January, 1976, during which time Jean had the opportunity to escort him to all his lectures and other engagements. After each event, it was never Michio who cut off the time given to the eager people who crowded around him. It was Jean, who was forced, with difficulty, to get Michio to his next appointment. At the IACVF convention in Los Angeles we had the privilege of further brief contacts with Michio, as did several hundred other people! (Chapter 6) We have frequently talked with his staff associates, in person and by phone, and none of them has ever reported impatience in Michio's dealings with others.

People we talk to about our cancer-curing experiences have trouble visualizing Mr. Kushi as anything but a physician. Because our story deals with Jean's return to health, our friends consistently picture a white-smocked doctor in a stainless steel clinic with white-uniformed nurses scurrying about. But we are describing a different kind of situation! To each friend we have to say several times, "No, it isn't *Doctor* Kushi!"

Rather, his appearance is perhaps that of a businessman — and indeed he happens to be a skillful businessman! His manner is quiet and receptive. No matter how long or how often you may have fractured the Laws of the Universe, or how many more times you will digress as you try to learn the macrobiotic way, Michio Kushi will accept you and *respect* you. "Ah, so — I understand!"

Mr. Kushi maintains a simple life style. The furnishings in the large rented house, which takes the place of the stainless steel clinic, consist of floor cushions and low tables. Side rooms have large old desks and chairs, typewriters, telephones, and stacks of papers. Someplace upstairs are living quarters for the family, and accommodations for a few students and visitors. Mr. Kushi has no flashy diamond rings, no automobile (he doesn't even drive!), no expensive gifts gracing his offices. A fat guru he is not. The admiration of his disciples goes far too deep for manifestation in any superficial "material things." And besides, they haven't got that kind of money.

For all that, we believe he is one of the intellectual giants of the century. His main mission is interpreting the Order of the Universe for the rest of us as we grope around trying to comprehend it. The fact that we recover from terminal illnesses in the process is coincidental.

Michio Kushi was born in Japan in 1926, to parents who were high school and university teachers and who later became involved in social concerns. He describes the family life during his youth as humble economically and socially, busy and studious. Their meals were simple, with grains as the main food. In his teen-age years he began to be aware of the intense social pressures brought about by Japan's involvement in war, and of the "high spirit and stimulated souls among the people."

When he was sixteen, he began visiting a shrine in Akita, a thirty-minute sunrise walk from his home. There he meditated, praying without desire, making himself "unified, clear and empty." During one especially early visit, a cosmic experience occurred which he describes very poetically.[1]

> I began to feel all my surroundings starting to shine in gold colors and when I noticed it more and more, the color became intense. Then the shrine disappeared and a bright light began to shine all over, and all space enveloped me and shone everywhere.
>
> I was utterly inside this golden light and I was breathing along with it. I began to know that this light is continuously shining and radiating, and being is nothing but this continuous radiation. I don't remember how long I was within it, but after this experience I almost could not breathe. I didn't know whether my heart was beating or not, and then, suddenly I started to awake and to realize that I was within this light. When I began to see myself, then gradually the light began disappearing, and after a while it completely diminished; I found myself climbing ing down the stairs to return home.
>
> While on the staircase, I saw in the dim light of morning, that all the trees and the grass were also shining in silver and gold colors, and that everything was being; everything was radiating light. I could then understand that everything is living, everything is breathing, including plants, grasses, trees, birds, and even houses, stones, and soil; everything without exception. Then I understood that life is nothing but light and vibration, or waves, and the universe is full of life, and is one continuity, yet is manifested in everything and every being.

When he talked about this awesome adventure to other people, "Some listened, some laughed, and some ignored."

So it became part, or all, of his being "to know that, while all things are one, there is, within that one, constant flux, constant motion." Throughout the remainder of high school, of university study in political science and law, and of military service, it was constantly in the back of his mind to find a vehicle to bring his insight to the rest of the world. In spite of personal poverty and hunger, he was able to see all the strife and suffering of war, for instance, as part of the universal pattern. He was to find his means of communication evolving out of a visit to an organization in Tokyo called the World Government Association. At their headquarters, several young students shared with him their dark brown bread.

"'Don't you think this bread has a wonderful taste?'

"I didn't think so, and thought rather that it was somewhat tasteless, but as a matter of courtesy, I said, 'Yes.'"

Strangely enough, these young people talked about food and cooking rather than world government. They introduced Michio to their teacher: Nyoichi Sakurazawa, whose name in the Western world was George Ohsawa. He asked Michio whether he had ever thought about attaining world peace through a "gospel" of proper food. Of course Michio was puzzled. Oshawa smiled and said, "Please come here often, eat our food and join in our study. Then you will understand." The main theme underlying the teaching was that world peace could be established only with the "biological reconstruction of humanity" *on an individual basis,* through daily life and diet. Ohsawa had come to this conclusion through about twenty-five years of studying the problem.

Ohsawa himself never spoke to Michio about food. It was always the view of the Universe he talked about — and of yin and yang. Now to Michio Kushi these terms would not have been foreign, as they are to most of us. (When our Japanese friends pronounce them they sound like "een" and "yahng." Oriental words are transcribed into our alphabet and spellings by sound, but the word "yin" is apparently "misspelled." These are Chinese terms — yin and yang — and we have checked them with highly educated friends of both nationalities. Neither nationality uses the "y" sound in "yin." The "i," however, is always pronounced like the "i" in "machine." Some of our American friends in the East West Foundation use the Oriental pronunciation and some say "yeen" and "yahng," which is what seems most natural to us. We just hope you won't say "yin" as in "sin" (oops!) and "yang" as in "sang.")

My husband has just pointed out that we're going to raise far more questions than we will answer by getting into this, and for once he's right. But, as he says, we hope in the brief discussion we can present here to arouse your curiosity enough so you will want to do your own delving into Michio's writings listed in the Bibliography.

First let's just try to describe by a few examples what yin and yang mean in our daily lives. The influence is inescapable. It is our origin, our continuing existence, and our exit, and it is with us, of course, whether we know anything about it or not. To make an extremely simple definition, yin denotes expansion, yang denotes contraction.

Did you ever wonder why most babies arrive at night? It's because that's the yin time, the time of expansion. OK, so if you're not into having a baby, how about this one: if you have something that hurts, why does it hurt more at night? Because that's when our tissues expand. Same reason you cough more at night if you have a cold. Same reason you can eat some foods for lunch that make you feel puffed up and uncomfortable for supper. The pupils of your eyes dilate (expand) when it's night, or dark.

Another thing: yin and yang constantly repel each other, as do like magnetic poles, but also attract each other, like opposite poles, antagonistic but complementary. This affects our everyday lives because, for instance, men (they are yang) and women (yin) are attracted to each other. Because when we eat too much of one type of food, we feel the need of an opposite type to counteract the effects of the first. Because the push and pull makes our hearts beat and our lungs expand and contract and our digestive system devote its rhythms to recreating us every day.

Moreover, yin *produces* yang, and vice versa, because of the repelling action. They are constantly changing places, constantly merging into each other, so that nothing is purely yin or purely yang. (Ohsawa declares that nothing is permanent "except change itself, the only constant."[2]) Cold expands and is yin, (water expands when it freezes); but cold makes *us* shiver and pull ourselves together. Foods *produced* in cold climates (expansive) are smaller and more compact (contracted). Fire, on the other hand, contracts and is yang (when you char the toast it's smaller than the piece of bread you ruined). But although fire is yang it *produces* heat-waves and smoke, which are yin. Hot weather (yang) makes *us* expand and sweat and feel fatter and lazier. (Thus, repose is yin, activity yang.) Foods produced in hot climates (yang) are larger and juicier (yin).

For a longer-range look at yin-yang influence, here is how Mr. Kushi describes its effects on his youthful activities. He says he was a yang person, born in May. (At first this seems like a contradiction, since May is the beginning of the yang summertime and should *produce* yin. But of course the yin-yang influence begins at *conception*, for that is when a person's life really begins. Thus a yang May birth would have been produced at conception in September, the beginning of the yin season of fall and winter. The pregnant mother's food, being also seasonal, would likewise affect the yin-yang characteristics of the child.) Because Michio was yang (active), he was often a champion in grammar school athletics and learning. But also because of his native yang (and because yin and yang are always changing places), in his teens he became attracted toward eating fruit and became less interested in physical activities. By sixteen, his intellectual interests shifted to the spiritual world, and this is the reason he was drawn to the shrine to meditate, as described above.

For a *colossal* view of yin-yang, we can again draw on material from Mr. Kushi's lectures and writings. Yin and yang govern the whole of creation, beginning in Infinity as two polar tendencies (positive and negative, contractive and expansive), from which stem all energy or vibration. Now all phenomena, we're told, are governed by both a yin force (centrifugal — spinning outward and/or upward, forming an enlarging spiral) and a yang force (centripetal — spinning inward and/or downward, forming a diminishing spiral). That's why yin is expansive — because something that spins outward grows larger; and the reverse applies to yang spinning: centrifugal and centripetal — these two forces are creating every phenomenon and every manifestation.

Besides the gigantic spirals throughout the spinning, whirligig universe, notice the spirals in sea shells, in whirlpools, and in hundreds of other things in nature. Three that we have heard about, but have had no chance to check out are rams' horns, spiral grooves made by a meteorite as it digs its crater into the earth, the spiral pattern made by a flock of pigeons as they land. Don't get impatient with this, because it applies directly to *us*: this is how we're put together — in spirals. For evidence, look at your finger tips, your ears, and feel the spiral in the "cowlick" on top of your head. Mr. Kushi can give many such examples, both internal and external.

Mr. Kushi teaches us that an essential characteristic of the constant change brought about by the relationship of yin and yang forces is this: "Since everything in the universe is eternally changing, and this change proceeds according to a certain order, the study of this order is the study of eternity, infinity, or God." (This universal process of change was called Tao (tah-oh or dah-oh) by Lao Tsu. We put this in only because you're going to come across it in your reading *before* you come across any explanation of it. Lao Tsu (Lah-oh-tsoo) was a Chinese philosopher (604-531 B.C.) who advocated a life of simplicity and selflessness. So now you can come back here to refresh your memory when you meet the frequent references to Tao.)

Incidentally, Einstein, Toynbee, and other such deep intellectual types base some of their theories on yin-yang principles.

These principles are also the foundation for the ancient Oriental art or science of medical diagnosis by observation. "Through the simple and practical technique of visual diagnosis it is possible to judge a person's internal condition just by observing his or her external features, without depending on expensive devices for internal examination." Here the law of opposites applies again — analyzing the inside by observing the outside. Furthermore, the facial features and the internal organs follow this same tendency, for the lower organs are represented in the *upper* part of the face, and vice versa.

For example, the condition of the bladder, located in the lower region of the body, appears in the upper forehead and hairline. Thus, when people drink excessive liquid, too much to be discharged normally by the bladder, this excess often shows up in the form of perspiration on the forehead.

Similarly, horizontal lines in the forehead indicate that the intestines are abnormally expanded. The central organs such as the liver, spleen, pancreas, kidneys, stomach and gall bladder are visible in the middle region of the face. For example, the region between the eyebrows corresponds to the liver. Vertical lines in this area indicate liver trouble, often caused by excessive intake of animal foods containing fat. The overall condition of the liver, spleen, and pancreas can be seen in the condition of the eyes. For example, a yellowish tint in the whites of the eyes indicates probable liver trouble.

The size and shape of the ears reflect a person's overall constitution. Traditionally, ears which reflected a strong native constitution began at the level of the eyes and extended to the level of the mouth. (The number of people with such ears is decreasing, indicating general decline in the biological quality of the human race.)... In addition to overall constitution, the centrally located ears reflect the size and condition of the kidneys, which are located in the middle region of the body. The condition of the kidneys can also be seen in the area underneath the eyes. Many people have what are called "eyebags" in this area. These indicate a yin, or expanded, condition in the kidneys, usually the result of drinking an excessive amount of liquid. Also, bags under the eyes may indicate the existence of mucus or fat deposits in the kidneys.

The bridge of the nose reflects the condition of the stomach, whereas the condition of the heart can be seen in the tip of the nose. An enlarged or expanded nose indicates that the heart is also enlarged or expanded, resulting in a tendency toward high blood pressure. A reddish color also indicates enlargement or expansion, which is caused by the expansion of the blood capillaries in this area. Either sign may result from excessive intake of yin such as liquid, sugar, fruits, animal fat, and dairy products.

Many modern people have a cleft on the underside of the tip of the nose. This indicates a lack of yang contracting power during the formation of the heart in the mother's womb. As a result, the left and right chambers of the heart are often not coordinating smoothly, and the heartbeat may be irregular.

The condition of the lungs can be seen in the cheeks. Reddish or "rosy colored" cheeks in adults are the result of blood capillary expansion, indicating that the lungs are also in a yin or expanded condition.

The mouth marks the beginning of the digestive tract, and its condition mirrors the condition of the organs of digestion. In the upper lip, we can see the condition of the stomach, whereas the lower lip shows the condition of the intestines. The region between the upper and lower lips at the corner of each side of the mouth reflects the condition of the duodenum. Ideally, the mouth should be tight, and both lips should be of equal thickness. An expanded upper lip indicates a weak, expanded stomach, while a protruding, swollen lower lip shows a similar condition in the intestines. Often, this is an indication of chronic constipation or diarrhea.

Using just these basic correlations, we can begin to judge a person's physical and even emotional condition.

Of course these paragraphs are only the sketchiest sort of illustration of the many facets of observation used in this art of diagnosis.

Additionally, yin-yang principles relate to all scientific disciplines (chemistry, physics, astronomy, biology, etc.), and in a number of specifics are contrary to present-day concepts, which are often formulated from experimentation using more extreme heat than necessary or more violent force than necessary, as with the cyclotron. We believe (my husband says) that more research and deeper comprehension will cause a change in scientific thinking, bringing it back into accord with yin-yang knowledge. For example, Michio believes that the old alchemy practice of transmutation (turning one element into another) is quite logical, for all elements eventually change into other elements. (I am getting this information — and I probably should leave it where it is! — from two *East West Journal* essays based on Kushi lectures on alternative science.[3])

Of the cyclotron, Mr. Kushi says,

> Modern science does admit the possibility of transmutation but only under very unusual — and expensive — conditions. ... Obviously that extreme, violent method is not the secret of transmutation employed in alchemy, nor can it serve as the basis for a natural technology.
>
> The elements evolved naturally, and are continously changing from yin to yang and back again. ....
>
> Nuclear fusion occurs readily throughout nature, because...the nucleus is not a closed system of stable particles, but is an open field of energy in continual change.

Here are random statements on this same theme:

> The simplest element, Hydrogen, turns into the next element, Helium, and so on by a natural process of growth, just as a one-year-old child turns into a two-year-old by invisible stages of change. The older child is different from the younger child, but...they share a continuous history, following one pattern of development.
>
> Alchemy...was known throughout the ancient world, in both the Occident and the Orient. In northern China, a tomb was recently unearthed which archeologists date around 1,000 B.C. Next to the person buried there, a metallic box was found. Analysis showed it to be an alloy of nickel with 70 percent aluminum. Aluminum does not occur in nature; its extraction from bauxite ore had only been possible in modern times after the development of high temperature technology, yet 3,000 years ago aluminum was produced by alchemy.
>
> Steel produced by alchemy is much harder and far more rust resistant than industrial steel. In India there is an ancient pillar of such steel, near Delhi; modern science cannot explain why it is completely rust proof or how it could have been made.
>
> Medieval alchemists were able to create Gold from Mercury, its neighbor in the periodic table. The intuitive powers of such men who could sense that similarity of gold and mercury puts us to shame.
>
> My teacher, Georges Ohsawa, transmuted Sodium to Potassium with the following simple apparatus. [The process is described, with diagrams.]

Using similar methods, we can easily create Iron, the basis of heavy industry, and Gold, the standard of monetary systems.* The alchemical revolution means the end of materialism.

Transmutation is a far more radical change than mere chemical combination. It's the difference between getting married and having a casual affair; you really have to change. There's no other way to create a new being.

It looks as if such theories are on the way to becoming reaccepted, for confirmation that there is truth in alchemy as a science is being sought by highly respected present-day scientists. After one of his 1976 tours of Belgium Mr. Kushi reported widespread use of macrobiotic principles, especially in Flemish areas. The University of Ghent, in coordination with a Flemish milling company, is trying transmutation experiments such as sealing grain and water in containers, first checking the element composition of the grain, water, and air. They put these mixtures in the sunlight to grow, and then discovered in the containers atoms which were not there before, as well as finding that the number of some atoms had decreased because they had changed into other atoms, the number of which had increased! Every time the experiments were repeated there was the same type of transmutation — under low pressure, low temperature, and low energy.

So there is no question of biological transmutation. That means not only in plants, but in our bodies, in all animals. That is a big shock to the modern way of thinking, to modern science, because present-day nourishment is based upon the assumption that the atom never changes. ...So they think what we eat — amino acids, elements, water, etc. — remain the same in our body. If transmutation is confirmed, then the present-day theory of nutrition becomes false.... If the modern theory of nourishment changes, that means also the modern theory of blood changes, because transmutation is being made into blood. Then that changes also the modern theory of cells. When biological and biochemical science change, so must mining and industry change, and so must the orientation of astronomy and all natural science change. So although this is but a beginning, it is going to be confirmed here and there by the application and understanding of yin and yang. This will change all of science.

*Following Ohsawa's example, Mr. Kushi has made small flecks of gold (laboratory tested) in his own kitchen!

An outstanding scientist who for years quietly carried out thousands of trials similar to those at Ghent University is Pierre Baranger, director of the laboratory of organic chemistry at the Ecole Polytechnique in Paris. In a 1959 interview for *Science et Vie,* Baranger boldly says that "we have to submit to the evidence: plants know the old secret of the alchemists. *Every day under our very gaze they are transmuting elements."* This interview was reported in the fascinating book *The Secret Life of Plants,* a *must* on your reading list.[4] By the time you read this part of this chapter in our book, you are supposed to be at least partly recovered from whatever illness you had. Therefore, for your exercise today, *run* — don't walk — to the nearest bookstore and get the *Secret Life* book. Devour Chapter 17 first of all: "Alchemists in the Garden," and then read the rest of the book. On page 290 you'll read that "By 1963 Baranger had incontestably proven that in the germinations of leguminous seeds in a manganese salt solution, manganese disappeared and iron appeared in its place."

In this chapter of *Secret Life* we become acquainted with the work of Louis Kervran, a native Breton who since early youth has been following and developing insights relating to transmutations and their bearing on agriculture and nutrition. The authors, who found Kervran to be "a pleasant and forthrightly cooperative man of seventy with a prodigious memory for detail," say that he is "now retired from his duties as one of France's more eminent professors in order to embark on the career of a determined alchemist." He has turned out one book after another dealing with the subject of transmutation. The first scientist outside France to "take Kervran's work seriously" was Hisatoki Komaki, a Japanese professor of science who abandoned his teaching to become head of an electrical company biological research laboratory. He "tied Kervran's findings into ancient Eastern cosmology and wrote to Kervran to say that the transmutation of sodium, a *yang* element, into potassium, a *yin* element, was of far-reaching interest," not knowing (and neither did the authors of *Secret Life!*) that Ohsawa had accomplished the same thing!

Russian scientists are likewise paying attention to Kervran. If we quote from page 301 of *Secret Life,* we could take Soviet scientist P.A. Korol'kov as their spokesman:

> The fact is that we are witnesses and participants in a scientific-technological revolution, …a radical revision, …of the basic status of an inherited natural science. The time has come to recognize that any chemical element

can turn into another, under natural conditions. And I am not alone in maintaining this. I know a dozen persons in the USSR who hold the same views.

Thus do the authors of the *Secret Life* book, with their own knowledge and that drawn from myriad other sources (an eighteen-page bibliography, no less!) display the same faith in the principles of transmutation as does Mr. Kushi.

One more interesting point I'd like to mention in connection with Order of the Universe philosophies is that years ago Mr. Kushi said the temperature of the planet Venus, deduced by means of yin-yang principles, was 800° centigrade, when scientists were saying it was −20° to −40° centigrade. With the Venus probe, Mr. Kushi's deductions were found to be correct!

That Mr. Kushi was accurate is not surprising to those who look at all things with an open mind. Minds are being forced open in the field of physics by "new" discoveries which are in line with the type of ancient knowledge we have been speaking of. Lately, some of the younger nuclear physicists have been arriving, sometimes painfully, at concepts which would have been inconceivable a few years ago. They are grappling with ideas which modern man can hardly imagine. An excellent source for further investigation of these statements is *The Tao of Physics,* by Fritjof Capra, Ph. D., a theoretical physicist at the Lawrence Berkeley Laboratory of the University of California at Berkeley.[5]

In a discussion of his book in the *East West Journal* of June 15, 1975, Capra says that we have been compelled to change drastically many of our basic concepts of reality — in matter, in time, space, and cause and effect.

> These concepts, however, are fundamental to our outlook on the world around us and with their radical transformation our whole world view has begun to change.
> ...A detailed analysis of the principal theories of modern physics shows that the underlying philosophical concepts are closely related to the basic ideas of Hinduism, Buddhism and Taoism. The material world appears not as a machine made up of a multitude of objects, but as a harmonious "organic" whole whose parts are only defined through their interrelations. The universe of the modern physicist, like that of the Eastern mystic, is engaged in a continuous cosmic dance; it is a system of inseparable, interacting and ever-moving components of which the observer is, him- or herself, an integral part.[5]

This insight compares with Mr. Kushi's account of his cosmic experience in the shrine at Akita.

Capra comments that both the physicist and the mystic "enquire into the essential nature of things." The mystic uses an introspective approach, whereas the physicist studies the material world; but they arrive at the same conclusion. Moreover, "the method of enquiry is thoroughly empirical in both fields. Physicists derive their knowledge from scientific experiments, mystics from meditative insights. Both are observations, and in both fields these observations are acknowledged as the only source of knowledge."

Capra says in his book that another important similarity, and a shared problem, is the difficulty of expressing that knowledge, since for both groups "all descriptions of reality are limited. ... As we penetrate deeper and deeper into nature, we have to abandon more and more of the images and concepts of ordinary language." (p 51)

He says also that Zen masters have used strange but carefully devised riddles to clear students' minds of lifelong patterns in order that they could begin to probe new truths without being disturbed by the fact that truth was hidden in "paradoxes which could not be solved by logical reasoning." (page 49) Scientists were up against a "striking parallel" at the beginning of atomic physics. "Every time they asked nature a question in an atomic experiment, nature answered with a paradox, and the more they tried to clarify the situation, the sharper the paradoxes became." (page 66) As in Zen, truth "had to be understood in the terms of a new awareness, the awareness of the atomic reality." (page 49)

The attempt to grasp this awareness "creates a true mental impasse." One of Capra's sources is *Physics and Philosophy,* written by the late Werner Heisenberg, whom Capra ranks with Einstein and Niels Bohr as "one of the giants of modern science who played a decisive role in the intellectual evolution of mankind."[6] Heisenberg vividly described his personal struggle in trying to fathom that mental impasse, when after seemingly hopeless late-night discussions with Bohr he went for walks alone, repeating to himself over and over: "Can nature possibly be so absurd as it seemed to us in these atomic experiments?" *(Tao of Physics,* page 50)

Capra avers that "whenever the essential nature of things is analysed by the intellect, it must seem absurd or paradoxical. This has always been recognized by the Eastern mystics, but has become a problem in science only recently." (page 50) An illustration of the origin of one such paradox is the elusive behavior of a subatomic particle, which "has tendencies to exist in various places and thus manifests a strange kind of physical reality between existence and non-existence" which cannot be described in conventional scientific terminology. (page 154) Another of Capra's authors, Robert Oppenheimer, makes this attempt at describing it: "If we ask, for instance, whether the position of the electron remains the same, we must say 'no;' if we ask whether the electron's position changes with time, we must say 'no;' if we ask whether the electron is at rest, we must say 'no;' if we ask whether it is in motion, we must say 'no.'"

Capra points out the similarity to this passage from the *Upanishads:*

> It moves. It moves not.
> It is far, and it is near.
> It is within all this,
> And it is outside of all this.   (page 154)

And Mr. Kushi, who finds no conflict in the paradoxes, calmly observes, "Infinity or God is expressed through yin and yang, or rest and movement." Mysticism has never had to bestir itself from the lotus position while science was struggling to find a way out of its turmoil. Transmutation, alchemy, and cosmic insights in the realm of physics may in time be relieved of the taint of seeming ridiculous, as science inclines toward returning to an attitude of wonderment and awe. This is what yin-yang is all about: all things in time become their opposites. Edward Esko, with his characteristic perception, weds science and mysticism as if there were no dichotomy:

> Ancient people considered all things to be a manifestation of spirit, and they lived accordingly. Science has developed in the opposite way, starting with matter as the basis of reality, and from there, has proceeded to uncover the world of spirit. Ours is a time of synthesis, in which both can be comprehensively understood, resulting in an appreciation of life in its totality.[7]

Jean has helped me close the lid on this Pandora's box by mentioning that we should save some space for Mr. Kushi's views on agriculture, which also bear little resemblance to what we consider orthodox. As an advancement beyond the organic gardening so popular today, he proposes *natural* gardening, which might be described as nature's organic gardening. He says it takes at least three years to prepare the ground or the environment properly to make it suitable for this type of agriculture. During this time no attempt is made to pull weeds, bring in compost, or control pests. (As a matter of fact, the lack of artificial fertilizer should lessen the damage from pests, according to Louis Kervran, who declares that even a limited use of these fertilizers has brought about one of the many consequences of biological imbalance: an increasing lack of resistance in plants to the pests which prey upon them.[8] In natural gardening, when weeds die down in the winter, seeds are scattered for low-growing weeds such as clover. Then vegetables or grains are planted that will exceed these weeds in height and will be compatible with the insects, soil, and general environment. Crops are not watered except in cases of extreme drought. The gardener merely picks the produce when it is ripe, being careful to leave enough seed to reproduce itself the next year. It is a lazy person's approach to agriculture, for plants that will not survive and grow this way should not be grown *or eaten* in this latitude.

Livestock would not be a part of natural agriculture, not only because of the harm in eating it, but because of the inefficient land use. From various East West Foundation publications we learn that it is generally estimated that each acre of land used for the cultivation of grains and beans can produce about eight times as much protein as that used for raising cattle or other sources of animal protein. The United Nations has recommended the wide-spread use of soybean protein, in the form of fermented products like miso, tamari, and tofu, as a possible solution to the world-wide food shortage. If we cut our meat consumption by only 10 percent a year we would save enough grain to feed sixty million people-type grain-eaters.

The East West Foundation is putting its philosophies to the test at Ashburnham, a 550-acre site about fifty miles from Boston. Home-sites are being staked out, the eventual objective being to have a small community with buildings suitable for teaching all the arts embraced by the EWF. Back to nature, anyone? Contact EWF!

The background for EWF is a large part of the background of Michio Kushi. The foundation for the Foundation was being laid, of course, from the time of Michio's first visit to Ohsawa's World Government Association. In 1949 he came to the U.S. and in 1950 began graduate work at Columbia University, supplementing his degree in law from Tokyo University. In 1953 he established a trading company, R.H. Brothers, Inc., to do business mainly with Japan, and followed up during the next eleven years with the establishment of six other Japanese gift stores and enterprises, including a restaurant, besides acting as the New York agent for two Japanese manufacturing companies. Also he gave weekly lectures in New York on

Oriental philosophy, culture, and way of life. By 1965 he had a wife and children.

An interest in helping a group of young people led the family to move to the Boston area, where Michio began lecturing, building up his following so that by 1975 there were about 500 active students in the Boston area, and several thousand in other areas of the U.S. and throughout the world. About fifty of his American students had by that time studied in Japan. During these ten years he also lectured at Harvard University and in many major cities throughout the country, and established Erewhon, Inc., a thriving natural-foods wholesale business supplying products to several hundred retail stores in North America and having a number of retail outlets of its own in New England, plus an affiliate company in Southern California. Also, he started two restaurants in Boston, and many others were established by students moving to other locations. The *Order of the Universe* magazine grew from a fledgling publication to a circulation of 3,000 by 1975, while the *East West Journal,* between 1971 and 1976, built up an international readership of 100,000 monthly. Between times Michio wrote a number of scholarly books, which are listed in our Bibliography.

Out of all this was born, in 1972, the East West Foundation for One Peaceful World. A tax-exempt educational and cultural institution with national offices in Boston, the Foundation has sponsored weekly seminars in Boston on the application of yin and yang cosmology to dietary practice; to the cause, mechanism, and possible cure of major illnesses; to art, history and social change; ancient and future worlds; natural agriculture and traditional food processing; religious traditions; Oriental medicine; man and woman; Oriental astrology and numerology; and physics, chemistry, and the natural sciences! In weekend seminars for medical professionals and students and the public (usually held at Statler Hilton hotels in Boston and New York) Mr. Kushi has lectured on Oriental medicine, including acupuncture, physiognomy (facial diagnosis), palm healing, shiatsu massage, the evolution of consciousness, and psychological development. Since 1974, such seminars have become international, with both Mr. and Mrs. Kushi making tours in Japan, Europe, and South America. Many more such tours are planned: East West Centers which can sponsor them are springing up all over the world. A partial list is in the Appendix; we say "partial" because keeping it up-to-date would not be possible without monthly revision.

Highly successful ventures sponsored by the Foundation have been annual ten-day seminars at Amherst (Massachusetts) College.

These deal with many facets of Oriental philosophy and culture, including macrobiotic cooking, and are taught by Mr. and Mrs. Kushi, by carefully trained associates on the EWF staff, and by outstanding guest lecturers. Longer-range courses have been presented at the University of Massachusetts in Amherst and at Chamberlayne Junior College in Boston, and are planned for other universities.

All this would not have been possible on such a large scale, of course, if some of the Kushi students had not decided to dedicate their lives, or at least a number of their years, to the organization and continuing operation of the EWF. All these people are now like graduate students, or indeed faculty members, of any institution of higher learning, each specializing in one or more facets of the Foundation's educational program. The extent of their achievements, judged from all indications we have seen, demonstrates outstanding teamwork, each person being a strong individual, but each giving selfless attention to the smooth functioning of the organization. More and more, we feel that we can turn to these capable young people for advice and thus save Mr. Kushi's time and energy. Closely allied to the Foundation is the outstanding *East West Journal,* for which editor Sherman Goldman assiduously guards and improves the fine quality he inherited from previous hard workers.

The major facilitator for Michio Kushi, however, is named Aveline Kushi, a tiny, smiling woman who is a giant in her own right. If you were a young kindergarten teacher only four feet-ten inches tall and weighing less than 100 pounds — and if home was a remote Japanese village set in very rugged mountains, a five-hour drive south of Matsue and a five-hour drive north of Hiroshima — would you have had the courage to leave that "poor but peaceful" home, all alone, with barely enough money to get to Tokyo, to go to a school there that you knew very little about? Aveline (Tomoko Yokoyama) had that kind of courage. She was largely inspired by a lecture of George Ohsawa in a village not far from her own. In the afterglow, she began making plans to go to Tokyo, and wrote to Ohsawa saying she would like to visit the school. But then without waiting for an answer, she resigned her job, sold everything she could, packed her few remaining belongings, and started out. Arriving in Tokyo very late at night, she managed to find the right address, which proved to be a large home. It was about five o'clock in the morning. One light was burning in an upstairs window, but rather than bother anyone at that hour in the morning Tomoko crouched down in the snow behind some bushes and waited till daylight. Then she washed her face with snow and went to the house, where she was welcomed by the other students. They told her that the lighted window had been in Mr. Ohsawa's room, for he frequently awoke about two a.m. to study till seven.

She stayed at this private school for about a year and a half. During this time a letter arrived from the U.S., which Ohsawa read to the students. It was from Michio Kushi, telling of his experiences and his dreams of widening the macrobiotic field in New York. By the time another letter or two had come to the school from this man, Tomoko knew that she had another star to follow. She worked hard enough and gained enough insight that Ohsawa felt she was ready to teach others — and, understanding her dream, he gave her a boat ticket to San Francisco and a bus ticket to New York!

She arrived in New York penniless, but determined. Then she located Michio Kushi. One marriage and five children later she was helping him establish Erewhon and the East West Foundation. The embryonic stages of Erewhon were nurtured in their own home, where they packaged bulk Japanese and natural foods for re-sale. In her own kitchen during these years, first in New York, then in Cambridge, Massachusetts, then in Brookline near Boston, Aveline taught many, many people the art of macrobiotic cooking, and she now does this teaching in the seminars in this country and on foreign tours. Her classes are sheer delight — incomparable, joyful, peaceful experiences! She can hold a large roomful of people, both men and women, spellbound during long sessions of speaking and demonstrations in food preparation.

And so the East West Foundation for One Peaceful World, a dream in itself, has made possible the fulfillment of other dreams for Michio and Aveline Kushi. In a newsletter of the Foundation, Michio describes the continuing goals:

> The global history of civilization over the past five thousand years is a record of technology's development, culminating in modern science. This long progress embodies the struggle of the human race to secure material well-being and peace for all.
>
> Now we see the beginning of a world community in which this dream can be at last fulfilled.
>
> However, numberless lives have been sacrificed through the course of that development, and we are experiencing a grave crisis on a universal scale in this century. We are confronted with recurrent, widespread famine; and, in the most prosperous and modern nations, an ap-

parent weakening of both individual and social health. Physiological degeneration, along with a decline in psychological and spiritual health, is manifest on a larger scale as the decay of society. We witness the continuous increase in chronic disease, mental illness, crime and drug abuse, the dissolution of marriage as an institution, and the steady decline of the traditional family unit. Amid this general corruption, education and religion seemingly have lost their ability to inspire and guide the human spirit. Finally, the degradation of the environment threatens to destroy the natural basis of human life, health, and future evolution.

Within this downward current there exists, as we are all aware, another motion which gathers strength, especially in the rising generation, toward the establishment of a healthy, emotionally sound, and spiritually aware humanity. The success of this reorientation in health and consciousness depends upon the degree to which our young people can come to understand the order of the whole universe. To realize their dream of a one-world community based on an unshakeably sound foundation, they will need the capacity to unify the fundamental complementary themes of man and nature, morality and technology, spirit and matter, ancient and modern, East and West.

The East West Foundation for One Peaceful World has been established, therefore, to offer all the encouragement and support we are capable of through education, material aid, guidance, and cultural exchange to further that constructive trend among the youth of this country and the world. Our activities will center on disseminating and implementing a sound and human technology for the biological, social and spiritual integration of all people. Our sole aim is to contribute toward the creation of one world where all may enjoy healthy, peaceful, and spiritually satisfying lives in mutual love, respect, and happiness.

Notes for Chapter 7

[1] See Note #1, Chapter 5.

[2] Georges Ohsawa, *Cancer and the Philosophy of the Far East* (Paris, 1963), ed. Herman Aihara, trans. Armand la Belle and Ralph Baccash (Binghamton, N.Y.: Swan House Publishing Company, 1971), p. 99.

[3] "The Industry of Love," *East West Journal,* 5, no. 2 (February, 1975), 22-26, and "Transmutations," *Journal,* 5, no. 3 (March, 1975), 34-35. From Michio Kushi lectures on alternative science delivered the preceding January at the East West Center in Boston.

[4]Peter Tompkins and Christopher Bird, *The Secret Life of Plants* (New York, N.Y.: Harper & Row Publishers, Inc., Avon Books, 1974), p. 290.

[5]Reprinted by special arrangement with Shambhala Publications, Inc., 1123 Spruce Street, Boulder, Colorado 80302. From *The Tao of Physics* by Fritjof Capra. Copyright 1975 by Fritjof Capra.

[6]Fritjof Capra, "Werner Heisenberg," *East West Journal,* 6, no. 3 (March, 1976), 36-37.

[7]Edward Esko, "Yin-Yang and the Spirit of the Earth," *Order of the Universe* magazine, 5, no. 10 (1977), 30.

[8]Tompkins and Bird, *Secret Life,* p. 298.

CHAPTER 8

Yin-Yang Principles —
Please Cooperate

Macrobiotic "postgraduates" — those who have learned to live in harmony with Universal Laws — possess an insight which requires concentration for the rest of us to attain. That is the attitude that disease — even cancer — is our friend and benefactor. It teaches us how to stay in line with yin-yang principles. In other words, how to flow with it: there's no use "pushing the river." If you try to ignore yin-yang principles, or rebel against them — *you* lose. You're as likely to give yourself a serious disease as you would be to be struck by lightning if you stand under a lone tree on top of a hill in a thunderstorm. This is as true for the human race as it is for individuals. In this chapter we can touch on how disregarding yin-yang requirements can bring about illness.

The flaunting of yin-yang rules to indulge the "sweet tooth" acquired by most people in present-day civilization has given the human pancreas a severe beating, especially from cancer and diabetes. Yet proper food can keep this hard-working organ safe.

As we get it, there are four types of sugar, or carbohydrates: glucose (in grains), lactose (in milk), fructose (in fruits), and sucrose (cane sugar). Various combinations of these make polysaccharides, as in grains, beans, and vegetables. Michio tells us that "polysaccharides are first decomposed by saliva in the mouth, then further broken down in the stomach, and then completely digested in the duodenum and intestines." Disaccharides — combinations of two sugar molecules — are found in cane sugar and milk. Monosaccharides are in fruits and honey; and they enter the blood stream so quickly that normal digestion cannot take place.

Our bodies need carbohydrates to make our energy, but polysaccharides are the type of sugar we should eat. Michio points out that grains are about 70 percent sugar and that while we are chewing them they become sweeter and sweeter. Carrots, parsnips, pump-

kin, and squash are also very sweet, because of a large percentage
of glucose (the most yang sugar).

Diabetes, of course, is one of the main afflictions of the pancreas. Michio describes how we eat our way into this predicament:

> In the pancreas there are isles. These isles have three
> different kinds of cells besides tissue cells. One isle is
> small, yang; another is a little bigger and more yin; and the
> other is neutral. The small isle secretes insulin and if the
> blood sugar is up, this hormone tries to make the sugar
> level low. The other more yin type of cell secretes anti-
> insulin, making the sugar level go up if it is low. This yin-
> yang balance controls the sugar level in the blood. But
> suppose the two combinations are not working well. Main-
> ly, the cause is that the small cells start to become bigger.
> If the ones secreting yang hormones are not working well
> and a more yin secretion comes out, the sugar level goes
> up, up. If the opposite condition exists, the sugar level
> goes lower. Both are not good conditions. What makes
> this small yang cell go toward yin? Yin type of food.
> So, we need to control yin type of food, especially
> carbohydrates. . . . .
> Drugs, alcohol, spices, especially hot spices — these
> things are much more yin than sugar. With drugs, a very
> little dose makes you high. Also, with spices, very little
> has a big effect. When we are taking these things, the yang
> organs change to more yin, expanding ones. Then intes-
> tinal juice, saliva, and hormone secretions become changed
> and we become more yin. Everyone has a different blood
> quality. Everyone's digestive juice has a different quality.
> Everyone's hormone quality is different, although a gen-
> eral standard is there. In this country, diabetic treatment
> by modern science recommends stopping all sugar — that
> means carbohydrates — and recommends animal quality
> protein. You can never cure diabetes this way, because
> protein is more yin than carbohydrate. . . . If you eat meat,
> this cannot help diabetes at all.
> Glucose is the yang carbohydrate among carbohy-
> drates. We also need more good minerals (salt), plus more
> yang types of protein and oil. Those things we should
> take. We must make our food category more yang. The
> patient should take grains, especially grains with more
> minerals — that means hard covers or skins — like millet,

yellow millet. He should also take vegetables which have more glucose and salt — pumpkin, acorn and butternut squash. Also, seaweed supplies minerals. Also good yang protein like aduki beans, and yang type of oil like roasted sesame oil — hard, leafy vegetables like carrot and daikon tops, with plenty of carbohydrate, fiber and minerals. Miso soup is also fine.

Teen-age diabetics are harder to cure: they have been eating badly since they were children and their systems are not strong. The total condition must be changed. This happens more and more because of sweets, soda. Their sugar is more milk, fruits, and honey every day, and disaccharides, ignoring glucose which is absolutely necessary to our bodies. After we eat any kind of food, suppose excess occurs. The body stores this excess in the liver for meeting future needs. The liver's storing ability is about 50 grams. It stores in the form of glucose polysaccharides. When needed, decomposition goes on and this glucose returns to the blood stream. In a similar way, when we eat, the sugar should be glucose polysaccharide form, which gradually becomes disaccharide and monosaccharide, and absorption goes on.

Further comments concerning diabetes are in Chapter 10, and Chapter 9 has more about sugar in it.

As regards blood pressure and cholesterol level, we can accentuate the positive and mention a Harvard research project with 210 macrobiotic followers, which was carried out between November of 1972 and February of 1973. The results, showing that both blood pressure and cholesterol levels were significantly lower in the macrobiotic people as compared to "typical" Americans of the same age, weight, sex, etc., were reported in the *American Journal of Epidemiology,* the *Journal of the American Medical Association,* and the *New England Journal of Medicine* (May 29, 1975).

Cancer, of course, is the disease which commands our main personal interest. We have tried to collect many of Michio's ideas on this topic, and the quotations on the next several pages, unless otherwise marked, are his.

We can see that America, along with our modern civilization as a whole, is now ending, as a result of biological degeneration, and that the time that is left has become very short. By the time the present generation of children become adults, we may witness the decline of our grandiose, modern way of life, which may be within the next

thirty, or at the utmost fifty, years. ...[We must] understand that no enemy or conflict exists, but that all factors
are proceeding in a harmonious manner, co-existing and
supporting each other. According to the modern view...
cancer is seen as an enemy which must either be removed
or destroyed, which view, in effect, separates the cancer
from ourselves.

[It should be seen, however,] as an attempt on the
part of an organism to create balance.

Present-day theory lists as possible causes of cancer a virus,
chemicals, X-ray, smoking, heredity, etc. In other words the tendency is to stand apart and blame some external factor. This is "dualis-
tic" — two entities, the accuser and the accused — and it is the
reason for the scientific dead end in regard to cancer, as well as
diabetes, emphysema, leprosy, arthritis, mental illness, the common
cold. Michio declares that we must learn to think "monistically" —
to realize that there is no difference between accuser and accused.
"Mea culpa." (page 48).

The macrobiotic idea is that *the body is trying to collect all
into one place the poisons from sugar, soft drinks, fruit juices,
animal products, etc., so that the rest of the body can function
smoothly.* As these foods have become more widely used, especially
in the last fifty years, cancer has increased at an alarming pace. If,
instead, we were eating according to the Universal Order — proper
foods, properly cooked — we would create a clean and toxin-free
blood stream which should not produce the excessive condition that
results in cancer. Cancer, our friend, is pleading with us to take note
of what we are doing to ourselves.

Remember that *cancer is a symptom of excess,* a warning to
stop overeating, or to stop overindulging in certain harmful foods.
(In *Cancer and the Philosophy of the Far East* Ohsawa describes it
(page 63) as "the storage of excess that explodes.")

Michio has reached the conclusion that there are two types of
cancer — a yang cancer for which we have stuffed ourselves full of
eggs and other dairy products, meat, and fish, and a yin cancer bubbling with soft drinks, spices, chemicals, citrus, sugar, fruit sugar,
honey, and maple syrup. (It happens that cancer, rather than being
produced by food, is a *continuation* of the food. Thus yin food *becomes* or *grows into* yin cancer, instead of manufacturing its opposite, a yang cancer.) Yang cancer is likely to localize in the
compacted organs, yin cancer in the hollow organs. The stomach,
being mostly hollow but having one contracted side, can have either

type; and some skin cancers may be yang even though they occur on our yin exterior. Yang skin cancers, appearing as small reddish spots, often derive from eating meat and eggs. Skin cancer "activated by exposure to sunlight" is also yang. Yin skin cancers may be a color similar to that of a combination of the milk and citrus which are likely to have caused them.*

Parkinson's disease also has two kinds of symptoms.

> One is like trembling in different parts of the body. When you go to fish-eating countries like Japan and the east coast of China, you see many people like this. This is more yang. The second kind is seizures like epilepsy. This is deeper. Coffee and hot spices make you tremble like this. This is yin Parkinson's disease, chronic, affecting more the brain nerves than the motor nerves.*

Leukemia is a "yin condition caused by foods such as sugar, and tropical fruits such as citrus, along with improper cooking and way of eating." Normally, "when we eat, food is digested and, in the small intestine, absorbed by the villi and transformed first into white blood cells and then red blood cells. If the white blood cells don't develop into red blood cells, their number increases, while the number of red cells decreases," resulting in leukemia.

As in some other areas, macrobiotic people have unorthodox theories in regard to the manufacture of the above-mentioned "toxin-free blood" which keeps us free from diseases. The inference in the preceding paragraph is that blood is made not in the bone marrow, as is generally believed, but from digested food particles in the intestines. Ohsawa tells that Professor Kikuo Chishima, a biologist at Gifu University in Japan, and his colleague, Professor K. Morishita, M.D., "succeeded in filming microscopically the transformation of digested food particles into blood, and that of red cells into proteinic cancer elements, ...clearly disproving the hypothesis that blood is manufactured in bone marrow — an hypothesis arrived at by observing the change of bone marrow in blood *in sick people.*"[1]

The significance of the last phrase is explained in an *East West Journal* article by Edward Esko ("Cancer — the Malignancy of What You Eat"), in which he states that Chishima's findings were supported by several leading biologists, especially Kryrikov and Lepeshinskaya

---

*A list outlining what to eat to counteract yin and/or yang cancer is in Chapter 13.

of the Academy of Medical Science in the Soviet Union. Says Esko,

> In a healthy and well-fed condition, the marrow of the long
> bones is filled mostly with fatty tissue, which originates from
> the differentiation of erythrocytes (red blood cells). In a
> malnourished state, the normal production of blood does
> not occur in the intestinal villi, but through a process of
> "reverse differentiation," whereby the fat cells in the bone
> marrow *change back* into red blood cells. Incidentally, the
> theory of the production of red blood cells in bone marrow
> resulted from a study conducted on pigeons that had gone
> without food for 11 days, allowing sufficient time for this
> reverse differentiation process to begin.[2]

We are sorry for the sick people and the hungry pigeons.

It goes without saying that the intestines can manufacture ener-
gizing, toxin-free blood only if we give them the right materials to
work with in the form of food selected according to yin-yang
principles.

Sometime we're going to have to tackle the battle of smoke,
and it may as well be now. Macrobiotic-ites say that the major cause
of lung cancer is foods such as animal fat, dairy products, and
sugar, "which," according to Michio, "produce a sticky condition
in both the blood stream and the air sacs within the lungs. If you are
eating well, you need not worry about smoking being a cause of lung
cancer. In fact, with a clean and healthy blood condition, smoking
can help to prevent lung cancer." (That's what the man says!) "If,
on the other hand, you are eating plenty of dairy food, sugar, or
animal fat, it may be better if you don't smoke."

Ohsawa, writing in 1963, said that everyone in London was
breathing contaminants equal to eighty cigarettes a day, so he
apparently believed that a city environment of this kind was as
threatening as cigarettes. He did not consider smoking to be injuri-
ous to health. Moreover, he declared that the medical profession
and the government were wrong to say, on the basis of "statistics
rather than logic," that smoking was probably the most serious cause
of lung cancer. Well...our personal opinions happen to be different
in this area. Since most people in Western civilizations have atrocious eating habits, we feel that the doctors and research groups are
right to keep saying that smoking causes cancer, even though, we
surmise, they don't know *why* they are right!

Muramoto, in *Healing Ourselves,* says that people who eat
badly and smoke are susceptible to lung cancer (page 120), but that
those who eat correctly and smoke *moderately* (our italics) will

probably not develop it. "Moderately," he suggests, and then shows that he is of the same opinion as Michio:

> The act of smoking disturbs the natural respiratory cycle by overstimulating inhalation. The tar and nicotine may adhere to the uric acid deposits in the lungs, thus making lung cancer a possibility. Uric acid deposits, however, are a result of excessive consumption of animal protein. Thus, while it is clear that smoking is not a good habit, smoking alone cannot be blamed for the lung cancer that is so prevalent today. The true cause, which makes this and all other diseases possible, is faulty diet. (page 47)

So again we're being warned about excesses. If you smoke, it looks as if you should not overdo on either tobacco or poor food.

We can use these discussions of cancer and diabetes as examples of the way too much wrong eating can cause almost any other illness, and we can see also that staying within sensible boundaries saves us from high blood pressure and other factors which relate to heart problems. It follows that this latter type of restraint helps us avoid other disease as well.

Now what about the effect of food on mental health and/or illness? Macrobiotic people believe that if we are eating correctly, our brains have a chance to function better. Michio says that food has a direct and definite influence on the brain, for from blood we receive inner vibrations that strengthen each region and function of the brain. We'll make an attempt to outline some of the information:

1. Poor quality liquids (soft drinks, alcohol, coffee, commercial tea, etc.) can cause negativity and loss of hope, while good quality fluids help develop cheerfulness, hopefulness.

2. Poor quality carbohydrates (sugar, excess fruit, etc.) can cause us to have feelings of uncertainty and cause many people to feel drawn to masters and leaders. High quality carbohydrates such as those in grains, vegetables, and beans allow us to develop the confidence to do our own pondering.

3. Poor quality protein (animal protein) causes unpleasant memories and nightmares to predominate. The good quality protein of beans, grains, and vegetables helps happy memories to remain uppermost in our minds.

4. Salt and minerals aid in the development of good memory, but please not the commercial sodium chloride with all minerals refined out! Use sea or solar salt, or miso or tamari. Don't eat too much (sound familiar?); eat yang foods; don't use much oil; use no

alcohol or sugar. Sugar destroys Vitamin B in the intestines, impairing the body's ability to produce betaine, the chemical which induces excitation in the nervous system. A high protein or high fat diet, on the other hand, upsets the relationship between oxygen inhaled and carbon monoxide exhaled (Respiratory Quotient), so that we would have to breathe harder to supply the body with necessary oxygen. This causes *over*-excitation in the nervous system.

5. To aid in developing intuition, eat less, eat regularly, use no dairy or animal food. Stay detached, develop acceptance, smile. Have faith in the order of the universe.

6. To develop imagination and clear away anxieties, eat brown rice, but little fruit or juices. Keep your hands cool and your feet warm, which may mean you'll have to cure sinus problems. The major organs involved here are the lungs and the large intestine, which may be helped by reading or singing in a loud voice. (These processes can also be aided by palm healing and Dō-In (doe-een) or shiatsu massage — a whole new ball game for which the rules can be found in books listed in the Bibliography.)

7. To improve intellectual powers, eat millet and other small grains; chew well; gargle with salt water daily; wear natural-cloth clothing and dress lightly.

8. To strengthen will power and eliminate fear (a delusion caused by poor cell quality), use less liquid. Treat kidney and bladder weaknesses by food (see Chapter 13) and by palm healing and massage. A valuable side-effect will be the clearing of the ear canals. Focus your attention on the region of the "third eye," in the middle of the forehead. If you are not familiar with techniques of this sort, information can be found in the reports of Michio's lectures. More readily available, at your public library, will be books on yoga. You can read just a few pages dealing with the third eye and the seven chakras.

Fear: this seems to be the main emotion that keeps human beings from realizing their potential. It also is one of the main obstacles in developing comfortable relationships with other people. After differing lengths of time for different people, proper food helps us begin to relinquish fears; and Michio has some suggestions for active mental and emotional cooperation in the process, which we will attempt to interpret.

It seems that just as good food sets up internal physical vibrations that aid the brain, so does it also maintain a blood quality that allows our internal compass to function properly, keeping us attuned to universal vibrations which come to our brains from outside our body and influence our emotions and our ideal visions. Our bodies are "charged electrical fields" aligned with these vibrations from the universe. If we can learn to become sensitive to these vibrations, we will begin to realize that each of us, in the largest sense, equals infinity, the universal and ultimate consciousness — the "I am" which is the cosmic element in many different religions.

When small problems seem to bury us, we should *try* not to face them on their level, for we will expend tremendous energy defending ourselves. Instead, we should practice rising above these problems, a difficult feat because much of our training has been in the direction of attack, or of suppressing our innate intuitive powers. The higher we rise above our problems the wider our perspective becomes and the easier the solutions become. Michio suggests that when we feel overcome by anxieties and frustrations we take five or ten minutes for quiet meditation, working to "feel" or recall our infinite origin, trying to become "empty," unattached. (Remember how in the shrine at Akita, just before he had his magnificent cosmic vision, he said he was "praying without desire," making himself "unified, clear, and empty"?) To receive vibrations for futuristic thinking — for long-range dreams — we should look up during meditation at an angle of about sixty degrees from an imaginary line directly in front of our eyes. For shorter-range hopes and wishes, try a thirty-degree angle. Looking *down* at a thirty-degree angle should bring pleasant memories to our meditation; but a sixty-degree downward angle exposes to the vibrations the area of the brain which deals with dark, unpleasant memories.

So — if we don't look down far enough to count our shirt buttons — meditation should help prepare us for overcoming our fears in our relationships with other people. Michio advises against allowing an over-accumulation of emotion to build up. We should get rid of emotions either by yin measures (language, talking) or by yang means (motion, exercise). We should keep in mind that we are the same as all other people — the same origin, the same destiny, the same infinite "I." When we look into the eyes of another person we are looking into a mirror. The only difference is that we each happened to create our separate bodies. In dealings with others we should practice developing patience, flexibility, acceptance. To avoid colliding with other thought streams, we should keep our thought stream flexible and maneuverable, like water, so that it can flow around obstacles. We should learn to be open and honest with each other. If there is temporary conflict, we should try to become in harmony with the adversary, learning to think, feel, and say, "I am the cause." If two people who are both practicing this technique meet, the argument would be very, very polite! But good food is the genesis for achieving this degree of mental and emotional harmony.

To a small minority of people is given the ability to achieve mental control over physical functions. In a report of one of Michio's lectures, when a student asked how some people could use psychological techniques successfully for development and change without a change in diet, Michio replied, "They are stimulating their endocrine and autonomic nervous systems by recalling and working on their emotions. This produces *physiological* changes in the blood and they are able to change mentally. All these changes have a *physiological* change as their basis." Perhaps this is the sort of conversion which takes place for those who use Dr. Simonton's techniques exclusively, as well as for yogis and the strong-willed people described in such books as *The Power of Your Subconscious Mind* (see our Bibliography).

The fact that so few people possess this self-cure attitude leads us back to the statement at the beginning of the chapter, to the insight that illness is our friend, for it tries to teach us to stop breaking universal laws. This key unlocks the door to solving health problems. But it also exposes the widespread and constant fear of illness which the human race has gradually allowed to become a dominant characteristic. The results of the submission to this fear are delineated by the author of the last — and very important — source we would like to share with you in this chapter.

Ivan Illich has written *Medical Nemesis.* He is a graduate of the University of Rome, and holds a doctorate in history from the University of Salzburg. Since 1964 he has participated in international research seminars on Institutional Alternatives. His erudite book was given royal treatment by the *East West Journal* in their March, 1976, issue, in the longest synopsis they had ever printed, and it is from this synopsis that we have taken our small bit of material.[3] As we understand it, one of the main thrusts of the book is the fact that we the people have forgotten all about the concept that each of us is a physician for his or her own needs. ["Physician, heal thyself!"] Each of us has been the cause of having doctors take over more and more in trying to accomplish healing by external forces. Again, *mea culpa.*

The *Journal* speaks of the "extensive documentation" behind the "tightly reasoned arguments that authenticate each point in the context of the complete book." One of Illich's contentions is that medical services have not been significant in producing changes in life expectancy, but have, rather, done damage to health: epidemics and diseases have always come and gone — and life expectancy would have increased — entirely outside the physicians' control. Yet because we are always so afraid we *will* be sick, we have demanded and demanded until the medical profession has tried more and more artificial means of "healing." We demand to have pain stopped before its meaning can be analyzed, fearing that whatever illness is about to grab us will be something we cannot cope with without the doctor's help. Illich declares that this is a feeling the patients bring on themselves, rather than being the result of any intention of doctors to "foist their ministrations" on people. Calling ours a "morbid society," he says further that people "subconsciously realize" that illness will relieve them of social and employment responsibilities they are apathetic about accepting. Even though they fear the illness, they don't want to have to do any of the work to heal themselves when sickness overcomes them. "Healing ceases to be considered the task of the sick."

These assertions tie in with our experiences with people who are afraid of getting well, or who want a pill or an injection to cover up their illness so that they can avoid becoming involved in any effort to cooperate in their own recovery. One way they go about it is to worry about each little pain or discomfort separately: "Doctor, I have a pain *here*. Give me something for *this* pain." So the doctor figures out what *this* organ does and selects some artificial chemical to supplement the natural chemical manufactured by the organ. In many cases it seems to help — till it causes a worse trouble somewhere else.

Oriental medicine, on the other hand, does not conceive of the body in parts, but considers each organ as part of the whole. A student was asking Michio whether mental depression might be related to Parkinson's disease. The answer was,

> In some cases...[along with] cramps, paralyzed parts, trembling, epileptic seizures, pounding of the heart, falling asleep easily. This is all paralyzing of the nerves. ... These things are the same sickness, appearing different ways. Doctors call them different names and treat them as separate sicknesses, but it's all one group of sickness. We have now in modern medicine several thousand names for sickness. ...For example, diabetics often develop eye trouble like glaucoma. These are two different sicknesses,

according to present-day beliefs. But these are the same sicknesses appearing in two different regions. You should treat it as the same sickness, same cause. If we had simplification of symptoms into groups, we would have twenty or thirty groups. Then divide these into yin and yang groups and suddenly all sickness would become so easy you could study it in one year.

So far in this book the emphasis has been on *us* — those of us who are living on this planet now, or who have recently left it because of illness. But what of the future generations? All people of child-bearing age (even those who believe that souls choose illness to repay a karmic debt) have an awesome responsibility to try to avoid inflicting poor health on their children and grandchildren. Michio knows that the 280 days an embryo spends in the womb form a telescoped repetition of the approximately 2.8 billion years of biological evolution. The embryo increases in size approximately three billion times, each day increasing roughly ten million times and passing through about ten million years of evolution. During pregnancy, the embryo is nourished entirely by the mother's blood, which is in turn synthesized from the foods she is eating.

One type of birth defect or "genetic" disease can be caused during pregnancy if the mother eats some imbalanced food or takes strong chemicals (including birth control pills!). If these are in the blood stream for, say, three days, it is equal to thirty million years of polluted environment for the embryo!

> A second type of genetic disease results from trouble in the genes themselves. For example, recently I heard of a girl who had been seriously practicing macrobiotics for several years giving birth to a deformed baby. What do you think caused this? In this case the problem was not the mother, but was the result of the father's past intake of drugs, which he was using at the time of conception. ...
>
> If the structure of the DNA existing in the reproductive cells is altered, which can result from taking LSD or other drugs, a baby born as a result of the fertilization of one of these cells will not be normal.
>
> Macrobiotic eating is the most fundamental way of curing both of these types of genetic disease, since it establishes a suitable quality of blood which nourishes the developing embryo, as well as securing the quality of both egg and sperm cells. *Ninety-nine per cent of what are termed "genetic" diseases could be prevented through macrobiotics.* (Italics ours)

If we could learn again to listen to the intuition of our infinite origin, we could break away from the fear of independent self-healing that has tricked us into the medical slavery which in itself is a violation of universal laws. And if we can release ourselves from drugs taken out of fear of peer pressure or whatever other reason, we can avoid binding our children with the same shackles.

Notes for Chapter 8

[1]Georges Ohsawa, *Cancer and the Philosophy of the Far East* (Paris, 1963), ed. Herman Aihara, trans. Armand la Belle and Ralph Baccash (Binghamton, N.Y.: Swan House Publishing Company, 1971), p. 76.

[2]Edward Esko, "Cancer — The Malignancy of What You Eat," *East West Journal,* 6, no. 1 (January, 1976), 36-38.

[3]Ivan Illich, *Medical Nemesis* (New York, N.Y.: Random House, Inc., 1976, Pantheon Books, 1976). (Book review in *East West Journal,* 6, no. 3 (March, 1976), 19-30.)

CHAPTER 9

Through Yin and Yang,
We Eat — to LIVE!

Having seen how ignoring yin-yang principles can bring about major illness, we can now take a sketchy look at the specific way these principles relate to food, and to the correction of imbalance if we choose our food in harmony with their influence.

In *Zen Macrobiotic Cooking* (one of the books used in Chapter 13), Michel Abehsera describes macrobiotics as "the traditional food of ancient Japan, now preserved fully only in the Zen Buddhist monasteries. ...Zen monks are the longest-lived and healthiest people in Japan, while, at the other end of the scale, Westernized physicians and restaurant owners [by proven statistics] die early."[1]

And this from Michio Kushi: "The practice of macrobiotics is the understanding and practical application of this [Universal] order to our life style, including the selection, preparation and manner of eating our daily food." The importance of food (granted its influence actually began, for each of us, generations ago) shows up in our original constitution, which, as we have seen in the previous chapter, is determined during the 280 days of embryological development. And we noted earlier (in Chapter 7) how the food our mothers ate during that 280 days, as well as the food we ourselves have eaten, shows up in our facial features.

Once we are ready to eat some food other than our mother's milk, the yin-yang principles should be taken into consideration, and of course ideally the young mother was following them during lactation. There's no need at all to panic about food selection, for it will be pretty much taken care of for you in the food program listed in Chapter 13. But since this program is based on yin-yang principles, you may want to know *why* you're advised to eat this way.

It has to do with the ratio of yin to yang which is observed to exist on the earth at the present time, and that is 7 to 1. We'll refer you to Mr. Kushi's writings if you want to get profound on this theory; but just as he could give examples supporting the "spiral" philosophy (Chapter 7), so there are many examples of the *7* to *1* ratio in such phenomena of nature as the distance *between* waves *(7)* in large bodies of water and the *height* of the waves *(1)*. (Care to swim out and measure?) As for us human beings, our hard heads (yang) are approximately one-seventh the size of our soft, pliable yin bodies (including our legs, of course).

Now — grains have an approximate ratio of seven parts of potassium (yin) to one part of sodium (yang), and therefore, in harmony and at peace with the Universal ratio, are at the center of foods we should be using. Foods with a higher percentage of potassium are more yin, and with less potassium are more yang. If we begin with grains and move toward yin, food categories are classified as follows: beans, then seeds, then root vegetables, leafy round vegetables (like cabbage and lettuce), nuts, leafy expanded vegetables (like kale and celery), fruits, maple syrup and honey, sugar, drugs. In other words, drugs are the most yin, beans and seeds the least yin. If we move away from grains toward *yang,* the classification is: fish, poultry, meat, eggs. *Within* each category of foods, there are yin-yang ratings, for which we'll refer you to the cookbooks, especially the Michel Abehsera *Zen Macrobiotic Cooking.*

In the selection of daily food, we try to maintain this 7 to 1 ratio of yin to yang. (Don't worry about it, for the balance will be outlined for you more or less automatically!) Since we're not supposed to eat very much meat, most of the yang quality has to come from grains, so that's one reason the percentage of grains in our menus is very high. The theory of using foods from our own latitude or seasonal belt also fits into the picture. Grains, which have adapted to all but the most extreme polar climates, can be eaten universally. Again we turn to Michio's lectures:

> People living in tropical climates traditionally eat a more yin diet than people living in cold northern climates. If we move from one climate to another, our method of cooking should also change, but always keeping whole grains and cooked vegetables as our principal foods, since they grow in almost all climates.
>
> [We could in a northern climate modify the ratio to 5 to 1 or in southern climates as far as 10 to 1. But] if we exceed this point of balance in either direction we begin to lose our adaptability to present-day earth conditions, and invite the possibility of sickness.*

---

*Michel Abehsera, in *Zen Macrobiotic Cooking,* writes (page 34) that excesses of potassium have been known to be poisonous. He relates that the Incas were said to have served eggplant and tomatoes to the conquering Spaniards to induce susceptibility to illnesses such as syphilis. Some foods are drastically off balance: potatoes have 512 parts of potassium to 1 of sodium; bananas have 850 to 1!

Within a particular climate, we experience various seasonal changes, and should vary our diet accordingly, depending primarily upon foods which are either naturally available during a particular season or which can be naturally stored. During the summer, fresh vegetables in the form of salad are naturally available, as are fruits, and they can be used from time to time as supplements, whereas in winter they are not naturally available. In traditional cultures vegetables were usually pickled in salt or stored in a root cellar for use in winter. Cereal grains, beans, seaweeds, and other foods which can be naturally stored in winter and summer should be the mainstay of our diet throughout the year. ... Nowadays, however, particularly in the modern industrial nations, most people eat a uniform diet throughout the year; for example, ice cream and citrus fruits are consumed both in winter and summer; and as a result chronic illness is reaching epidemic proportions.

In an address at the United Nations on February 10, 1978, Michio gave considerable emphasis to the importance of eating foods according to environment and season, such information being especially relevant for an audience drawn from all parts of the globe.

When selecting and preparing our foods, individual differences need also to be considered, with variations according to age, sex, amount of activity, occupation, original constitution, previous eating patterns, and social environment. (These minor differences are the reason that someone who is ill should get individual information from Boston or some other macrobiotic center listed in our Appendix.)

Another basis for the theory of 7-to-1 food selection is the formation of our teeth:

We have eight front teeth primarily for use in cutting vegetable foods; four canine teeth for tearing animal foods; and twenty molars for grinding grain. So, twenty-eight of our teeth are for chewing vegetable foods, whereas four are for eating animal foods, in a ratio of 7 to 1. Thus our proportion of animal food to vegetable quality food can be about 1 to 7.

(With vegetables are included grains — the "most modern species of vegetable life.")

Now there's also an important theory that we should eat primarily those meats which are biologically as far removed from us as possible. Therefore, since fish pre-dated mammals in time of creation, fish should be the principal meat in that 7-1 ratio (provided we're well enough to eat fish). Besides that, fish are less yang than other meats. And, just from a purely personal standpoint, we don't feel that it's too inhumane to eat fish, because they eat each other, and because their mamas simply lay eggs and swim merrily away without forming any emotional attachment to their offspring.

We can put aside the dice game now with the notation of another reason why, in general, consumption of animal foods should be small. Grains and vegetables remain in the stomach for about two to two and a half hours, whereas meats remain up to four and a half hours. Decomposed amino acids (now with a yin *effect,* although the meat originally was yang) are finally released into the blood stream, "altering its delicate balance." Excess protein from meat is discharged in the form of body hair, or else becomes fat which is stored first in the inactive or adipose regions and then in and around the vital organs, often causing them to become enlarged and hardened. "Furthermore, in the intestines, the putrefaction of animal protein is destructive to beneficial bacteria which synthesize the vitamin B complex utilized in the metabolism of carbohydrates and in the synthesis of glutamic acid in the brain." This would be an appropriate place to note that Ohsawa points out (and we know that Michio concurs) that females have a greater capacity for protein-production than males and must therefore remain stricter in their abstention from animal food.

Almost all nutritionists stomp on the macrobiotic diet as lacking in protein — a total misconception! Of course, the diet *is* an altogether different world from everything they've been taught, but it definitely has its own built-in protein, requiring only that our wayward bodies take time to adjust to utilizing it adequately. Grains, beans, and miso are especially rich in protein; buckwheat contains more of it than eggs, and both aduki beans and soybeans contain more than beef or eggs. Moreover, it's a very high quality protein. Likewise, the mb diet is rich in calcium, another worrier for nutritionists. (Check your macrobiotic cookbooks for details on protein, calcium, iron, etc., including comparison charts.) They also stew around about vitamin C; but this is more dependably supplied by the mb diet than by the presently acceptable "orthodox" diets which require the addition of citrus fruits. Brown rice and other grains are the only foods in which vitamin C is not destroyed by cooking. Our raw vegetables, also, have plenty of vitamin C as does bancha tea. Michio points out that the reason the scurvy-racked British sailors of the past century needed C so urgently was that they were doing hard physical labor in a salty ocean environment, and eating primarily salted meat!

A very important way to help our bodies acquire balance — and this also bewilders nutritionists — is to limit our intake of liquid, drinking only when we are honestly thirsty, to avoid *drowning* our kidneys. According to Oriental medicine, everything we do in Western customs and Western medicine leaves our poor kidneys gasping for air. They're awfully sturdy and hard to kill, or they'd be dead — and we along with them — years sooner. Instead, we demand medicine and kidney machines (guilty again!) and hang on miserably, clobbering them — and *us* — with blow after blow. They're only about the size of our ears, and weren't *intended* to filter gallons of liquid daily or be coated with and invaded by fat and mucus. Our bad habit of drinking icy liquids is also terribly harmful to our digestive system. The beverages we *should* drink are listed in Chapter 13.

Once we recognize the importance of balanced food selection, and reassure ourselves that the food contains proper nutriments, what's the best way to extract and utilize those nutriments? The macrobiotic slogan might be, "Chew, chew, and chew again!" (And again and again — till there's only cream left in your mouth. Make it 100, 150, 200 times if necessary.) Pull lots of saliva into your mouth as you chew: you'll have lots of it with these foods. It's your first agent of digestion, and it's free — what a bargain in effective medicine! In Chapter 12, we'll have some little household hints on how to make time to eat this way. It's also best to remain active after eating, in order to receive the most value from our food. Michio says we should not eat for three hours before retiring for the night, for if our food is not used up through activity, it accumulates as excess through the body. If you are insufferably sleepy after a meal in the daytime, take a nap sitting up.

A sad consequence of being out of balance, and a major curse of the human race, is obesity, imprisoning its victims in a vicious circle of self-hatred, self-pity, and defensiveness. If you look back through the last few paragraphs, you will see that for most people the powers of correction are inherent in the macrobiotic program: if you don't eat meat, you don't have the excess protein to store in the wrong places. If you cut back on liquids, you don't have all that expansiveness running around in your tissues. (Usually less liquid implies less salt in your food, to avoid thirst. Meat and eggs are among foods that seem to demand salt, and cheese is usually made with too much salt; so you've eliminated some big problems already by limiting the amounts of those things.) If you chew as well as you should, you feel satisfied with less food, and if you stay active after eating you don't have excess to store.

For those who are fearful that rice will make them gain weight, we have this information from Iona Teeguarden and others (page 16 of *Freedom Through Cooking,* used in our Chapter 13): "The outer layer of grains contains proteins, a little fat, minerals and vitamins — including thiamine (B$_1$), without which carbohydrates turn to fat, stored in the body. With thiamine, carbohydrates are used up to give us energy."[2] Of course, you have to use the *rest* of the macrobiotic foods — you can't just add brown rice to what you're already eating and expect it to help you lose weight!

Another way macrobiotics helps in losing weight is in forbidding the use of sugar, for it also causes fat storage. Thus, by forgoing the extreme yang of meat and eggs and the extreme yin of sugar you can attack your excess padding with a double whammy! (After you read in the next few pages the terrible things sugar does to people it will seem much less attractive.)

In some extreme cases we have known Michio to keep people on a restricted food intake for ten days to lose weight (Chapter 12); but we feel sure that, for most people, following the regular macrobiotic program will be sufficient to normalize weight, and we have seen it happen with many of our friends. This means you never count another calorie, and if you follow the above suggestions you can usually lose weight without being hungry. You can eat till you feel satisfied, although *never* uncomfortably stuffed. So you need not feel frightened or threatened by the macrobiotic program.

As we mentioned earlier, fasting is not especially recommended as part of the macrobiotic way, and not in connection with weight loss. If occasional fasting appeals to you, here are some hints, indirectly quoted from Michio: In fasting, one must never suddenly stop eating, but must gradually reduce the quantity of food at each meal and then reduce the number of meals each day to one. The usual moderate amount of liquid must be continued. Select foods that will assist in neutralization — vegetables are best. Fasting must be accompanied by activities that calm the spirit, such as meditation and breathing exercises. Daily activities should also accompany fasting. Then return gradually to regular eating habits. For a ten-day fast, take twenty days to resume normal eating. As for the business of eating brown rice exclusively, Abehsera in *Zen Macrobiotic Cook-*

ing (page 97) quotes Ohsawa himself: "One should never eat only rice without consulting me or some friends who know about it. You must eat and enjoy food. To eat only rice is a big decision."

Lurking at the farthest yin end of the yin-yang scale, next to drugs, is the sugar-demon. We used to say, "Sugar — yummy!" Now we have to learn to say, "Sugar — yukky!" We'd better take a careful look at this ogre, which must have been put on this planet to test our character and make it difficult to maintain our balance.

We've already had some discussion of Michio's advice on sugar in Chapter 8; now here's what he has to say in more specific terms:

> When refined sugar enters the stomach, it causes what is known as a "sugar reaction," whereby the stomach is temporarily paralyzed. As little as one-fourth of a teaspoon of refined sugar can cause this. Since refined sugar is strongly alkaloid, the stomach secretes unusual amounts of acid in order to make balance, which, if repeated over a long enough period, can cause eventual ulceration of the stomach wall. Our blood normally maintains a weak alkaline condition, and when strongly alkaline refined sugar is introduced, what is known as an "acid reaction" takes place, causing the blood stream to become over-acidic. To compensate for this our internal supply of minerals is mobilized so as to restore a more normal balance. The minerals in our daily food and in our normal body reserve are sufficient to meet this situation if it arises now and then. However, if we are eating refined sugar every day, this supply is not sufficient, and we must depend on minerals stored deep within the body, particularly calcium in our bones and teeth. If this continues for a long enough period, the depletion of calcium from the bones and teeth results in their eventual decay and general weakening.
>
> Excess sugar is stored in various places within the body, first in the form of glycogen in the liver. When the amount of glycogen exceeds the liver's storage capacity of about 50 grams, it is then released into the blood stream in the form of fatty acid, which is first stored in the more inactive places of the body such as the buttocks, thighs, and mid-section. Then, if the intake of refined sugar is continued, this fatty acid becomes attracted to the more active organs such as the heart and kidneys, which gradually become encased in a layer of fat and mucus, which also penetrate the inner tissues of these organs. This of course weakens their normal functioning, and when excessive enough, causes their eventual stoppage. The grow-

ing consumption of refined sugar in modern nations can be seen in the increasing incidence of such degenerative diseases as heart disease, which two out of five people in the United States are now suffering from. Refined sugar also directly affects our thinking abilities, through the destruction of the intestinal bacteria which are responsible for the synthesis of B vitamins necessary for the synthesis of glutamic acid which is directly involved in the mental activities carried on in the brain. A lack of this component can result in a lack of memory and ability to think clearly. [Compare with the identical effect, mentioned above, that meat consumption has on the brain.]

In general, the intake of refined sugar, which is highly processed and a refined product of tropical climates, results in an overall *yinnization* of our physical and mental condition, particularly affecting the para-sympathetic nervous system, and the organs which it governs, such as the small brain, which become inactive and in some instances paralyzed. This is what causes "sugar-reaction" in the stomach, mentioned earlier............

Sweeteners such as honey and maple syrup have an effect similar to that of refined sugar, although to a lesser degree, and should be avoided as much as possible in daily use. They cause an obscure type of thinking, more doubt and "mist."

If you're not completely convinced after all that, we strongly recommend that you read William Dufty's *Sugar Blues,* in which he paints a terrifying picture of the toll sugar has taken in the human saga. In colorful style and great detail, using carefully selected and hard-hitting source material, he enlarges upon the same sort of baleful symptoms Michio has just outlined. Dufty tells that in his earlier book, *You Are All Sanpaku,* he had quoted this wide-sweeping opinion from Ohsawa: "Western medicine will one day admit what has been known in the Orient for years. Sugar is the greatest evil that modern industrial civilization has visited upon the countries of the Far East and Africa."[3] (Unfortunately, its use became very general in spite of such warnings.)

Dufty slaps down the "quick pick-up" people commonly think they get from sweets, calling it the deception of "empty or naked calories," because the let-down which follows leaves us with lower energy than before (page 29, page 100). He also declares that our "immunizing power" becomes more limited, "so we cannot respond properly to extreme attacks, whether they be cold, heat, mosquitos, or microbes." (page 101) (This reminds us that somewhere in Michio's writings we have come across the encouragement that if our blood is macrobiotic and not sickeningly sweet, insects will not bother us!)

Sugar is preparing our children and young people for a terrific burden of ill health. Some parents who are beginning to get wise to this fact have reported noticing a marked difference in the behavior of their children after reducing or eliminating their sugar intake. An increasing number of counselors dealing with "juvenile delinquents" (as well as with mental patients) are recognizing the relationship between sugar and "obstinate behavior." Dufty substantiates this trend by recounting that in the 1940's the late endocrinologist, John W. Tintera, chanced on to a relationship between sugar and behavior in young teen-agers, when he "rediscovered the vital importance of the endocrine system (especially the adrenal glands) in 'pathological mentation' — or brain boggling." (page 48) Patients being tested for hormone imbalance were found in glucose tolerance tests (GTT) to show the same symptoms as persons whose systems were unable to handle sugar. Among the early adolescents in this group it was found, by rechecking earlier records, that similar indications were present at birth and in the early childhood years! (page 49) The indications became more marked as the age of "juvenile delinquency" approached. Tintera declared that periodic GT tests during a child's life could save countless hours and dollars spent probing the child's psyche and home environment for causes of maladjustment (page 49). After much frustration, he finally was able to persuade enough medical people of the validity of his theories so that most doctors now urge a GT test before any other psychiatric tests are begun (page 50).

There's one more point we'd like to bring out. Dufty discovered that many doctors, especially French doctors, know that sugar causes menstrual cramps. He quoted one French doctor, a Dr. Victor Lorenc, who found in 1911 that a woman of thirty, hooked on sugar, realized that her painful discomfort disappeared when she abstained from "this murderous food," as the doctor described it. After that time the doctor observed "many analagous cases." (page 161) Perhaps "many" doctors do recognize this type of sugar reaction, as Dufty says; but if Dr. Lorenc knew it in 1911, *every* doctor in the world should have known by 1912 how to rid women of this monkey. Mr. Kushi places much of the blame for this difficulty on animal products. During a question and answer session following his

February 10, 1978, address at the United Nations, he was speaking of hormone imbalance and said that if women plagued with this problem would stop eating meat for one or two months they "would be surprised to see how completely menstrual cramps disappear."

We hope we have compiled in this chapter evidence to show that many imbalances which cause us poor physical and mental health can be corrected simply by *omitting* harmful substances. This knowledge should make it less difficult to give up those poisons, and easier to accept the shining offer of the soothing — but perhaps at first restrictive — foods chosen for us by macrobiotic principles. Luckily, as people become more and more attuned to correct balance, many of them have less desire to stray toward the extremes of yin and yang — especially when it becomes obvious how many troubles they bring on themselves by indulging in those extremes.

We can call on Ohsawa to summarize matters for us in this advice from *Cancer and the Philosophy of the Far East* (pages 61-62):

> [This] is the conclusion I have reached after fifty years of studying and teaching the Unifying Principle of the philosophy of the Far East. ...It can enable you to immunize yourself your entire life against any disease...Refined sugar and excess animal protein are the two main causes of all our misfortunes!
>
> 1. Suppress sugar completely from your diet. [We imagine that if he were making this list in 1977 instead of in 1962 or earlier he would include the suppression also of all chemical additives.]
> 2. Learn that it is possible to live without being carnivorous.
> 3. Eat primarily whole grain cereals, vegetables, beans, and seaweeds, all as unrefined as possible.
> 4. Eat as little as possible of other foods.
> 5. Keep liquid down to a minimum.

Now that we've tried to show why we eat the way we do, we'll try to tell you *how* to do it in Chapters 12 and 13. We hope you'll find you like the ideas, for the more you learn to live with these principles, the less conflict you'll have in your lives. So — instead of crying, "Stop the world — or the universe — I want to get off!" simply relax and go on spinning.

P.S. We hope we can learn to follow our own advice!

SEQUEL: I'M STILL EATING —
AND LIVING BETTER THAN EVER

(JK)

In the matter of "relaxing" and of "following our own advice," there was a period when I relaxed *too* much. As regards the business of eating to LIVE, I began, about the end of my third macrobiotic year, to live it up a little too far away from center too soon, although I didn't stray anywhere near either of the yin-yang extremes we just spoke of. Telling you about this time of digression (transgression?!) will give further examples of the process of discharging explained in Chapter 5, will show the closely woven interplay between food and state of health, and will have the incidental result of up-dating my own schedule of recovery.

You may have noticed that several times since 1973 I had thought, because of feeling so well, that I was beyond any more symptomatic annoyances. In Chapter 2 my wife stated, for example, that there had been no chills and fever for eleven months. But then, as I mentioned in Chapter 5, similar spells later recurred periodically as a liver discharge. At present (September, 1978), it has been so long since I had anything like that that I have almost forgotten what it was like.

To continue the story, we have to return to the seminar mentioned in Chapter 6. This seminar was called "A Wholistic Approach to Cancer and Major Illness," and was sponsored in Boston March 5-12 ('77) by the East West Foundation. On March 9 there was a day-long conference with invited medical authorities: "A Nutritional Approach to Cancer." I had the privilege of attending that conference as a guest of the East West Foundation, so that I could be one of those who described the amazing benefits derived from the macrobiotic life. An eminent guest lecturer was Hideo Ohmori, a very highly respected Japanese macrobiotic authority from the George Ohsawa Foundation in Tokyo. Our good friend Mari Samuelson went to Boston for the entire week of the seminar to attend classes and to be one of the translators for Mr. Ohmori's lectures and for most of his private conferences. She had told him about my experience with cancer. When he first saw me he told Mari I "looked fine," or however you say it in Japanese. But by late afternoon, having lost sleep for a couple of nights getting my work

ahead in order to be off-campus for a short while, having had the
plane trip out there and a long day of meetings, I was feeling tired.
Ohmori happened to take a closer look at me then and told Mari
I was definitely anemic. (Michio was so much involved with the conference in the brief time I was there that he did not see me again
after I became tired.)

The dessert for supper was apple pie, which looked very
tempting and seemed harmless enough, being non-sugared, non-
chemicalized, non-spiced, lightly sesame-oiled pie made at the
Seventh Inn Restaurant managed by macrobiotic disciples. But Mr.
Ohmori saw me eating it and was horrified. Later I learned that
anemia is a yin blood condition, so no wonder the yin fruit-pie
"binge" shocked him. *My* only reaction to that dessert was a feeling
of contentment.

I had not thought about my physical condition not being the
best, but now I reflected that I had taken a lot of freedom with diet
since the good blood test in July of '76 (Chapter 5). In August Mary
Alice, Mari, and I had gone to California for three weeks of vacation prior to the IACVF convention. During that period of travel it
was impossible to eat strictly according to regulations, and anyway
I didn't think I needed to worry about departing temporarily from
my diet of nearly three years. On two occasions we celebrated by
eating "health-food" ice cream. (Michio says that ordinary ice
cream is the most dangerous and unhealthful food of all, and I
suppose the "natural ingredients" kinds are almost as harmful.)
After coming home, I continued my habit of eating cheese once or
twice a week ("occasionally" was allowable); but the amounts were
small and the cheese was made from the milk of "organic" cows and
was free of chemicals. Perhaps two or three times a week I ate generous portions of fish, which was permissible in smaller servings. I
ate fruit pie, often as much as three or four large pieces a week. But
the fruit was dried (less yin than fresh fruit) and was apples or
pears, which would grow locally. No other unapproved ingredients
were used. Shortly before going to Boston I had celebrated Ivan's
birthday — two evenings in a row! — with large portions of salmon,
which would probably be OK once or twice a year, except that I
followed it with health-food ice cream. I suffered no ill effects the
first night; but the second time resulted in what I thought was a
stomachache, violent but brief, with chills and fever afterward. My
wife, who sometimes can match a caustic tongue with a bluenosed

attitude, made the observation that my body was finally getting smarter than my brain and could now give me macrobiotic back talk when I fractured the rules to that extent. Probably my pancreas was telling me it didn't want to go back to the former overtime working conditions.

So some groundwork had been laid for my fatigue that evening in March before the boom fell on the piece of apple pie. And for a while I had to go back to restrictions even more stringent than those of my first macrobiotic weeks. Mr. Ohmori told Mari that he would recommend a very yang diet for a while. One thing I should eat was koi-koku twice a day. This is carp fish with only the gall bladder and intestines removed, cooked six to eight hours with an equal amount, or more, of burdock root, and with used bancha tea leaves and twigs to soften the bones, scales, and fins, so that every bit of the fish can be eaten. This recipe is in macrobiotic cookbooks. In spite of the awful sound of it, it makes a very rich, delicious, and healthful food. Incidentally, the Landes story in Chapter 14 relates how it brought a dying dog back to life!

Mr. Ohmori also suggested using several teaspoons a day of miso tekka, a yang condiment (which perhaps might be found in Oriental food stores in large cities), and two small cups a day of umeshoban tea (see Chapter 13). He said I should abstain from all fruit, all sweeteners, cheese, raw vegetables, nuts, sunflower seeds, and even oatmeal (the most yin of grains); and I was to eat larger proportions of grains and less of cooked vegetables.

I followed these instructions for about three months, and I *did* feel better. As I said, I hadn't noticed not feeling well when I went to Boston in March, but I remembered I did seem to tire more easily than before. Now, during the three months of yang eating, my endurance returned and was better than ever. (You remember that in January of 1976 Michio had sent me back to the drawing board to get over a similar washed-out "wintery" condition.) I now work longer, play piano better, sleep less, jog a couple of miles a day, climb four flights of stairs "on the double" again, chin myself 15 times, do 28 push-ups, and take care of plenty of heavy-duty yard work. From now on I'll be more likely to set a good example and avoid over-indulging in favorite foods. After the three months, I returned to the more balanced type of diet Michio had given me, for a too-yang program continued indefinitely could cause other problems.

As one more illustration of the way things seem to fall in place for us, a few days after I got home from Boston a young-at-heart doctor (a different one from the one in Chapter 5 who had asked me to have blood tests taken) became warily interested in my pet pancreas. He phoned and said he had read the Sherman Goldman interview in the *East West Journal* and would like to make some tests, as he wasn't sure the case was as unusual as it sounded. Thus I unexpectedly acquired a doctor who could authorize blood tests, which of course gave Western medical verification of Ohmori's visual diagnosis of anemia. Very significantly, the tests also showed that my out-of-bounds eating had taken its toll in other ways, for the alkaline phosphatase and SGOT readings, normal the previous July, were now both very high. The CEA, while it would indicate to macrobiotic people merely that I was still discharging cancer cells, and therefore would be no cause for anxiety, was viewed with great suspicion by my new medical friend. He was very doubtful when I told him that in a few weeks I could improve those results. So he was all the more impressed and *much* interested in the case again when one month later the readings were already considerably better — and for the next test some weeks later were completely normal again!

A young surgeon with a similar interest phoned from a distant state and said that, having read the *EWJ* interview, he would like to examine me on his way through Muncie to move to a new location. He thought, too, that there could have been a mistaken diagnosis. But now that both doctors have checked further, they seem sure that the tumor was malignant, and in a very deadly area.

I'm hoping, of course, that their interest will continue, and will be "contagious" for other doctors. The fact that my tests react like a thermometer to slight deviations or excesses in the diet proves, it seems to me, the strong influence that food has on our bodies. Actually, the *continuance* of an excess could be fatal for some patients. Also, since my *main* deviation was too much fruit — albeit dried, local-type, cooked, and considered by its "consumer" to be safe — I now feel as if I have unwittingly demonstrated the insidious toxic effects of fruit which macrobiotics warns against. The Garden of Eden apple was perhaps symbolic of the lesson that we should eat sparingly of *all* fruit! I also hope the fact that I have more than once brought unfavorable tests back under control by simply cutting out minor infractions will help prove to skeptical friends that this diet program *does* work. Some of our case histories in Chapters 14 and

15 also present this type of evidence. These small-scale deals, plus the large-scale government research, should sway at least a *few* of our on-the-fence observers.

Notes for Chapter 9

[1]Michel Abehsera, *Zen Macrobiotic Cooking* (New York, N.Y.: Avon Books, 1970; Fourth Printing, 1971), p. 9.

[2]Iona Teeguarden, *Freedom Through Cooking* (Boston, MA: Order of the Universe Publications, 1971; Oroville, CA: George Ohsawa Macrobiotic Foundation, 1978), p. 16.

[3]William Dufty, *Sugar Blues* (Radnor, Penna.: Chilton Book Co., 1975), p. 60.

CHAPTER 10

Alternatives — There _Are_ Other Ways

(JK — plus MAK)

While I still have the floor from having made the comments in the sequel to the previous chapter, I should mention a few matters of a different sort which need clarification before you read the next few chapters. I must add a reminder asking you to understand that we are strictly amateurs in the health field and that you should regard our statements for what they are: those of well-meaning but non-professional adventurers, statements that are unproven as far as scientific testing goes. All the ideas have worked beautifully for us and the other friends whose case histories are in this book. _However, since our beliefs appear to most doctors, nutritionists, and scientists to border upon absolute madness, the reader must realize that his or her decision to follow in our wake is one in which he or she assumes in full whatever risks there may be._

Our first reaction to the question, "What risks would there be?" would be to say, "None, really." But when we give that a second look, we have to say that there _are_ risks involved, the most likely one being, probably, that the patient will not take time to thoroughly understand or carefully follow the macrobiotic dietary instructions. Even _that_ point we have to qualify by saying that the significance of meticulous study is _our_ sentiment, for I'm sure that most doctors would declare that almost everything about the program is questionable if not downright nonsensical, and hence not worthy of _any_ attention, either careful or careless. Therefore, please realize that from our standpoint you "proceed at your own risk," as it were. We are sharing our story, despite lack of scientific proof, because of sharing also the attitude of IACVF President Joseph Kosarek expressed in his message quoted at the end of Chapter 5, and because I am sure I would not be alive today if we had not taken the risk of trying an uncharted course by departing from the conventional medical route. I believe that, in my own case, my decision to cancel chemotherapy treatments was a big factor in the success of my recovery. All my friends thought I was making a serious mistake in not taking the treatments in conjunction with the diet, in order to have *two* avenues leading to possible safety. But I chose instead to heed the macrobiotic theory that chemicals tend to counteract the beneficial effects of the food. (However, this theory also holds that if a patient is afraid to put aside the radiation or chemical therapy, he or she is still much better off accompanying the orthodox treatment with macrobiotic food rather than conventional food.)

So, in this matter the patient must make a very important decision on what course of action he or she will take, for either way could be fatal. *Again we must warn that our approach, in spite of **our** confidence in it, is still unproven. Moreover, an additional hurdle is that the macrobiotic program requires responsibility and participation on the part of the patient, a self-discipline that many will not be able to maintain for a long enough time to effect recovery. This in itself is a risk, for **halfway** macrobiotic measures have little chance of controlling cancer.* In making a decision, if you are a cancer patient, you may consider it advisable to ask your doctor to check recovery statistics for orthodox treatment of your type of cancer, for some types have apparently responded very well to such treatment. Include in your research the degree of response for a degree of disease-advancement comparable to your own.

As for inattention to detail in following the macrobiotic diet (since we consider that it *is* worthy of close study!), we are appalled by the fact that many people who are terminal cancer patients, after supposedly reading instructions, are still extremely casual about and ignorant of what they can and cannot eat. For a patient fighting for his or her life to spend so little time studying the foods which are forbidden is a form of suicide. Frequently, people express surprise a month or two after saying they are following the diet: "You mean I can't eat *eggs?*" or, "I can't drink *orange juice?*" We think that eggs are probably the most dangerous food that most cancer patients can eat. And oranges are considered macrobiotically to be suitable only for people living in hot climates, and only in limited quantities at that. (These views are unsupported, of course, by any scientific proof.)

It is both an advantage and a disadvantage that cancer (looked upon by macrobiotic proponents as a friend and as one cure for civilization's ills) sends signals to people that they are doing something wrong, often giving them time to "mend their ways," if they will but pay attention. We believe that the macrobiotic way of avoiding all harmful foods, including eggs, makes the cancer warning an ally rather than an enemy. On the other hand, the period of grace can cause terminal cancer patients to feel quite complacent, for they may not become ill for some months no matter what they do. They think that if they need to correct their habits they will gradually realize it and will have time to make adjustments. What often happens instead, we believe, is that suddenly they find themselves in great pain and suddenly very ill. At this point, the ball game may be over. They are returned to the hospital, given drugs (partly because of the pain), and, in our opinion, have much less chance for recovery from then on.

If, by contrast, a patient does conscientiously try macrobiotics before an illness becomes too critical, blood tests authorized by a physician can be a good indication of progress or lack of progress. As you might expect, our viewpoint (again unsupported by scientific proof) is that if the results of a test are unfavorable the patient probably was not making complete use of the diet, either because of lack of study or (as we pointed out early in Chapter 5) because of cheating or even over-zealousness. Blood tests can also be enlightening if people are adhering conscientiously to the diet but are having a a trying time with "discharging" toxins stored up from years of improper eating (details in Chapter 5 and in the Sequel to Chapter 9). The tests can show that various symptoms are caused by recovery rather than by regression. And they can place in a similar rosy light the weight-loss bugaboo so worrisome for patient, doctor, friends, and family — but not upsetting to people who are used to macrobiotics, for most conformists become very thin, I emphasize *very* thin! I am still (after more than five years) forty pounds lighter than at the time of surgery. Since weight loss is a characteristic of cancer, it does seem frightening to the newly initiated. But my wife, with Cancer only in her horoscope, dropped from 105-109 down to 83, and this sort of loss seems to happen to most macrobiotic people. We become resigned to the fact that we weigh what we're supposed to weigh — and most of us, like most of you, started out with a shocking amount of excess. There may be some risk if a patient tries to counteract the weight loss by over-eating, in spite of the frequent warnings in this book and elsewhere against such indulgence.

Another hazard is that if you are eating strictly macrobiotically, but have not been doing so for a long enough time to trust the philosophy, you may feel you should still take vitamins or food supplements. You may worry that the food alone could not have all necessary nutrients. This is understandable; but macrobiotic "old-timers" tell us that since our food *does* have all vitamins, proteins, and other essential elements, you may upset your own digestive balance by adding artificial vitamins and supplements. (No scientific backing here, either!) Let me illustrate food value with just one example: *our principal beverage, bancha (kukicha) tea, contains, according to Japanese government figures, more than six times as much calcium as milk and more than 2½ times as much Vitamin C as orange juice, in addition to its digestion-easing enzymes!* [a]

On the other hand, if you are eating a typical American diet, then vitamins and supplements *may* be beneficial, our macrobiotic experts say. Please keep in mind, though, that *a food program based on the most healthful foods nutritionists and doctors can think of will not cure or control cancer.* This is probably the reason these professionals consider as preposterous the claims that any *other* diet — such as macrobiotic — can control cancer. They no doubt feel that if a healthful diet were the solution, cancer would have been eliminated long ago for those willing to eat healthful foods. You may want to review our Chapter 6 and check current professional dietary opinions against the government reports on the relationship of diet and major disease. It seems to us that most doctors are not making use of this government information.

Geared to offset eventual danger to our health, as well as contributing to our day-to-day digestive comfort, is the adjustment of food to climate, season, and altitude. As described early in our Chapter 9 and at the beginning of Chapter 13, we use "heartier," more robust foods and cooking methods for colder temperatures, lighter or more delicate foods and methods for warm temperatures. Eating locally grown food is highly important to help us adapt to our local environment.

Having revealed the ominous side of my nature by listing these hazards, I can now return to our dual authorship so that Mary Alice and I can *both* cheerfully tally some of the different ways you can take chances. As firmly as we believe in the macrobiotic approach to health and life, we must recognize that people do recover from illness by using other methods! If we're going to support freedom of choice, we should mention a few other routes that seem to have merit. Of course in the process we also give the reasons we prefer the macrobiotic way! From the vantage point of our own learning during the past few years, we ourselves would not adopt *any* of these alternate systems, for no other seems to us to be completely adequate. We feel that no choice should be decided upon without first making a detailed study of macrobiotics. In our opinion, the "yin" qualities of most other programs could lead eventually to health complications other than the original one, as discussed briefly later in this chapter. Also, we have seen examples where cancer returned when a person for one reason or another rejected the macrobiotic way which was bringing about obvious improvement and changed to another type of cancer program.

Another observation we'd like to make is that we came away from the convention of the International Association of Cancer Victims and Friends (Chapter 6) with a heightened appreciation of the *simplicity* of the macrobiotic approach. All the others sound to us as if they are overly entangled with supplements, vitamins, enemas, and a confusing maze of other impedimenta. We are sure we'd get badly mixed up and take the wrong pill at the wrong time for the wrong reason. Then we're worried about all the raw food and the juices consumed by our new friends. But since some of them are equally worried about us, with our cooked food and limited liquid, everything balances out nicely. There is common ground, however, in that followers of the several systems we describe all manifest a great deal of self-discipline and determination, all reject radiation, chemotherapy, unnecessary surgery, meat, quantities of dairy products, and food additives, preservatives, and other chemical additives.

You will find that the standard answer of medical experts is that these unconventional treatments are often not harmful in themselves, but that they lull people into postponing orthodox medical aid until too late. Yet more and more we learn that even some members of the medical profession are beginning to realize that these methods have limited value. Experienced macrobiotic proponents consider that chemotherapy and radium, as well as much of the accepted surgical treatment, seriously impede the effectiveness of proper food program, for the body's natural ability to create balance will have been impaired.

The latter viewpoint seems to be substantiated by the research of Dr. Hardin B. Jones, professor of medical physics and physiology of the department of medical physics at the University of California at Berkeley, one of the best known statisticians in the medical field. We first learned about him when a friend gave us a clipping from the September 1, 1975, issue of MIDNIGHT,[1] stating that Dr. Jones had for twenty-three years traveled world-wide, collecting data on cancer. His research showed that people who refused treatment for cancer lived longer than those who used medical treatment. "Beyond a shadow of a doubt," he says, "radical surgery on cancer patients does more harm than good," destroying the body's natural defense mechanisms and causing the disease to spread throughout the body and gain other footholds. He has little or no confidence in radiation and chemotherapy.

About a year after we read that clipping, we were in California for the cancer convention we told you about in Chapter 6. While there, we phoned Dr. Jones to ask more details about his findings, and received very cordial consideration. Later he mailed us a copy of his March, 1969, address to the American Cancer Society, along with a copy of a paper presented to the biology section of the New York Academy of Sciences in February, 1956. One determines from Dr. Jones' statements that published statistics are likely to be altogether misleading, as when those for cancer include many easy-to-cure skin cancers and others which were formerly not reported at all, but do *not* include the count of people who die before "controlled" tests are completed, for they did not finish out the term of the test!

Dr. Jones believes that

> With every cancer patient who keeps in excellent physical shape and boosts his health to build up his natural resistance, there's a high chance the body will find its own defense against the cancer. He may have many good years of good health left. He shouldn't squander them by being made into a hopeless invalid through radical medical intervention, which has zero chance of extending his life.[2]

(Many of our friends have been able to "boost their health" through macrobiotics.)

Two people who suggest boosting health by a method with which they have had success are (M.D.) John A. Richardson and Patricia Griffin, R.N., who have written the highly significant new (1977) book *Laetrile Case Histories*. Mrs. Griffin is the wife of G. Edward Griffin, mentioned in our Chapter 1 as the author of the two earlier volumes, *World Without Cancer,* praised by Dr. Richardson as a "masterpiece of research."[3] Reading these three books is practically a requirement for being well-informed about alternatives to orthodox medical treatment.

All of these authors had also "discovered" Dr. Hardin Jones and his quotations from MIDNIGHT. More about his statistical studies can be found in "The Hoax of the Proven Cancer Cure," the chapter written by Mr. Griffin for the Richardson book. Also quoted is Dr. James D. Watson, Nobel Prize winner in medicine: "The American public is being sold a nasty bill of goods about cancer. While they're being told about cancer cures, the cure rate has improved only about one per cent. The grim cancer statistics are about as bad as ever." (Richardson, page 64) Dr. Watson's declaration is supported by quotations which Griffin selects from professional medical journals to show that although radiation has been used extensively for decades its clinical benefit is still dubious. Two of the quotations are these: from Dr. Phillip Rubin, Chief of the Division of Radiotherapy at the University of Rochester Medical School: "The clinical evidence and statistical data in numerous reviews are cited to illustrate that no increase in survival has been achieved by the addition of irradiation." (p. 57) And Dr. Vera Peters, radiologist at the Princess Margaret Hospital in Toronto, says, "... there has been no true improvement in the successful treatment of the disease over the past thirty years." (p. 58)

As for chemotherapy, the *Textbook of Medical-Surgical Nursing* (1970) states that "As yet no drugs are available to cure most malignant tumors." (Richardson p. 63) And Griffin cites sources which reveal that because of toxic side-effects, chemotherapy could actually *produce* more cancer than it *cures*. (Richardson p. 61) He devotes several pages (59-63) to other dreadful suffering which chemotherapy causes.

Yet, in the light of Griffin's research, it would seem that statistics are slanted in favor of these treatments. As one example, he illustrates manipulation of statistics by revealing that clinics often accept only those patients who have a good chance of survival, sending poor risks elsewhere to die. He denounces the American Cancer Society as "an organization that annually produces tons of literature containing exactly the kind of erroneous statistics" described by Drs. Jones and Watson (p. 67). "The 'proven cures' of the American Cancer Society do not exist. ... Undoubtedly they are useful for fund-raising purposes but they cannot be supported by the scientific record." (p. 71) (It is worth noting that the above assertions concerning the ineffectiveness of radiation were made by Drs. Rubin and Peters in speeches to the Sixth National Cancer Conference (1968), sponsored by the American Cancer Society and the National Cancer Institute!)

Dr. Richardson, having watched with puzzled regret during part of his twenty years of practice the negative rather than positive results of surgery, radiation, and chemotherapy on many of his patients, leaped at the chance to investigate the qualities of an "in-nature" substance such as Laetrile (also called amygdalin and Vitamin B_{17}). Through pleasant personal contact and in-depth study of the 1923-1952 research of Dr. Ernest T. Krebs and sons ("father and brothers" of Laetrile) Richardson became convinced of the non-toxicity of Laetrile (page 25), and was fascinated by the prospect of treating not just isolated "lumps and bumps" but the entire patient (page 11). (Compare with the macrobiotic "wholistic approach" to cancer and *all other diseases.)*

As we understand it from sources prior to the Richardson book, the way Laetrile works is this: the contact of Laetrile with the cancer in the body releases hydrocyanic acid from the Laetrile, destroying the cancer cell. Normal cells have an enzyme, Dr. Richardson learned from his Krebs research, which converts the cyanide into harmless or even vital substances. As is the case with the macrobiotic diet, even in advanced cancer cases Laetrile apparently decreases pain.

The Richardson book, while admitting difficulties and certain weaknesses, still makes a very convincing argument in favor of Laetrile. Their difficulties parallel those of the East West Foundation, and of chiropractors whose patients got well but didn't bother to report their improvement to those responsible for it! In previous chapters, we pointed out this type of indifference on the part of "beneficiaries," although most chiropractors and the Richardson Clinic would have kept careful records, thus making it somewhat easier to locate people again if need be. (The EWF is only just beginning to keep track of friends who visit there.) Other Richardson difficulties, also similar to those *we* have observed, were described by Mrs. Griffin: some people ask their doctors about the unorthodox route and then reject it; others are afraid to try anything "experimental;" others fear that if they must have a special diet or follow an unusual routine their employers will find out they have cancer and will consider it risky to award them promotions.

The weaknesses Mrs. Griffin mentions also resemble those of EWF: the Richardson Clinic, as it now practices, is very new. They began using Laetrile in 1971, but it was 1973 before they began to handle a heavy case load. Still the *number* of people treated — some 4,000 — is very impressive, and they were able (by dint of much effort) to locate and up-date records of about 250 of them on which to base their book.

Because of their newness, they have few cases of the magic five-year-or-longer survival. But, Mrs. Griffin notes, "The literature of orthodox medicine is loaded with studies involving only one or one-and-a-half-year survivals." (page 120). Moreover, she points out that many of their clients were in such critical condition that it was a "major victory for Laetrile" that *any* of them should be alive after even a year or two. The case histories presented in their book demonstrate, however, that these people are not only just alive, but are remarkably well. Mr. Griffin bolsters his wife's contention about the chances for their critical patients with somewhat unspecific, but probably not unrealistic, figures. For cancer victims with advanced, metastasized cases which doctors have diagnosed as terminal, there is a 15 percent chance of survival if the vitamin therapy (Laetrile) is used. Orthodox treatment offers one-tenth of one percent for a five-year survival!

Now the East West Foundation case histories also are not long-term, although the way of life behind the recovery of the people described is in accord with ancient principles.

As macrobiotic boosters we are surmising that the main ingredient of the Laetrile success is the diet that accompanies it. Wouldn't you know we'd think of it that way! Mrs. Griffin says that when she first aligned herself with the Laetrile work she thought that that substance itself — the "magic bullet" — was responsible for the results achieved (page 122). Even that attitude was a big reversal for her, for she declares that as an R.N. she naturally believed that *if* cancer *was* essentially a deficiency disease, responding to supplements like Laetrile and enzyme tablets, medical research centers would have tested it and introduced it "properly" to the public. She avers that the "hardest pill for many professionals to swallow is not the vitamin pill. It is the thought they have been wrong and, further, that they and their colleagues have strongly criticized those who have been right." (pp. xvii-xviii) (We are grateful to have from a person of her calibre this corroboration of similar statements in our Introduction and in Chapter 3.) But before long Mrs. Griffin came to the realization that Laetrile could not stand alone. "It appears that the cancer patient is no more likely to respond to Laetrile alone than is the severe diabetic likely to be symptom-free by taking insulin and then consuming banana splits, whipped-cream pie, and soft drinks. *I had to conclude that, for the so-called terminal patient, adherence to the diet is literally a life or death requirement.* (Italics ours)

The diet is principally fresh fruits, vegetables (70-75 percent of which are eaten raw), seeds, nuts, and grains. Excluded are animal foods, including dairy products, coffee, alcohol, sugar, and tobacco. Massive doses of Laetrile (partly by injection and partly by mouth, plus apricot kernels, plus pancreatic enzymes, plus Vitamins B$_{15}$ and C (750-2000 mg daily!) are taken.

Well, we would consider this a "yin" diet, and yet it does cut out both *extremes* of the yin-yang scale (see our Chapter 9). Commercial chemicals are also eliminated because of the use of fresh rather than processed foods. With those elements plus animal products off the list, the diet should, according to our macrobiotic learning, bring improvement, for it would promote the removal of many toxins from the body, thereby creating a neutralized condition which would clear the way for the possible relief of both yin cancer and yang cancer. Of course we feel it would be better to get the enzymes, protein, and vitamins from more grains, seaweed, and fermented soy products, rather than from the synthetic supplements. (Miso, seaweed, umeboshi plums (Chapter 12), and the outer coatings of brown rice all are rich sources of B vitamins.)

We'll venture an amateur guess that yang cancers would respond more readily, and for a longer time, to a high yin in-take than would yin cancers (Chapter 13). We will also hazard the opinion that a program this yin may in time bring its own problems. At first, as we said, it will neutralize toxins; but once neutralization is attained, the continuation of this type of food leads into a danger zone, perhaps causing a weakening of the yang organs — heart, liver, sex organs, etc. Mucus deposits may begin forming, and arthritis is a likelihood. (Please check, for instance, Michio's descriptions of the harmful effects of fruit sugars, in Chapters 8 and 9.) In his address at the United Nations, mentioned before, Michio explained that people are attracted to the raw food diets because of the fact that they are the opposite of the animal products their mothers probably ate during pregnancy, and which they themselves no doubt ate while growing up. "But," he said, "two to five years of eating only these other extreme foods will make them develop the sicknesses opposite to those common among people eating excessive amounts of animal foods. In individual consultations, I have met thousands of people who have developed skin diseases, vaginal discharges, headaches, and so forth because of this type of vegetarian diet. When they return to a more balanced macrobiotic diet, all these sicknesses disappear."

We must not put away the Richardson book without touching on one of the main reasons for writing it — to bring to public attention such interferences as the sudden raid upon the busy little office where the case load had increased beyond expectation through word-of-mouth recommendations of patients whose illness had greatly improved.

> Uniformed officers surrounded the building and, *with guns drawn,* nine men and one police matron burst through the front door, flashed a search warrant at the receptionist, and pushed their way on through the clinic itself. I was thrust against a wall and frisked for a concealed weapon. ...I was informed by Inspector Jackson, of the California Health Department, that I was under arrest for violating the California "anti-quackery" law...(Richardson pages 14-15)

The officials ransacked his office, refused to let him contact his attorney or his wife, and took him to jail past the TV cameras which had been covering the raid. After four hours he was released. Another of his chapters quotes his self-defense at his trial.

Like Dr. Max Gerson (an earlier "renegade" mentioned several times before in our book, whose workable theories have been adapted to a number of current unorthodox cancer-treatment methods), Dr. William F. Koch (discoverer of Glyoxylide), Dr. James R. Privitera (Laetrile),[4] Dr. William D. Kelley (in our Chapter 2 and elsewhere),[5] and other medical professionals who have pulled away from traditional thinking, Dr. Richardson has had to fight for the right to continue his practice. He and Drs. Kelley and Privitera, among others, in 1977 were still facing legal restrictions. In similar vein, eminent scientist Linus Pauling, for all his prestige and his Nobel prizes in science and peace, was not able to obtain funds to continue his research in diet-cancer relationship. For further details of the experiences these people have had, read the Richardson-Griffin books, and supplement them with the older, but partially updated, *Cancer Blackout Amended* of Nat Morris (see our Bibliography).

An attitude which Ivan Illich would approve of (our Chapter 8) is evinced by the innovative do-it-yourself cancer cure of E.L. Buckner (Chapter 6), described by his wife Ruth in a letter to us dated November 13, 1975:

> Last January my husband was diagnosed as having cancer of the prostate. He was sent home for radical surgery, pain pills, and a not-too-distant death. All of this he rejected and became his own doctor. Since he is a research biologist, he began intensive research in the field of cancer and nutrition. We eliminated all of the following: sugar, white flour, all refined and packaged foods, coffee, tea, and all foods containing preservatives, additives, artificial colors and flavors. My husband is sure it is this last group that destroys the cell and damages the gene.

We include only whole grains, fruits, and vegetables, either raw or very lightly cooked over low heat. We use cheese without color added, raw milk and a little meat. My husband eats 75 apricot kernels a day and takes Hydrozene sulfate, a mild non-toxic fungicide. He has gained weight and is in better health than in years.

I am most interested in the program you were taught in Boston. Perhaps we can improve our methods. Surely we can gain new wisdom. ... My husband is convinced the reason this nation has the highest incidence of cancer is due to the refined foods and the junk put in the foods most people buy. We are the victims of the manufacturer who wishes to give his product shelf life. By all means buy G. Edward Griffin's book *World Without Cancer*.

This was, of course, the letter which led to our going to the IACVF convention the following fall. On July 13, 1976, Ruth wrote that Buck had just had another medical checkup from which all tests came back normal, showing bones healing, cancer contained and decreased. His doctor would not investigate any offbeat cures, most certainly not any dealing with nutrition. Yet he was amazed and delighted with Buck's progress and told him to continue his project.

The large number of apricot kernels he takes would warm the hearts of the Laetrile enthusiasts. Notice, too, that Buck cut out all foods with chemicals of any kind, and refined foods. But he does eat a lot of cooked food, which is "non-Laetrilian," some dairy products, honey, any vegetables he wants, and plenty of fresh fruit, all of which is "non-macrobiotian." (True, he does live in fruit country.) He enjoys life thoroughly. In June of '77 we phoned to bring ourselves up-to-date and found that he is in great shape. He is now "tuned up" to the point where he can't eat sugar or food chemicals without feeling the effects, but with all the variety he has, he doesn't *need* to deviate!

So impressed were the rest of the family with Michio Kushi and his philosophies expressed at the convention that they are leaning strongly toward macrobiotic ways; and Sandy and Ed (Chapter 6) even opened a large, deluxe natural-foods store in Los Angeles! It was so successful during its first eight months that a branch store was added (see Appendix). Sandy told us that they carry many macrobiotic products and EWF literature, and stay in touch with Roy and Marijke Steevensz of the Los Angeles East West Center. Many people tell the store employees that they are grateful to have easily available the foods which had improved their health or had even cured them of this or that serious illness.

The optimistic mental attitude which is crucial in the recovery from all illness is given its greatest emphasis by Dr. Carl Simonton (Chapters 1, 4, 8, 11 and 12). As with other systems involving some effort on the part of the patients, Dr. Simonton and his associates have some difficulty finding many who will stick to their total program. But those who do "not only do exceptionally well in the management of their disease but are also able to maintain or improve the quality of their lives." Out of one group of fifty people, they had 70 percent who worked at full-time employment and participated fully in leisure activities.[6]

For a blow-by-blow account of the extent to which attitude and iron will can reinforce mental power, you should read Norman Cousin's story of his twelve-year struggle with, and victory over, a near-fatal collagen illness. This is in his *Saturday Review* of May 28, 1977: "Anatomy of an Illness." The persistence he exhibited leaves one with a feeling of wonderment. Soon after being stricken, unable to move, informed by his doctor that he might have one chance in five hundred of surviving, his reaction was, "I felt a compulsion to get into the act." Dr. William Hitzig cooperated sensibly and sensitively with him in trying daring, but carefully conceived, theories. Cousins learned that adrenal exhaustion and impaired oxygenation are factors in collagen breakdown, and learned from the Hans Selye *Stress of Life* that adrenal exhaustion can be caused by emotional tension, as from extreme frustration or suppressed rage. The book detailed the negative effects of negative emotions on body chemistry. By reverse logic, Cousins reasoned that positive emotions should have positive results — and he found that *ten minutes of "belly laughs,"* as from comic movies or from jokes read by obliging nurses, *would provide two hours of narcotic-free sleep.* Moreover, the *effects were cumulative.* From this first stirring of hope, it was "many months" (he is not specific) before he could reach up for a book on a high shelf, but he was able to go back to work full-time. When the article was written, he was pain-free, even for certain sports, except in his knees.

What if he had known about macrobiotics — would it have shortened the recuperation to a fraction of that time? One can only conjecture, but judging from the benefits we have personally observed for arthritis and multiple sclerosis (diseases in the collagen category), we would consider it likely that he could have been greatly helped. That he placed faith in the value of nutritious food was shown by his lament over the quality of hospital food: "No wonder the 1969 White House Conference on Food, Nutrition, and Health made the melancholy observation that the great failure of medical schools is that they pay so little attention to the science of nutrition."

Mr. Cousins offers us this conclusion — and he certainly proved the truth in it by the depth with which he played his role: "The will to live is not a theoretical abstraction, but a physiologic reality with therapeutic characteristics." This ties in with Mr. Kushi's assertion (Chapter 8) that some people have the ability to put mentality to the same *physical* use as beneficial food. It is also borne out by the belief of Ana Aslan, one of Romania's leading endocrinologists, whom Mr. Cousins visited, that "there is a direct connection between a robust will to live and the chemical balances in the brain."

While on the subject of alternatives, we would like to speak to arthritis sufferers for just a moment before we close this chapter. People will be telling you, as they do us, about a "Chinese diet" for arthritis that is "just like" ours. Of course, they'll tell us that the Laetrile diet is just like ours, too, and the same for other diets. Any time brown (or even white!) rice is involved, or unrefined flours or fresh vegetables, we hear the same thing. Usually we find there's too much fruit, too much liquid, too much raw food, etc. But we decided to investigate the "Chinese diet."

It resulted from the work of Dr. Collin H. Dong, M.D., of San Francisco, who is indeed Chinese. His theories were recorded in book form *(The Arthritic's Cookbook)* by one of his grateful patients, Jane Banks, who in two weeks experienced almost complete freedom from pain, followed by gradual disappearance of the arthritic swelling. Dr. Dong himself had had a crippling case of the disease which developed insidiously during the busy years of medical training and practice when he ate the well-balanced, brain-washed food of modern advertising.[7] He emphasized that *it was a food balance that would meet with the approval of nutritionists and doctors as being properly healthful.* In regard to healing his sickness, he declared that out of Western scientific knowledge "all the expertise had failed me." (his page 3) His childhood culture had included a diet of meat, fish, vegetables, rice, and fruit, but of course no preservatives. While this childhood pattern was considered generally acceptable, we took note of the fact that his father and all the children in a large family had various food allergies, summed up by Dr. Dong with the statement that "Allergy to food has been chronicled in Chinese medical literature for centuries." (page 4) He returned to that early diet and then experimented with omitting medications (especially *aspirin*), then with leaving off one food component at a time, finally settling on fish, vegetables, and rice (probably white rice!). (page 6) The "metamorphosis" of the next few weeks led to an almost complete "remission" lasting for thirty-one years (sounds like a *cure* to us!). (page 5)

Mrs. Banks fills in with other details: elimination of all fruit, and of tomatoes, vinegar, chocolate, soft drinks, dairy products except egg whites (somewhat close to being "just like ours"). So with that diet, plus the usual "chemical therapy" (he is not specific), plus a warning of the dangers of *all* food additives, Dr. Dong began making recommendations to his patients. Out of thousands of cases of rheumatic diseases, he obtained a remarkably high percentage of remissions from pain and misery. Again there's no way to know for sure, but we wonder whether with macrobiotics his percentage would have been higher and whether for himself he could have said "complete" remission instead of "almost complete." For he does allow yin foods such as avocados, eggplant, potatoes, beets, coffee, tea (artificial coloring in commercial teas!), margarine (coloring), mushrooms, some herbs, white rice, white flour, soda water (!). Mrs. Banks says, "Honey is a fine food." (Fine for *bees,* Mr. Kushi once told us, while permitting small amounts occasionally for us healthy people.) Mrs. Banks also says that "sugar is, of course, perfectly acceptable." (!!!) (page 26) (William Dufty's *Sugar Blues* had not yet been written.)

So, arthritic people, if you try this program and are still aching, you might consider eliminating these non-macrobiotic items. Then you would be macrobiotic, provided you added other grains, seaweed, miso, and a few beans. But even if Dr. Dong and Mrs. Banks don't eat seaweed and miso, we think they deserve unlimited praise for the valuable work they have done.

Dr. Dong is saddened by quotations which show that the Arthritis Foundation publishes misinformation just as do the cancer organizations (page 7). But he finds satisfaction in the supportive encouragement of the thousands of patients to whom his guidance has brought "dramatic relief," and in the fact that young long-haired interns are shaking up attitudes in the usually stuffy medical meetings (page 9). These hopeful signs finally gave him the incentive to write his book, which he had postponed for years because he "did not have the courage to fight the medical establishment." (page 6) You will no doubt want to check also his second book, *New Hope for the Arthritic* (see our Bibliography).

Notes for Chapter 10

[a] This type of information will be expanded by further macrobiotic reading, as, for instance, learning that sea "vegetables" (seaweeds!) abundantly supply iodine, iron, calcium, potassium, magnesium, phosphorus, sodium, and Vitamins A, B_1, B_2, B_{12}, C, D, and niacin, besides being high in protein.

In regard to using artificial vitamins and food supplements, we believe that there should be much more research to clear up the confusion even in present-day orthodox medicine and nutritional theory. Some studies we have read about indicate that, for all their "well-balanced," supplement-fortified diets, many, if not the vast majority, of "healthy" Americans — even nutritionists! — show areas of deficiency when given exhaustive blood, urine, or hair analysis tests. Research should also be carried out during the time of adaptation to the macrobiotic food program, when people are likely to worry about "discharging," various symptoms of which (skin irritations, temporary intestinal irregularities, visual adjustments, dental problems, etc.) are discussed in this book. Michio Kushi, reminding us that some vitamin and mineral deficiencies are common until people learn macrobiotic balance, says that *it may be wise for a short while to add a* **natural** *(not* **artificial***) form of food supplement.* "Such additions, however, should be gradually decreased as understanding and balancing of food factors more nearly approach macrobiotic well-being. Eventually, all these supplements should be eliminated because all living beings can secure their health and well-being through a normal way of eating, breathing, and carrying out activities and other life phenomena."

[1] "Cancer Cures *More Deadly* Than Disease," MIDNIGHT, September 1, 1975.

[2] *Ibid.*

[3] John A. Richardson, M.D., and Patricia Griffin, R.N., *Laetrile Case Histories* (Westlake Village, Cal.: American Media, 1977), p. 6.

[4] *Ibid.,* p. 43.

[5] *Cancer News Journal,* a publication of the International Association of Cancer Victims and Friends. Write to the IACVF at 7740 West Manchester Ave., Playa del Rey, CA 90291, if you wish to ask for the most recent information on Dr. Kelley's legal situation.

[6] From "Statement of Purpose" prepared by the staff of Oncology Associates directed by Dr. O. Carl Simonton (radiation oncologist), M.D., D.A.B.R., Fort Worth, Texas. (See Appendix).

[7] Collin H. Dong, M.D., and Jane Banks, *The Arthritic's Cookbook* (New York, N.Y.: Thomas Y. Crowell, 1973), p. 3.

CHAPTER 11

So You Have Only a
Short Time to Live!

(J K)

Always before, this crushing news belonged to someone else, and you thought, "How awful," and "What a shame," and things like that. Now suddenly it belongs to *you,* and as the meaning of it begins to sink in, "What a shame," is no longer equal to the situation.

Well, what can you do? In this book we have related my experiences in curing "hopeless" pancreatic cancer, as well as similar stories of other people. If you're willing to accept the humble offering of our experience as a guide, *let's get busy.* We were lucky blunderers, but if we could have gone through it in the light of all the practice we've had, we don't think things would have been a lot different. Just easier. And making things easier for you is our goal in compiling this book.

The application is not *only* for "terminal" patients, of course, nor for cancer only. The *urgency* may not be there for other cases or other illnesses, but the prospect of a wretched existence certainly is. All we can do is tell what we would do to wipe all this away, with the gentle reminder that what we would do is based on what we *have done,* and on what many hundreds of others have successfully done.

If you began reading with the first part of Chapter 10, as suggested (at the end of our Introduction) for those who are in a state of crisis, you'll have to follow the pointers in our next few paragraphs more or less blindly, and some names and ideas will be unfamiliar, till you carry out our second suggestion to read certain other portions of our book. As you read, you will find that *you definitely are not to feel sorry for yourself,* so you may as well drop that feeling immediately. You have work to do which doesn't permit any time for moping around. We believe, as a result of reading we have done, that by mental attitudes and the food they eat *people give themselves cancer* or whatever illness they have — and therefore they can jolly well rid themselves of it. It will take some effort, but that's all to the good.

As a starter, don't feel you must necessarily have a great amount of rest; exercise as much as you can. Walk. Walk. And walk some more — even if it's only around the bed.

One of the first things we'd do would be to make bright-colored cards saying, "From this day on I am no longer ill. From now on all symptoms and sensations I have are manifestations of recovery. No matter what else I may be doing, *healing is progressing every minute of every day and every night."* Keep one of these cards in your pocket. If you're able to be up, paste one on the mirror in the lavatory. If not, have someone write it large enough for you to see it somewhere near your bed. *You have to become a pioneer at heart, with determination, courage, confidence, and conviction. This is no time for submission or passivity.*

Here's one adapted (very freely!) from Dr. Carl Simonton: "My basic defense mechanism repels all abnormal cells presented to my body — bacteria, viruses, and all others." This was taken from an article in *FATE* Magazine of December, 1975, entitled "The Role of the Mind in Cancer Therapy."[1] Dr. Simonton uses "destroys" instead of "repels," but we like the feeling that all little antagonists are *repelled* before they can get close enough to need to be destroyed. Also, he is likely to speak of an "immune mechanism," which may appeal to you more than the "defense mechanism" we use. (We like the *active* connotation of "defense.") We are sure Dr. Simonton won't mind our making such good use of his idea in our own words. Thank you, Dr. Simonton!

What else should you do right away? Check our Bibliography and order *The Will to Live*. The Joseph Murphy *Power of Your Subconscious Mind* also has many affirmative statements you can use for daily reminders (Bibliography).

Michio Kushi (the guiding light of our entire recovery campaign) says that, especially in the recuperation of a cancer patient, mental attitude is very important — that the patient "must maintain a happy, positive attitude, and forget about the cancer." In his opinion, as long as appetite and the ability to digest food remain there is always the possibility of recovery.

Envision yourself as completely cured. Never again envision yourself as being ill.

There are a few paragraphs and a couple of chapters in our book you probably should read next:

Chapter 1 — Dr. Simonton's techniques, near the end of the chapter.
Chapter 4 — first seven paragraphs.
    If you decide to work at macrobiotics read Chapter 5 (first half, especially concerning "discharging").
Chapter 6 — Government Reports.
Chapter 7 — read about one-fourth of the way into the chapter, ending with "the 'cowlick' on top of your head." Also, enjoy Mr. Kushi's hope for the future, at the end of the chapter.
Chapter 8 — through the comments about leukemia.
Chapter 9 — entire chapter, including the Sequel.
Epilogue

Then you'll need to know what you can and cannot eat, where to get the food, how to prepare it, and — yes — how to *eat* it, if you'll pardon our getting personal. Most of this information has been scattered throughout the book, but it is so important for you to have it easily available that we repeat it all in one place at the beginning of Chapter 13. For, as crucial as mental attitude is, the use of proper food is even more essential to this way of staying well and/or getting well. We each have our original creation, but through food we are *re*-created each day we live, and we may as well re-create something strong.

It may begin to seem as if there is nothing else in a macrobiotic life except food and eating. But before long you come to realize that the food is only the key to unlock the gateway to any ideal we want to accomplish, from healing a single invalid to building the One Peaceful World which is the goal of the East West Foundation, Mr. Kushi's ever-growing, non-profit organization. The essence of that goal is that while food is only a key, it's the *only* key that fits!

We can mention here some surprising things to show you how much power we believe this food has. Now that we have been macrobiotic for five years, we feel *well protected against ever having any major illness.* That may sound extreme, but we firmly believe it. Even if it should happen sometime not to remain true, it's certainly a great feeling to live with. As a matter of fact, it's a part of the Order of the Universe philosophy that if human beings are the ultimate manifestation of the spiral of creation, they are responsible only to that Universe and cannot be devoured by any other living thing within it.

Mr. Kushi tells a revealing anecdote illustrating the protective power of brown rice. During World War II he was a guard at a train station in Tokyo. A trainload of miserable refugees from the atomic blast on Nagasaki came into the station. From them he learned that St. Francis Hospital had been in the center of the explosion and was destroyed. *But the hospital staff seemed not to be suffering any ill effects.* He learned that the personnel had been eating brown rice, miso soup, Hokkaido pumpkin, and other vegetables, and that the only person who became ill was a priest who had come from Europe and was eating cheese and white bread. Michio attributes the protection against Strontium 90 mainly to the phatin or phatic acid in brown rice, acting "as a buffer which neutralizes and eliminates toxins."

In *Cooking for Life,* Michel Abehsera relates what must be the same incident, through a quotation of Dr. Tatsuichiro Akizuki (M.D.), whom Michio also mentioned. The date was August 9, 1945.

> ...the hospital I was in charge of at the time was located only one mile from the center of the blast. It was destroyed completely. My assistants and I helped many victims who suffered from the effects of the bomb. In my hospital there was a large stock of miso and tamari. We also kept plenty of brown rice and wakame. So I fed my co-workers brown rice and miso soup. I remember that none of them suffered from the atomic radiation. I believe this is because they had been eating miso soup.[2]

Apparently Dr. Akizuki was not so well-informed as Michio and did not realize that, although his total food program was an excellent one, it was the phatin in the rice that provided the particularly protective quality.

A faculty member in the health science department at Ball State University asked Michio this question: "If the macrobiotic system makes people well and keeps them well, how do they die?" Obviously pleased with the question, Michio answered that they finally die a *natural* death — no reason why it should not be after 120 years or more. But more often, having attained what they consider a ripe old age, they feel that they have rounded out most of what they want to accomplish here, and besides, many of their friends have died. So they get their affairs in order and announce to living friends that they will soon be taking their leave. And then some morning they just don't wake up. The longevity of residents of Vilcabamba in southern Ecuador and of the Hunzas in Pakistan, whose life-style is austere and whose food is simple, attests to the actuality of such a way of living and leaving.

People ask, "How soon will I know whether this macrobiotic

business is going to help?" Our reading and our experience with many new friends tell us that there are frequently hopeful signs within ten days. You may read that George Ohsawa declared that "any illness can be cured in ten days." Now while I feel that Ohsawa deserves a vast amount of credit for introducing the macrobiotic philosophy to the West, it seems to me that he does get carried away sometimes and makes exaggerated claims for the program. Immediate benefits of various kinds seem to occur, of course, from a change to macrobiotics, and I had this type of experience myself; but ten days is too early, certainly, to speak of a "cure" or even a control of the illness. But there is no escaping the constantly increasing volume of evidence that health and hope are here.

So come along. We hope you can see that macrobiotics is a pretty safe umbrella to be under! Remember you *count on* being well. And with this in mind, one practical plan we want to suggest quickly is that if you and your employer are willing for you to work even part-time, *don't give up your job* (unless, of course, that's part of your problem!). If I had believed in traditional medical methods and doctors to the extent that most patients do, I would have been so sure they were right that I might very well have sold our home, resigned my position at Ball State University, and spent much of our savings enjoying my last few months.

In that event what a bewildering realization — at once joyous and nightmarish — it would have been to begin to comprehend that I wasn't going to die, that I was going to be healthier than I had been before surgery! In one sense such a development would be exhilarating news indeed, but in another it would be tragic. Our home and our superior collection of rare evergreens and Japanese maples plus our five hundred roses (many of them imported) mean a great deal to me. Also, my piano teaching and my recitals at Ball State have been most rewarding. To suddenly lose all of this, and most of my very good retirement plan only nine years from retirement, in addition to my position as a full professor, would have been a loss of very serious proportions. All because of a mistaken belief that I was going to die! However, I think my doctors did me a service to tell me openly what my chances were. They, naturally, did not know about the macrobiotic approach, and the rules of Western medicine as it is known and practiced today said that I had *no* chance of survival. The fact that my doctors were so positive about my limited future made it easy to skip the chemotherapy and go for broke on the possibilities offered by macrobiotics.

On the other hand, we have known a number of patients who

haven't been told their illness is terminal. Their doctors admit that their situation is very serious, but the patients are encouraged to believe that the doctors can save them. (For example, we learned of one woman whose doctors told her that cancer of the pancreas responded very well to chemotherapy! By the time her family chanced on to macrobiotics, almost a year later, she was sleeping a drugged sleep of some twenty hours a day: the disease was simply too far advanced, and it was not possible to feed her properly.) In *some* instances a hopeful prognosis would be the best procedure, as some few people can recover by *believing* they will recover. But probably most patients will see no reason to take an active part in their own recovery unless a doctor outlines a specific regimen for them (see the Ivan Illich discussion in Chapter 8). Patients who don't know that they are definitely terminal can see no purpose in trying a macrobiotic diet, with the self-denial it entails, because they believe their doctor is going to save them. If he can, then well and good. But the resulting complacency, without the need for struggle in order to recover, is likely to be their undoing.

We have a tragically appropriate illustration of this situation. A man and his wife came to see us about his cancer of the pancreas because a friend of ours had told him of my good luck. After our conversation, we thought he had decided to try the diet, but we were mistaken. His doctors had not told him, nor apparently even his wife, that his condition was terminal. The surgeon had said to him in a cheerful manner after telling him of the cancer, "We'll get the very best man available for your radium treatments." The patient took this to mean that they could cure him so he felt no necessity for trying the diet. Some few months later, riddled with cancer and suffering unendurable pain unrelieved by narcotics, he hanged himself in the hospital.

But as we were saying, if you are one who, instead of a misconception, has had to face the announcement of imminent "finality," our third recommendation (after you start your active pursuit of optimism by means of your bright reminder cards, and then read a few key passages in our book) would be to hold on to your job if at all possible.

Finally, we hope you'll be willing to try macrobiotics, for this is mainly what restored health for me and for all the other people we'll tell you about. Study our next two chapters on preparation, stock up on the food, and begin practicing cooking and eating. Then you can read the rest of this book as you eat and get well. But one of the main things we've learned is that most of you are not convinced.

If not, please read a few of our case histories of people with serious illness.

A striking contrast to the defeatism of those who seem to want to be ill is the exuberance of the people whose stories are in this book. One of the most gratifying facts about our adventures in macrobiotics in Muncie is that in a high percentage of cases where a person had a receptive mental approach, and seemed to follow the diet assiduously, the reward was extraordinary success. We hope that the case histories provide evidence and inspiration, and that the information in our next two chapters will allow you to begin to understand the macrobiotic program. As we have said, we can only tell you what *we* would do, in the light of our experiences and of our interpretation of macrobiotic philosophy, for we feel sure in our own minds now that this way of life offers optimism and excellent possibilities for good health.

In the event you want to join in the optimism and want to telephone the East West Foundation at this point, you could dial direct (1-617-536-3360) between 10:00 a.m. and 5:00 p.m. EST or EDT, depending on the season. Probably it would be best, the first time, to speak with the executive director, who is always more than willing to answer questions. He or she can tell you whether you should have a meeting with Michio or one of his associates, and if so, can tell you how to arrange it. If you are too ill to travel very far at first (or if on the other hand your condition is not overly serious), the director may suggest following the information given in our next two chapters, adding modifications which you can practice on your own until you are able to visit Boston or perhaps an East West Center nearer to your home. These Centers are becoming more numerous and the friends who manage them are becoming more knowledgeable. But do please check by phone first, because you know how quickly lists can change and be out-of-date.

If a trip to Boston is the decision, transportation and the motel bill will be your main expense. If your home is not near one of the Centers where you can get follow-up help, it may prove most practical for you to stay in Boston for a while to absorb some instruction on food preparation at one of the several macrobiotic student houses in the area, or by joining one of the regular classes in cooking presented by the Foundation. Besides that, someone on the Foundation staff can help you select books to buy and take home, as well as a few kitchen items that may not be available elsewhere, such as one of the special small graters the Erewhon store carries, to prepare finely-grated daikon, ginger root, etc.

After your first trip, any time you feel puzzled or insecure about anything, the staff at the Foundation office, long-time disciples and students of Michio's, will be most happy to answer your questions by phone, asking his help if necessary. Sometimes people like to make a second trip to Boston after following instructions for four to six months, but that is often unnecessary.

If you are not ill but want to become macrobiotic to prevent illness and to ward off the common infirmities of aging, then let this book be your guide as much as possible. One of our reasons for writing this chapter and the next two was to save Michio and his staff unnecessary questions. Be sure, please, that you're not going to ask questions that are answered here. But for information which you feel we have not given clearly, or for questions which may be unique to your own problem, don't hesitate to call the Foundation.

Now we're going to assume you have either seen Michio or some other macrobiotic friends and are ready to join the rapidly growing throng who think they've found the road to the best way of life. It's still a rocky road, but part of the philosophy is that overcoming hardship is great for us. It develops strong character. It's not easy to adopt a single-minded, non-deceptive discipline in eating. Not to cheat in the food department — being honest even with yourself — requires unusual courage. But do try to be as conscientious and diligent as possible. Very often the personal suggestions you are given apply to your day-to-day comfort, such as ease in digesting your food, as well as to recovery.

One thing that helped me get through the months when I had to be strict — or *else!* — was to think of the short length of time a forbidden food is enjoyed. This was the key to a concept that helped me avoid eating things I knew I should not have. If you estimate how long it would take to eat a piece of pie, for example, and then just for that short amount of time *make yourself abstain,* in one sense the problem is solved. If the piece of pie is consumed in five minutes, then five minutes' pleasure is all you get out of it. Once eaten, the pie gives you no pleasure, but does do your body much harm. So after only five minutes of abstinence you feel the same as if you had indulged, but you don't suffer the consequences. In other words, *be disciplined for just five minutes.* We don't eat the pie because we are hungry — we eat it because we enjoy very much the five minutes of pie-eating. If we honestly are hungry after the five minutes, we can eat more of something else that's not harmful. We should be able to stand almost anything for very short intervals! This is the kind of reasoning I had to use in my early macrobiotic months and each time I got off the track thereafter, innocently, unintentionally, or sneakily.

Another trick is to imagine that that is the last piece of pie and it's the favorite kind of your son or daughter. You just couldn't eat it and deprive your child, could you?

(Or could you?!)

We hope you will soon develop a strong affinity for macrobiotics. Talented followers soon lose interest in harmful foods and find them unappetiizing. They may find some former favorite foods even repulsive. Unfortunately, I am a good macrobiotic follower in theory but my guts place me with the bad guys. I still consider milk shakes, cream pies, strawberry shortcake, swiss steak with potatoes and gravy, and other such temptations awfully attractive. In general, though, I don't miss meat very much, and I am now having broiled or baked lean white fish a couple of times a week, occasional chicken or turkey, and some cheese.

While I still am not repelled by "orthodox" foods, I would not under any circumstances consider going back to my former way of eating. Regardless of what certain nutrition experts may say about food additives being harmless, we believe that such ideas are untrue — that these chemicals do lead, for many, many, people, to long-term health troubles. And I would not want to eat foods containing sugar, now that I know how harmful sugar is for both mind and body.

Happily, you'll soon discover that you can notice the natural sweetness inherent in certain foods, such as carrots, if they are of good quality, and especially in squash and parsnips. The sweetness in vegetables and grains, of course, is high on the "approved" list. Dried [non-tropical-unless-you-live-there] fruits, when boiled to be served with rice or other grains as a pudding, or thickened with arrowroot for a pie or cobbler with whole-wheat crust, need no sweetening at all, and most people can have these things in very limited quantities within a few months.

I'm trying to point out that this way of life soon won't seem as grim as it might on your opening encounter with it. My wife has felt from the first that this food program is not a penalty but an opportunity. She would have had me think all along not whether I liked this food, but whether I was worthy of being associated with it! And indeed it wasn't long — through good fortune which we'll share with you in Chapter 13 — before we learned that this food can be made so delicious that you can hardly stay away from it!

As we mentioned earlier, striving to overcome all kinds of obstacles is beneficial to our health. Because of that, the fact that you have been working hard to achieve macrobiotic success, and have been eating the nourishing food as you carry out the rest of your recuperative efforts, you are on the way to recovery. Next you'll be like all the other macrobiotic neophytes who worry that they will have a difficult time socially if they can't eat and drink what their friends are having. I can't quite identify with that problem, but I honestly believe that even those who are at first bothered by it will soon get used to the idea.

For carry-in dinners or other such occasions where the atmosphere is informal you can take a brown rice and vegetable casserole. Use some lentils or beans as one of the ingredients if you haven't had your 10 percent yet for that day, and plan things so that you've already had miso soup for an earlier meal. Ordinarily, good raw vegetables will be someone else's contribution to the dinner, and you can eat a variety of those. Take your bancha tea in a thermos (glass-lined, not plastic — bancha tea *recoils* at the idea of being stored in plastic!). Then you will have had your "universal balance." Admittedly it's enough to unsettle the most resolute stoic to be near the temptation of fried chicken, apple pies, and chocolate cakes at one of these gatherings and not succumb! Just don't get close enough to get a whiff of the desserts, if that's your nemesis. Keep thinking you don't want to make your liver, or pancreas, or kidneys, or whatever, work *that* hard. Think how you've been brave for several weeks now and you don't want to blow the investment you already have in this thing. Then, think that in six months or a year you'll be well, instead of sick or dead, and can occasionally have small servings of these luscious items, partly because you will have learned to surround all food with ten parts of saliva and thus protect your grateful internal organs to some extent. In time you'll be able to make "safe" desserts from macrobiotic ingredients and can look a little less longingly at that chocolate cake.

Formal banquets pose a problem, of course. Our solution has been to go late to these occasions, in time for the speaker and the rest of the program. Since we are in a university milieu this arrangement has no embarrassment for us, but I can see that in some professions it might cause consternation.

As for parties, you're mostly among friends who already know your situation. You can either eat some of your mb desserts before you go, or, as suggested above, when you have advanced to the point of being allowed a little fruit and finally a touch of cinnamon, you can take along some samples of your oatmeal-raisin-apple juice-cinnamon cookies for yourself and others. Other people are usually curious about what life is like for macrobiotics, and my wife (who delights in counting *my* blessings!) reminds me that I've derived miles and miles of conversation at parties and elsewhere while describing our new life style. Frequently now, when we go to a party we omit the eating and drinking and turn our attention to enjoying the party. Socializing should not be based exclusively on eating and drinking anyway. If you skip the food and don't enjoy the party, then you haven't much of a party!

If you have a position — such as some sales or executive positions — where eating and drinking are a key factor, you have a tough decision as between recovering from your major illness or keeping your job and hanging on to life as long as you can. Personally, knowing what I know now, I would change jobs, even if I wanted to follow macrobiotics only for the reason of maintaining good health.

Not being the type of person for lodges, country clubs, or veterans' organizations, I have not had to face the dilemma of taking bancha tea to functions of that sort. But I imagine that would be a bit too much!

Having described to you the possibilities for a wild macrobiotic social life, I may as well discuss eating while traveling. On our second visit to Boston we asked Michio how to handle this. He said that for a few days (or even weeks if you are not ill) you can manage by eating as macrobiotically as possible, avoiding meat, rich desserts, milk, eggs, coffee, etc. Of course, one cannot stay very close to a macrobiotic diet when eating in restaurants, for chemicals and sugar are in everything (just as they are in canned or packaged foods from the grocery). Green beans are traditionally [over] cooked with ham, spices are in most foods, sugar is in vegetables and soups, and sometimes even raw vegetables are sprayed with a compound to keep them fresh-looking. Macaroni is made of pasty, dead white flour instead of whole-wheat flour and the cheese on it is full of preservatives, besides which it's often too salty and peppery. (But I still enjoy it!) Fish is easy to come by in restaurants; but of course 90 percent of the time it's breaded and fried. Once in a while you can find it broiled or baked. If so, go ahead and enjoy the inevitable butter sauce with paprika and parsley! However, do put lemon slices and tartar sauce off to one side rather than on your fish. Also, sort out pieces of tomato and other forbidden items from your fresh vegetables, and don't regress to the extent of using salad dressings. (By now you've discovered that vegetables have a flavor of their own which shouldn't be ruined by dressings.)

Happy is the traveler who locates an occasional natural-foods restaurant near his pathway! Listings of these oases are sketchy, but we plan to include some information about them in the Appendix.

Before too long you begin to feel uneasy about putting ordinary-type restaurant contaminants in your digestive tract. If you're traveling by car, you can do quite well at avoiding a large percentage of harmful foods. Some macrobiotic recipe books list things to make to last for a few days. During a three-weeks' trip to Florida, we took along an electric cooker (most motel rooms have several Formica-top surfaces) and a generous supply of raw brown rice — plus, of course, a large sieve for rinsing it. Just before the rice is done, some frozen or finely chopped fresh vegetables can be added. This you can fix in the motel room for dinner, and what's left will stay fresh in the cooker during the next day's drive (especially if an umeboshi plum is dropped in on top of the rice). We also boiled water in a Corning Ware electric coffee maker (with the coffee mechanism removed), transferred the boiling water to a granite casserole pan and finished cooking miso soup over canned heat. (Miso and seaweed travel quite well.) Then we could make bancha tea in the coffee maker and have it with us all the next day in a glass-lined thermos. (Don't fix the miso soup in the coffee maker or your precious bancha tea may have a soupy flavor.)

Of course, for this kind of routine, you need more time in motels, but that provides a welcome opportunity to catch up on reading, correspondence, and swimming! Moreover, following such a travel plan will require a minimum of transition for your digestive system when you return home.

One other curiosity I had was in regard to the macrobiotic diet for people who engage in very strenuous physical activity. For example, weight lifters eat enormous amounts of food, particularly meat. Michio's answer was that for such a person up to 15 percent of the diet could be fowl, and of course white fish may be eaten (shellfish only occasionally, however). (Methods of cooking, just as for everyone else, should be baking, broiling, or boiling, as fried foods soak up too much oil.) Thus, if you want to eat more fish or fowl — become a weight lifter!

Most of us, though, will not be placing that much emphasis on physical prowess. But to help you maintain the degree of good health you have now found practical for yourself, we pass along these "Standard Suggestions," slightly reworded, from the East West Foundation:

GENERAL WAY OF LIFE

1. Let us live happily without worrying about our condition, and let us be active mentally and physically.
2. Let us be grateful for everyone and everything, and let us pray before and after each meal.
3. Please try to sleep before midnight, and get up early in the morning.
4. Please avoid any synthetic or woolen clothing worn directly on the skin, and please avoid using many metallic accessories on fingers, wrists and neck, keeping such ornaments as simple and graceful as possible.
5. Please chew very well, at least 50 times or more. [While you were recuperating, remember, the number of "chews" was two or three times that many.]
6. If your condition allows, please go outdoors often in simple clothing, possibly barefoot. Walk on the grass and soil, even one-half hour, every fine day.
7. Please keep order in the house, beginning from the kitchen, bathroom, bedroom and living rooms, to every corner of the house.
8. Begin and maintain active correspondence, extending love and friendship toward parents, brothers and sisters, relatives, teachers and friends.
9. Do not take long baths or showers unless you have been taking too much salt or animal food in the past.
10. Rub and massage the whole body with either a hot damp towel or a dry towel, every morning or every night before sleeping, until the skin becomes red. At least do the hands and feet, each finger and toe.
11. Please avoid using chemically perfumed cosmetics and try to use all natural ones. For care of the teeth, use dentie* or sea salt to brush them every morning and night.
12. If your physical condition allows, please do actively any exercise. It is especially good if your daily work involves exercise, and you may participate in other forms such as yoga, martial arts, and sports.

Before turning to the specifics of actually working with macrobiotic food, we'll close this chapter with George Ohsawa's evaluation of the qualities of a healthy person. In time we are all supposed to be able to attain these qualities:

---

*Charred eggplant and sea salt. (We'll whisper in your ear that we, personally, don't like it!)

1. No Fatigue — Having worked through the night you can leap to work again the next morning.
2. Good Appetite — You can thoroughly enjoy the simplest food and take deep pleasure in but a drop of water.
3. Good Sleep — Your sleep is deep and you enter it within minutes after putting your head on the pillow. You neither thrash about nor dream, and you can awake spontaneously at a predetermined hour without the help of an alarm clock. You awake fully refreshed after four or five hours' sleep.
4. Good Humor — From morning until night, living is a joy for which you feel deep gratitude. You fear nothing and are grateful for everything. Out of misfortune you create joyful promise and opportunity.
5. Good Memory — You never forget and, as you age, your ability to remember the names of an ever-increasing number of friends improves.
6. Good Judgment and Smart Action — You make all decisions confidently and quickly. Your movements are swift and graceful.
7. A Striving for Justice — You keep your promises and are always faithful. You neither lie nor deceive, and you value deeds above words. You live an unselfish life in pursuit of beauty, truth and justice. Living this way you are happy.

Macrobiotics gives us high goals to aspire to!

Notes for Chapter 11

[1]O. Carl Simonton, M.D., D.A.B.R., "The Role of the Mind in Cancer Therapy," FATE, 28, no. 12 (December, 1975), 37-48. (An address delivered at the Fall, 1972, Symposium ("The Dimensions of Healing") of the Academy of Parapsychology and Medicine, presented at Stanford, Berkeley, and Los Angeles, California.)

[2]Michel Abehsera, *Cooking for Life* (Binghamton, N.Y.: Swan House Publishing Company, 1970; New York, N.Y.: Avon Books, 1976), p. 82 in the Fourth Printing.

CHAPTER 12

Prelude to Reprieve

(MAK)

Now we are confronted with the actual preparation of macro-biotic food and building of menus. You have a loved one who is ill — and *you* are elected to reverse the course of the illness.

I hope all good cooks and all people who know macrobiotics will skip most of this chapter, because I need to talk to the people like me — the people who have never really cooked before, who don't like cooking, who are dreading the prospect of having to learn, but who are determined to do it anyway to restore health to the loved one. It may not look like it right now, but besides healing the other person you'll come out of this much stronger yourself. Fortify-ing the line of thought from the previous chapter that great effort aids health, we have Mr. Kushi's statement from a recording called *Spirals of Everlasting Change* (out of print) that "difficulty is the mother of our development." And George Ohsawa, having quoted Hans Selye (author of the famous *Stress of Life*) to the effect that one never becomes diseased if the interbrain (thalamus and hypo-thalamus) is in good health, declares in his own *Cancer and the Philosophy of the Far East* (page 104) that extreme difficulties, especially from childhood, strengthen the interbrain and the sym-pathetic nervous system. So aren't you the lucky one, to be facing difficulties?!

A woman who has not developed cooking skills is not much better off than a man who may have to take on the task of caring for a sick family member. Also, a woman cook nowadays is likely to have to continue with a job just as a man would. In this fix, I think I would advertise for help from a young person who likes to do natural-foods cookery. It seems to me that a majority of young people now have their heads on right and are way ahead of the rest of us who got a late start on sensible value judgments. Such a per-son would have only a minor transition to make to do macrobiotic cooking — usually simply learning which foods, spices, etc. to *omit*.

Macrobiotic people feel that men should learn to cook just as women should — and from an early age. Mr. Kushi says so, right there in the report of one of his Boston lectures in the fall of 1975: "I would like to urge boys to please learn cooking. ... Unless you know how to cook, you cannot make anyone better and you are still children of macrobiotics, not masters. If you learn to do this, you will establish your mastership of your biological destiny." In our little restaurant the men — all of whom are strongly masculine (so strong, in fact, that they can afford to be both gentle and genteel) — soon attain a level on a par with the ladies in cooking skills. And the manager of the incomparable Seventh Inn in Boston (the East West Foundation restaurant) is Hiroshi Hayashi, a high-art chef who also frequently teaches macrobiotic cooking. So there's nothing effeminate about learning it. This is such hearty food anyway that it is quite compatible with masculinity.

Women's libbers may have a bad time with some of the philosophy. Some of the written material describes the reverence accorded to women, as creators of life when their children are born and as the daily *re*-creators of life through their cooking. They are described as superior in most ways to men and are held in the highest possible regard — as long as they stay in the kitchen. It's like the cartoon in which a beautiful young woman says, "First he puts you up on a pedestal, and then he expects you to dust it." However, we find that in current macrobiotic centers there is, instead, a complete and natural sense of equality and partnership. So try to keep your hackles down, ladies, if you read the overly chivalrous put-down about how heavenly you are. In up-to-date macrobiotics the men can be heavenly, too! They can't bear the babies but they can help keep that all-important RE-creation going through cooking.

If you're a libber and a career woman and suddenly have an invalid on your hands — well, I hope you have the stamina to handle two careers at once, for your healing project is a new career. You're probably the efficient type who can soon get on top of the cooking duties.

This statement would apply also to mothers whose career is raising several small children. This marvelous food refrigerates well, so that cooking can be done for several days and re-warmed for meals, with much mixing and matching for variety, so that after the original cooking it's almost as instant as the ghastly instant junk-food that was a major contributing factor to the illness and your present dilemma.

As I mentioned, dear Cook, if your circumstance really does

not allow time for all the cooking, advertise for that young person to help. Such a one could cook your supply of rice, beans, and ban-cha tea, for instance, and bake your unleavened bread. This plan will be infinitely less costly than medical and hospital bills, and of course we believe that it has a better chance of effecting a recovery.

If you're as smart as I think you are, you'll change to this food program yourself, mostly to prevent future illness, partly to identify with your invalid and as a result strive harder to make her-his food palatable and varied, and partly to simplify menus. (This will bring about changes in your own body, eventually for the better; so read up on "discharging," elsewhere in this book and in referred sources.)

If you have children, there may be problems with bringing them around to this type of food; but if you can gradually work it out with them it would start counteracting some of the poisons they've been soaking up from present-day commercial foods. If you have to do both macrobiotic and "worldly" cooking for an extended period of time, I don't even want to think about it!

If you have teenagers I hope they will cooperate in the care of the sick person by helping with the cooking, and by studying the philosophy (see sources in the Bibliography) and reporting to you and the invalid. This will save you time and perhaps would help "convert" the youthful members of the family. They can assist also with such essentials as massage (see Bibliography) and ginger com-presses (Chapter 13). The family, even rather small children, *and the invalid, too,* can participate in such tasks as sorting rice and beans, and stirring foods while they simmer, for these are tedious but neces-sary jobs. Speaking of tedium, there are the obvious chores of dish-washing and housekeeping that teenagers and pre-teens can help with, for curing a serious illness, like other lofty goals, is a challenge which requires many commonplace building blocks. In homes as well as small restaurants like ours, the whole operation would soon grind to a halt without the dishwashers and cleaners.

The brochure describing courses for work-study programs at the Seventh Inn Restaurant states that "dishwashing is fundamental in learning the importance of order and cleanliness, without which the Art of Cooking cannot be mastered." I'm also thinking of those ads titled "First Movement," showing a picture of a burly custodian moving a concert grand piano onto a large stage. Without his work, there couldn't be much of a concert. So the whole family can keep in mind that even the "chores" are more significant than they are in ordinary circumstances. For your merry little band, the various parts add up to Saving a Life. If all of you love your invalid, helping her-him with both easy and difficult work is your present Ideal.

If you're tackling the job alone, there are going to be lots of hours alone, with quite a bit of time waiting for food to come to a boil or to thicken. Failing to oversee it attentively can mean a boil-over or scorched pans to clean up, annoyances to be avoided be-cause they take still *more* time. So here are some things to do. First, read — and for me the most valuable books to read and underline at this stage (with one eye and ear on the bubbling kettles) are the DeLangré Dō-In (doe-een) books. (Order them as soon as possible — Appendix.) Make lists of the exercises you can do while baby-sitting with the cooking. There are many! And you'll benefit greatly. One I especially like to do is to grasp each finger separately with the other hand, pulling till I can feel it in the wrist. Then I go back and pull hard on the very tip of each finger. I fancy this will help prevent arthritis. If you already have painful, arthritic hands, might *gentle* pulling gradually improve the condition? I don't know. But after you eat macrobiotically for a while the pain should gradually disappear.

Also, stretch your legs one at a time, stretching hard and point-ing the toe hard as in ballet class. Then alternate the weight back and forth from one leg to the other as if you were walking. These things counteract the fatigue of standing, making the standing it-self therapeutic.

Do breathing exercises: high "shoulder" breathing (Oops! Jerk the lid off the spaghetti!), middle-chest breathing with shoulders down, and belly breathing. To borrow from the wisdom of our Sum-mit Lighthouse friend mentioned in Chapter 1, the healing, re-juvenating *prana* (life force, vital energy) one can take in from yoga-type breathing is available instantly and constantly to all of us. We need only to practice accepting it. DeLangré, yoga books, and Sum-mit Lighthouse pamphlets (Bibliography) have exercises you can adapt into a collection of "breathing exercises to watch the cook-ing by."

You can do some of your eating while you cook, so that you can chew until each bite is creamy. Don't just "piece," but eat a real serving of something. (OK, macrobiotic friends, I *told* you not to be reading these pages! One is supposed to be more spiritual and more creative by not eating while cooking. But at meals, because of serving others, you may not have time to sit down long enough to chew thoroughly, and it's pretty hard to be creative or spiritual if you're not taking time to get all the elements in your diet, or if you're eating too fast.)

Another way to turn your time in the kitchen to good advantage is to meditate à la Simonton. Read up on his methods in our Chapter 1. If you have a chronic physical irritation, you can learn to imagine that white corpuscles are dispersing it as surely as soapsuds are cleaning your dishes. Work on psychological hangups the same way, with imagined Universal vibrations (which you can learn to make *real*!) bringing calm, and in the same rhythm carrying away the hangups.

Some months after our first trip to Boston I commented by phone to a husband-manager of one of the student houses out there that one of the disadvantages of the macrobiotic program for those of us out here in the hinterlands was the time required for cooking. He countered with, "Oh, it doesn't take that long. My wife prepares a dinner for twenty or more people in a couple of hours every day." I walked around under the rug for a while after that, till I began to remember how things were the few days we were in Boston the first time, when I watched the cooking to learn how to do it. Not to discount in the least the skillful task these ladies perform each day, I remembered that during that couple of hours, all children were kept out of her way, and other people answered the phone and did not interrupt her unless a question was absolutely essential. Food was usually prepared in the simplest, most monastic form, which is fine as long as you're in that kind of a milieu. But when you get back here in the world, you're going to have to invent lots of variety and not have plain rice, plain miso soup, and plain beans day after day. So far as I know, in Boston others besides the Cook did the marketing, a student cook prepared breakfast (the only other meal), and I know others washed the dishes. Everyone went to Mr. Kushi's lectures, and our Cook took care of her own family throughout the rest of the day; but I don't think there were any civic committees or other such complications. So then I felt better. It's tougher out here away from "Mecca," but you can learn to handle it. Our case histories have some hints as to how some of your predecessors worked things out.

Before turning to the actual recipes, I'll mention some random bits of information I've culled from here and there, in most instances without remembering the source. If, through your reading, you come across some inaccuracies in these statements please just lay it to the fact that I haven't been macrobiotic long enough to have a perfect memory!

Pronouncing Oriental words. There's a kind of easy-going system of transcribing oriental words into our alphabet, in which the letter *a* is pronounced *ah, e* is like the long *a* in *same, i* is like *ee* (miso=mee-soh), *o* is *oh, u* is *oo, ai* is *ah-ee* (daikon=dah-ee-kahn), *ei* is *ay-ee* (seitan=say-ee-tahn). The letter *g* is hard, as in *go* (even before an *e,* as in aburage: ah-boor-ah-gay; and before an *i* as in mugi: moo-gee, with the *g* hard as in *go* — not moo-*jee*. Ginseng root, frequently mentioned for its medicinal properties, is pronounced with a soft *g* (*j*in-seng), but it is Chinese rather than Japanese.) The combination *ch* is pronounced as in *church; s* like the *s* in *so.* As for accents, all syllables are nearly evenly stressed.

Other miscellaneous items: aduki, azuki, and adzuki are one and the same little bean. "Shoyu" is another name for "tamari." "Nituke" is the same as "nitsuki." A macrobiotic oddity, at least for me, is that the term "noodles" usually designates whole-wheat or soba (buckwheat) spaghetti.

Soybeans are too oily and too yin for frequent use. (If they are eaten, they must be soaked 24 hours and slow-cooked two days.) Therefore, the Japanese use them mostly to produce *miso* and *tamari. Miso* — 3 kinds, all made with sea salt: hacho (red miso), our favorite of the misos, being somewhat stronger in flavor than the others, is made with soybeans and sea salt, aged together 3 years; mugi is made with soybeans, barley, and salt, aged 18 months; and kome combines soybeans, rice, and salt, aged 6 months. Miso is a valuable source of high-quality protein, amino acids, vitamin B-12, enzymes, and lactic acid bacteria which aid in digestion. Likewise, it increases the availability of protein in other foods. *Tamari* is the liquid by-product of miso.

Umeboshi plums — small plums preserved 3 years in sea salt. Used to help keep other foods fresh longer. The juice from boiled plums is used in salad dressings. For a medicinal use, see Chapter 13.

Surprisingly enough, according to Iona Teeguarden in *Freedom Through Cooking,* we need less salt in summer than in winter. (I'm sure her sources are reliable, and macrobiotically it makes sense, since both salt and the summer season are yang. But it is contrary to common present-day beliefs.) Children need less salt and more liquid than adults. You know by now that the color of the urine, which should be that of light beer, indicates our proper quota of salt (if darker, too much salt; if lighter, not enough). Also, healthy males should urinate only four times in 24 hours, females only three.

Water — In most places tap water isn't yet *really* unusable for cooking and drinking, especially since we should drink very little of it anyway. But if you prefer buying bottled water, do make it spring water rather than distilled, which has some valuable minerals removed. Michio says that it lacks life-giving forces: seeds, for instance, will not sprout and grow so well in distilled water as in tap water.

Oil — Try not to use over two tablespoons per person per day, and use sesame or corn oils only, for others are too yin.

Tahini — "Peanut butter" made out of sesame seeds, so that it's much less harmful. Still, use sparingly, especially if you have a problem with mucus. And, it would comprise part of your day's quota of oil, already!

Carob — "Fruit" (actually a long bean pod) of the carob tree. Roasted (in dessert recipes) it tastes like chocolate, but without the latter's harmful properties. Unroasted it tastes like apple butter. Very good, but yin — use sparingly.

Sweets — Read Chapters 8 and 9 and throw away every grain of sugar in your pantry. (Sorry to inform you also that according to William Dufty, on page 259 of *Sugar Blues,* brown *and* raw sugar are merely refined sugar with molasses added!) Iona Teeguarden on page 8 of *Freedom* echoes a summary of Mr. Kushi's warnings against sugar: "Its extreme acid-forming nature causes temporary paralysis of the stomach, stopping digestion. Unable to neutralize it, the duodenum lets sugar pass through. To digest sugar the intestines must then use much of the body's mineral reserve, and this leads to tooth decay and weak bone structure."

Honey is not much better (too bad!), but maybe you can use it to ease your family away from sugar. As soon as possible shift to *pure* maple syrup (purchased at a natural-foods store), although it's only slightly less objectionable than honey. The price will also encourage the frugal use of this commodity! We asked Mr. Kushi how soon most people could use rice honey and barley malt after beginning the macrobiotic food program. He gave a *very* reluctant "maybe" to our "What about six weeks?" As for how much, just one teaspoon a day of one *or* the other! The flavors are so mild that a teaspoon is hardly noticeable. Barley malt syrup helps a little in baking. The least objectionable sweetener is blackstrap molasses, the flavor of which, in our opinion, would deter anyone from using large amounts in baking! You can cook dried fruits (but not *tropical* ones unless you live in such a climate) and purée them in the blender to make desserts, although Mr. Kushi isn't too happy about that plan, either. Baking the purée into unleavened breads (Chapter 13) is a little more acceptable.

We probably should insert another reminder of the harmful effects of ice cream (boo-hoo!). It has *everything* wrong with it — sweeteners, dairy products, liver-paralyzing iciness, all held together with chemical poisons. In Chapter 13 we have some recipes for summer desserts which will be somewhat of a balm to soothe this difficult abstention.

Meat — Increase servings of grains, while decreasing the size of servings of fish and chicken (white meat, being less oily, is preferable). Rather than the gross hunks of meat we are used to, try using small pieces of fish and chicken in casserole dishes whenever the family will let you get by with it. Eventually, the men in the family can have fish two or three times a week, those doing physical labor needing it more often. Chicken or turkey should be served only once every three or four weeks. Women need very little meat, for remember that their bodies manufacture more protein than men's bodies do. Children and very elderly people, especially, need no meat.

Cheese is the only dairy product we can use, and the only cheese we use in our area is made by Eilers Cheese Market in DePere, Wisconsin, whose cattle are fed organically. We order forty pounds of cheese at a time for our restaurant; but perhaps you could interest some neighbors in going together to order the minimum shipment, first phoning Eilers to find out what the minimum would be (address and phone number in the Appendix). But use as little as possible to flavor your casseroles. We read in a Kushi lecture that people who eat *large* amounts of cheese stutter, or at least do not speak smoothly. It does form mucus, of course.

Grains contain minerals and protein, the richest being oats, whole-wheat, and buckwheat. Oats are highest in mineral salt, with barley second. Buckwheat is the richest of all grains in magnesium, calcium, and amino acids; its protein more than equals the best animal protein. It also has enormous quantities of vitamins B_2 and E. Somewhere I read that it is good for the lungs. Usually it is used in the form of flour, or as kasha (also called buckwheat groats), which resembles the "Grape Nuts" commercial cereal. We'll have recipes in the next chapter. Of course brown rice is the most perfectly balanced of all grains. This we must have at every meal!

Coffee — I, Mary Alice Kohler, was an addict! I didn't drink more than two or three cups a day, but it was certainly a prime enjoyment, and it seems downright unfair that something so dark and so concentrated as strong black coffee could be tropical and yin! But it is, and according to all our experts it's harmful to us. (Read how Jacques de Langré rails against it on page 67 of his second book of Dō-In.) Anyway, after I was macrobiotic for a while, I was relaxed enough that coffee didn't keep me awake at all. In fact, being yin, it made me very sleepy. But I found a stealthy way to beat the desire for the kick that the coffee flavor gives: use it for a mouth wash! Rinsing my teeth with it after meals makes my mouth feel as if I've drunk a cup of coffee, but I haven't damaged my insides. I'm sure that even at today's prices it wouldn't be so expensive as the bottled anti-freeze sold for mouth washes and gargles. While we're in the lethal department, don't use instant coffee even for a mouth wash. I tried it and just having it in my mouth made me feel sick. It's solid poison. This is gossip, but a friend of ours knew someone who worked in a factory making instant coffee who said that no one there would touch the stuff because of all the toxic chemicals they saw being added to it. It's not gossip but a fact that it made me feel nauseous.

Vinegar is used only for washing windows.

Some macrobiotic cookbooks recommend ways to work gradually into this food program, unless serious illness demands a quick change-over. But they do urge *immediate* rejection of red meat, sugar, tropical fruits and juices, coffee, and commercial tea, as well as getting away from chemicalized foods, meaning everything canned and packaged, just as soon as you can manage it.

Lunch boxes — Macrobiotic lunch boxes, for Occidentals, are admittedly a bit of a problem. We'll have a few suggestions in the next chapter. Inventing variety in lunch-box foods for your wage earner will take some ingenuity. As for school-age children, I hope you can train them to make this food a matter of pride for themselves, and of interest and curiosity for other children. "My mom can show your mom how to fix this stuff and then *you* won't have to eat food with chemicals in it." Hopefully, your teenagers will pack their own lunches using macrobiotic foods. Of course, some of the time, "out with the gang" will leave no choice but junk foods, and there's no use in their worrying about it. They will just have to figure that they're getting a lot less junk than their peers (unless they can convert them!). I hope, though, that they can always order toasted cheese (unavoidably colored and preserved, of course), or even hamburgers (phew!), in preference to hot dogs, which are not merely no-no's, but never-nevers. To counteract toxic effects, train your family to eat some brown rice when they get home if they have had to eat restaurant food.

Preserving vegetables — People ask whether they can use vegetables they canned or froze themselves, after having grown them in their own gardens. The answer is that the East West Foundation hierarchy looks down somewhat on both of these methods of preserving. Of course you should use what you already have on hand. But wouldn't you know they believe that drying is superior to canning or freezing! They think that a "root cellar" is a good idea, for many of the "approved" vegetables do keep a long time in that kind of a location. That's not a very practical idea if you live on the thirty-first floor of a high-rise apartment, especially if you had a crop failure in your window-box and if the janitor is crotchety about letting you dig a cellar under the elevator shaft. But if you do live in an area where it would be possible to convert some neighbors and build a cellar, the EWF would consider it an ideal setup. Meanwhile, what else can you do but use your own products? But macrobiotic or not, don't use any preservatives in canning or freezing. Most of you will probably have to buy vegetables the year around at the supermarket or produce stand, hoping they're not plastic-sprayed to stay beautiful-looking. Even this is probably preferable to canning or freezing, as they are really supposed to be given their first cooking in your soups and casseroles. If you can ever find a market that leaves the tops on vegetables, *that's* the place to buy. Those tops are loaded with nutrition.

Obesity — If you have an overweighter, eating this food right along with the rest of the family may help this difficult problem automatically, although the chubby one may feel more threatened than the others by any tampering with the beloved food umbrella. Perhaps if you form the habit of using the term "food program" it might be less irritating than "diet." If the overweight member really does yearn for slenderness, and has been discouraged previously by diets that didn't work, he-she might try a couple of weeks of a crash program Mr. Kushi has been known to suggest: breakfast — one rice ball wrapped in nori, a few sips of bancha tea; lunch — two rice balls wrapped in nori, bancha tea; supper — one cup of miso soup, rice (probably one cup), vegetables (one-half cup), aduki or garbanzo beans (three or four tablespoons), bancha tea. Try this bravely for a couple of weeks, then eat like the rest of the family for a while, then another couple of weeks of the crash program. Muramoto suggests that a good food for weight losers is kanten, a seaweed which makes gelatin (recipes in the next chapter). It has no fat or protein, but has a large mineral content. Losing weight probably takes more courage than recovering from any other illness, but it will be facilitated by the following activity: chew-chew-chew!

As a matter of fact, train all the members of your family to swallow only rice *cream,* vegetable *cream,* bean cream, bread cream, and all other kinds of cream they manufacture themselves by chewing each bite until it is liquid. Then *sip* drinks, don't gulp them. When any one of you is eating alone, if your time is as limited as ours, or if it gives you the fidgets to sit there and grind away for so long, do some of your reading while you eat, pausing once in a while for a grateful thought. Strict macrobiotic disciples would say that the eat-read combination is poor advice, but maybe they are not as busy as you are. (Or they might approve if you're reading East West Foundation literature!) *We* say that if it takes reading — plus the occasional pause to acknowledge how lucky you are to have such supreme food, and to hope that you can turn it into a life of value through service — then go ahead and read. It's a lot better than swallowing bits of food instead of cream.

You may become so enamored of this way of life that you may even be able to talk a few of your friends into trying it. And you may begin to think that *everybody* is going macrobiotic. So I feel that somewhere in this book we should mention a "state of the economy" impact. It may occur to you to wonder, "What am *I* doing plugging this kind of food? Our family income depends on soft drinks!" Or on the dairy industry! processed foods! cattle-raising! pharmaceutical products! sugar! liquor! And on and on. Well, relax. Even though there's constantly more interest in the effects of diet on health, the [slowly] increasing number of people who take it seriously is going to remain a very small minority for a long time. It's going to be years, if ever, before the natural-foods way makes a dent in the economy. Years from now people will still be wanting to take vitamins and supplements to counteract the bad eating they don't want to give up. Years from now people will still be picking up their sacks of oranges and bananas from the grocery check-out and wading out into boot-top snow!

And yet — how wonderful it would be if enough interest *should* develop that more grains would be grown, that some processors would begin adding a line of non-poisoned food, that fewer people would be sick!

Meanwhile, all of us who have decided to let good food come to our rescue can turn our attention to the actual handling of it.

CHAPTER 13

From Invalid to Gourmet

(MK, with the help of Jean, Mari
and the Harvest Moon Cooks)

In order that you can have everything about using our kind of food in one place, we'll repeat the list of foods that are off limits, as well as the basic foods allowed in the macrobiotic program. It must be kept in mind that location (even altitude!), climate, and season have a direct bearing on the selection and preparation of our foods. As we have mentioned before, especially in the first few pages of Chapter 9, we should eat only those foods which do grow, or *could* grow, in our own latitude. However, this principle must be modified by the fact that there are "pocket areas" on this globe where the climate is drastically different from that of the surrounding territory, as with the Bodensee area between Germany and Switzerland. People who live outside that vicinity, even at a distance of only a few miles, should not indulge in the tropical foods which grow there. Fruits, especially, should be used sparingly everywhere, for reasons clarified in the brief discussion of types of sugar at the beginning of Chapter 8. Ideally we eat, in small amounts, only those fruits which grow locally, and in season or dried. Juices of fruits or vegetables should be taken only very occasionally, in small amounts. Macrobiotic cookbooks, and pages 58-66 of Michio's *Book of Macrobiotics* (see Bibliography), provide guidance on this topic, until your own intuition can take over. (For an interesting touch, see the Postscript at the end of the Landes story in Chapter 14.)

People always counter with, "What about brown rice? *That* doesn't grow here." Usually it's only because it hasn't become our *custom* to grow it. Some varieties, with proper water conditions provided, will grow almost anywhere on the North American continent. (The East West Foundation is experimenting with rice cultivation.) The outstanding *preservation* quality of brown rice should also be considered, for this gives it almost a world-wide habitat. Rice that has been planted after being discovered in Egyptian tombs, closed up for centuries, will still germinate! Dried seaweeds have this same quality of endurance. Thus rice and seaweed could be transported anywhere without the spoilage that afflicts other alien foods — and seaweed, as a matter of fact, once grew right where you are sitting, wherever you are!

Here follows a list of harmful and beneficial foods, eating habits, and general use of foods.

Harmful: all meat, all dairy products, all sweets (meaning honey and natural syrups as well as sugar), all chemicalized foods, all refined foods, all canned foods, spices, yeast, herbs, mushrooms, nuts (temporarily, for recovery from many illnesses), all fruits (including bananas and avocados), all fruit juices and vegetable juices, soft drinks, coffee, tea, and these vegetables: potato, tomato, eggplant, asparagus, spinach, beets, and sweet potato.

Beneficial: grains, making up 50 percent of the food eaten (may be more than 50 percent but never less). The principal grain, of course, is brown rice, but also good are millet, barley, corn, wheat, buckwheat, rye, oatmeal, kasha (also called buckwheat groats), bulghur, wheat flours and other grain flours (unrefined), whole-wheat and buckwheat spaghetti or noodles. (Note: of the *grain* percentage, the amount of ground or cracked grains and cereals should be about 15 percent of the total daily *grain* intake, as compared to 85 percent *whole* grains.) Cooked vegetables, all except those listed in the preceding paragraph, comprise about 25 percent of the *total food:* and, unless your macrobiotic friend suggests otherwise, an additional 5 percent-10 percent of your food may be raw vegetables. Frequently, half the amount of cooked vegetables may be pumpkin or winter squash (see next paragraph). Beans, principally azuki, garbanzo, or lentils, should make up 10 percent of the total, while the 5 percent miso and 5 percent seaweed (see below) will usually be used in soup. At the end of meals, the beverage will be bancha tea, which may be taken during the day if thirsty; but in general drink only as much as you need to satisfy thirst. Take no other beverage, although if you are unusually thirsty, you may sip a little cool or room-temperature water. *No ice,* if you respect your digestive system, especially your liver.

Cooked or raw, or as a "boiled salad" or pressed salad (see recipes, below), the vegetables we can use most frequently are winter squash (acorn, Hubbard, or butternut), pumpkin in season, carrots, parsnips, daikon, turnips, radishes, burdock, cabbage, Chinese cabbage (bok-choy), Japanese cabbage, onions, scallions, broccoli, lotus root, Brussels sprouts. Leafy vegetables for regular

use are kale, parsley, watercress, dandelions, greens of root vegetables such as turnip, carrot, and daikon, Swiss chard, head lettuce
or leaf lettuce. If you are in good health you may occasionally use
string beans, peas, celery, snow peas, and taro potato in small
amounts. For information about the more unusual vegetables on
this list, as well as some hints on handling vegetables, see later in
this chapter.

A good friend who previewed our manuscript came up with
some specifics we hadn't thought of. "What's the status of peanuts,
tuna and salmon, bibb lettuce?" she queried, and sent us scurrying
to the phone to confer with Ken Burns, the East West Foundation
authority on plants and agriculture. Bibb lettuce? It's o.k. Rhubarb?
Unapproved — contains much potassium. Being very yin, it has in-
filtrated the American diet to counteract the flavors of heavy meat
eating. In April and May in temperate areas a Japanese knot weed
may be used. It's about one-fourth as strong as rhubarb. What about
chicory? It's related to the dandelion and may be used occasionally.
Extremely yang, it strengthens the heart and weak, thin blood.
Peanuts and peanut butter? Small amounts occasionally — hard to
digest. Shellfish? Oil is very hard to digest. Tuna? Salmon? Both
yang — o.k. for a very short while for recovery from a yin illness.
(We'll remind you that if canned, these fish no doubt contain preservatives or other contaminants.) Watermelon and cantaloupe? A
few bites in season are OK and refreshing. Also, while varieties of
winter squash are highly desirable, summer squash such as zucchini
and cucumber are, although not prohibited, undesirable. What about
wheat germ and bran? They are generally avoided because of not
being *whole* foods.

We may eat two or three meals a day, eating as much as desired but not overeating. Do not eat snacks between meals, and
never eat for three hours before the night's rest, for the inactivity
tends to cause fatty deposits to collect around vital internal organs.
Do not take a nap for one hour after meals; if unbearably sleepy,
nap sitting up.

A couple of years after Jean's recovery, we put together some
primitive suggestions about the rudiments of using macrobiotic
food. We have found these helpful for people who come to ask us
how to get started. Again we hope that macrobiotic experts will look
the other way while we repeat some of this material to help new-
comers out of their bewilderment.

The pantry may be stocked with these flours: whole-wheat,
whole-wheat pastry, corn meal, small amounts of buckwheat, rye,

and brown rice flour, small amount of oatmeal powder, small amount of arrowroot flour, small amount of kuzu (a starch-like thickening agent helpful to digestion — see end of chapter). Flour loses its freshness quickly, so until you know your way around, buy it in relatively small quantities. Grains and cereals are brown rice (lots of it), lesser amounts of sweet brown rice, barley, millet, less of soft white wheat, kasha, bulghur, oatmeal, wheat flakes, whole-wheat and buckwheat macaroni and spaghetti ("noodles"!), packages of wheat gluten. Beans include azukis, garbanzos, and lentils, with occasional servings of pintos and kidney beans, and even less frequent use of limas and black beans. Also on hand are miso, tamari, various seaweeds, including kanten (agar agar), sesame seeds, sunflower seeds, sesame oil, corn oil, small quantity of safflower oil, tahini, raw carob powder and roasted carob powder, almonds if you can have them, corn-barley malt syrup and pure maple syrup if allowed, and bancha tea (kukicha). Get the twig tea, by the way, not green bancha tea, although if only the latter is available, you can roast it and it will be preferable to any *other* kind of tea. You're likely to want to get into doing your own "sprouting," for which you'll need alfalfa seeds, mung beans, wheat berries (hard red winter wheat), and a few soybeans, plus Mari's instructions later in this chapter. All the above products are available at "authentic" natural-foods stores.

If you live in or near a large city, try to locate an Oriental food store. During much of the year you may be able to buy daikon and gobo (burdock root); in season there should be Japanese cabbage and snow peas. (It's easy to grow your own snow peas, Japanese cabbage, and daikon, remember — see Appendix for seed source.) In addition to miso, seaweed, umeboshi plums, lotus root (NOT canned!), and such (usually available now also in many natural-foods stores), you can often find tofu (some natural-foods stores are equipped to handle this perishable bean curd), konnyaku (a funny, tough, gelatinous stuff which Mari says acts like a "vacuum cleaner" for the stomach), gourd strings, dashi iriko and chirimen iriko (little fishes), bonita flakes or shavings, soybean sprouts, and somen (thread-like whole-wheat or buckwheat spaghetti for occasional use — highly recommended by Jean Kohler for "dressing up" soups). These packaged items are usually safe to buy, whereas you need to be wary of other things. Aburage (fried bean curd) and transparent noodles are nice, but are likely to have had "hidden" chemicals used in some part of their construction, so that even if you could read the labels you couldn't be sure of "purity." Chinese package foods, according to Mari, always contain monosodium glutamate or preservatives, whereas Japanese products almost never do. The latter usually have little stickers listing ingredients in English, although even here you may have unlisted preservatives, as in the oils, for instance.

Seventh Day Adventist stores frequently have bulk grains, flour, and beans, and may order other things you need. Trustworthy products are Erewhon (Kushi's brand), Eden, Arrowhead Mills, Lundberg, and Deaf Smith, that we know about in our area.

If you can't find any source at all, you might try getting a group of people to use at least some of these foods, form a co-op, and order wholesale from Eden Foods, Ann Arbor, Michigan (see Appendix), or ask them about another wholesaler nearer to your location. They might arrange shipping with some trucking firm. None of this is easy, we know.

We took information on tofu, daikon, burdock root, and taro potato to the produce manager of a locally owned supermarket chain, and dangled before him the prospect of fairly good (and hopefully increasing) sales to friends interested in natural foods. He was able to locate these items, and the experiment is working well so far, whenever these root vegetables are in season in California. (The manager prefers to use the Japanese word "gobo," incidentally, for who would buy burdock root after having spent part of a recent holiday hacking a burdock bush out of his alley?)

As for kitchen equipment, the macrobiotic cookbooks have lists from which you can choose what you want. You don't really need everything they list. We don't have a suribachi, for instance, because we prefer "finger-crumbled" seaweed as a condiment; and since we get plenty of salt in other ways, we'd rather use toasted sesame seeds to sprinkle on foods instead of making gomasio. We haven't needed a suribachi for anything else, but most good cooks have them. You can't get along without one or two good vegetable-cutting knives, available at natural-foods and Oriental stores. They are better if they're fairly heavy. You'll need a wok; stainless steel is fine. And with that you'll need an oil skimmer. A fine-grater is essential, especially for daikon and for ginger root and taro potato for compresses (see end of this chapter). We wish everyone had one of the dandy little graters available from the *East West Journal:* they are very fine, easy to clean, and have their own little tray to catch the "gratings" (see Appendix).

If your family is one hundred percent macrobiotic, the food budget is going to be considerably less than for your present program. Estimates have ranged from one-third of the previous budget to three-fourths as much, the latter probably being more realistic. If you want to be austere to the point of saintliness, and if you can work out a co-op system with some friends, then you could pare the food costs to an incredible minimum. But if you add the gourmet touches which make life fascinating, but still gastronomically safe, you can, of course, turn the food budget into somewhat of a luxury.

We hope you understand that we are not trying here to write another cookbook. Those listed in our Bibliography have much more information then we can possibly include, and there would be no point in duplicating what they do far better. Our purpose is to outline what to eat if you've been told you have a serious or potentially serious illness. This the cookbooks do *not* do, for they are written from a considerably freer overview which assumes good health.

Before we begin, let us point out one little item that most of you know, but may need to be reminded about: as you work with this food be careful not to lick your fingers or sample your creations with the cooking spoon! Instead, keep a separate tasting spoon handy and drop food into it from the cooking spoon. Also, if you need to sniff food to check flavor or freshness, inhale and then move the pan or bowl out from under your nose or turn your head to exhale, rather than snorting back into the food. No insult intended, but your saliva or your breath (life-saving though they are for your own needs) will initiate food spoilage! You're now working with food that has not been impregnated with preservatives, and it does, therefore, require more solicitous treatment to prevent spoilage.

Now we can introduce you to sea vegetables (seaweeds), which are essential for minerals, trace elements, youth, and from which we usually make —

Soup stock: Break off a 2-in. square of kombu for each two people. Rinse quickly under running cool water and put it in about 1 C of cool water in the pan you will use for soup. Soak 5 minutes, bring to a boil, reduce heat and simmer about 20-30 minutes. People don't usually eat the kombu if it's *dashi* (stock) kombu, for it's tough and rubbery. (More tender varieties, if well-cooked, are eaten in stews and other recipes.) Leave dashi kombu in the liquid and add whatever other ingredients you want for the soup — no off-limits vegetables, of course. You can make any kind of soup you like, using the kombu water as part of the liquid, and miso (see below) as the flavoring. Usually Miso Soup is best if it is kept uncomplicated — say, with burdock (see below), onions, and carrots, plus perhaps turnips *or* parsnips *or* kale *or* cabbage. Or else make it mostly onion soup, if your family likes that. Or bean soup. Or simmer some lentils for 15-20 minutes before adding vegetables. You can add cooked grains to any soup, simmering them with the soup toward the end of the cooking time. (Miso and kasha, however, don't like each other, flavor-wise!) We like to put in some uncooked oatmeal at the beginning of the cooking time, to make what we call "cream of Miso Soup." Also, whole-wheat or buckwheat spaghetti or macaroni are very good to use in soups, with fine-chopped green onions as an almost necessary companion. If you're going to have a soup that requires long simmering, it's best to have pasta-type things cooked separately and drop them into the soup just before serving, at which time it's also a delight to add chopped uncooked watercress.

More seaweeds: Let's get used to another valuable seaweed — wakame. To make stock out of this, you would break off about 8 strands 2 or 3 inches long and dip them up and down a few times in a bowl of cool water for a quick rinse. Put them in your soup kettle and soak till very soft in 2 quarts of cool water. Bring this same water almost to a boil. (Watch it — it boils over easily!) Lift out the wakame with a fork or chopsticks and save it. (You can refrigerate some of the stock, including some of the wakame, if you don't want to make that much soup right now.) Make the soup, chop the wakame into smaller pieces, and put it back into the kettle when the soup is done. For a few weeks, when seaweed was new to us, we soaked and then cooked a large amount of wakame for about 5 minutes and made a kind of paste of it in the blender. Then each time we made soup we stirred in about 2 T of the paste per cup of soup. If your family objects to pieces of chopped seaweed, you can try the paste method at first, being careful not to make it so strong they they say, "This tastes fishy!" (You can gradually increase the amount till someone does say that, and then you'll know how much *not* to use!) Before long they will probably be enjoying the flavor of the seaweed liquid or paste, and then you can try the chopped pieces. That seaweed flavor grows on you — we can eat it now till our eyes slant, relishing large pieces in soup or casseroles, or eating softened, uncooked wakame with other salad vegetables. (P.S. Eating seaweed will take a lot of the "gray" out of your hair, if you're using other good foods along with it.)

Another way to serve some seaweeds, which surely must be delectable for everyone, is to toast them just a *few* minutes in the oven (don't scorch!) and then crumble them over rice or other food. They impart a salty flavor which is particularly welcome to those who must use a low-salt intake. We like wakame best for this, although kombu, with a somewhat stronger flavor, is also o.k., as is dulse if you like it. (That's pronounce "dullss," which our dictionary says is Irish. The Oriental word is a long one meaning "Buddha's ear"!) As we mentioned a few pages ago, you can crumble these toasted seaweeds with your finger tips or in a suribachi.

Thin sheets of the seaweed called nori can be toasted in a few seconds in the oven and crumbled over food, with a sprinkle of tamari if desired. (Our recipes include one telling about wrapping Rice Balls in nori.) For me, nori has a definite (and delightful) tea flavor. You'll just have to try each kind of seaweed to learn which ones you can get used to and finally enjoy. Later on we'll describe some ways to make the seaweed hiziki turn into a real treat.

More toasting: While we're toasting and roasting, let's list the other foods which need this treatment. They are tahini, seeds, nuts (go easy on these — almonds are probably the best kind for us), bancha twigs (or leaves if you can't find the twigs), solar salt or sea salt (see below), and grains that may be a bit stale. You can roast things a few minutes in a dry heavy skillet, stirring until they become aromatic or lightly browned. For an easier method, when you have the oven hot anyway, tahini can be roasted in an oven dish, 10-15 minutes at 325°-425°. Spread the dry food on sheets of aluminum foil and roast 5-10 minutes at 325°-425°. Check after 5 minutes (the tea and seaweed, especially, are likely to scorch), and stir from the outside edges inward; then flatten out the foods again and finish the toasting process. Take out the seaweed and tea first, then the others as they turn light brown and/or aromatic. Be sure all foods are *thoroughly cool* before storing.

Salt: Solar salt is taken from the Great Salt Lake in Utah, and has all the properties of sea salt, which comes from the ocean near France at three times the cost. Only a pinch is added to cooking, more to yang-ize food, I believe, than for flavoring. As a condiment, it is used (sparingly) at the table in gomasio, which your macrobiotic cookbooks will describe for you. Of course, tamari and miso are our main sources of salty flavor.

Now we can take a look at the use of some other foods which may be unfamiliar to many of you.

Burdock: This common weed, surprisingly enough, is a valuable food which we should have almost every day (although less often in hot weather) for its great benefit to our skin and its help in purifying our blood and in balancing our intake of oils and other yin foods. Ken Burns tells us that it has the ability to concentrate the strength of the body toward the solid organs such as the liver and kidneys. As a bushy plant, it has been the target of much verbal abuse because of its burs which get all over our clothes when we take a walk in the country, or anywhere else that weeds grow. The one that has the large, puffy burs, and leaves like rhubarb leaves, except dark green — that's burdock. It's a biennial, and the first year is the best for digging the long roots, if you can learn to recognize it before it bears flowers and burs. Early the second year is also an ideal time to collect the roots, but after the flowers and burs appear the roots begin to get too tough and "woody." Going deep enough to get those roots is a challenge!

We discussed above the possible places to buy burdock. So if, one way or another, you can get these roots, rinse them (but don't scrub the hide off!) and sliver them as if you were sharpening a pencil. Sauté the slivers and put them in the soup, along with other sauteed vegetables you have decided to use. *Macrobiotic recipe books have instructions for cutting and sautéeing vegetables in the proper order.*

If you can't find fresh burdock, try to find dried burdock at a natural-foods store. We use a heaping T for each 2 servings. You can simmer this separately for about 15 minutes and strain the liquid into the soup, or you can tie the dried burdock in cheesecloth and simmer it with the soup. If you have time (or, if not, here's a good project for the invalid or one of the kids), pick out the spongy pieces of burdock (which are like walnut nougats!) and add them to the soup, discarding the "woody" pieces.

Dandelions: These are not exactly unfamiliar, but the extent of their value to us as food is not adequately recognized by most of us. Again we are indebted to Ken Burns for the information that the roots and leaves of the often-scorned dandelion have, like burdock, the energy to counteract strong yin. We questioned the danger of sprays in collecting dandelions to eat. Mr. Burns' reply was that meadows are rarely sprayed; and of course you would know about your own lawn and those of your neighbors, as well as the vicinity of organic gardens. He says also that present-day sprays are very unstable, and are destroyed by cooking, or even after a while by sunlight. Thus we can have the assurance, also, that supermarket vegetables are made safe by cooking. Check our recipe section for the method of cooking dandelion greens. A few cooked greens may be added to Miso Soup to lend the same type of rich, dark flavor as burdock.

Lentils: I wasn't acquainted with lentils, but probably most other people are. They're one of the three principal macrobiotic beans, and the nice thing about them is that they cook in 35-40 minutes, after rinsing in a large strainer but without previous soaking, and have a distinctive peppery flavor to lend to soups and casseroles. They seem to be everyone's favorite! Use a cupful of lentils to 3-4 cups of water, or more if you want to store the liquid for soups and gravies. Don't waste time or money on red lentils. They're expensive, they cook to a mushy consistency, and they don't stay pink anyway.

Daikon: This is a large — sometimes enormous (as big as your arm!) — white Japanese radish. Sliced (julienne style) and cooked with other vegetables, or cooked in 1-inch cubes with rice, it has a sweet flavor. We sometimes fine-grate daikon and put it in miso soup at the same time as the miso. Also — 1 T of fine-grated daikon + 1 t of tamari = presto! Horseradish! Healthy people can use this whenever they wish such an accent, especially to offset the oil in tempura or possible toxins in fish, and it's a great aid to digestion in certain types of cancer. But you need to learn from a macrobiotic friend whether it fits your type. Everyone who can have a garden should grow daikon radishes, for lots more of them are needed than are available. A source for seeds (Johnny's Selected Seeds) is in the Appendix. Dried daikon, which you can sometimes buy, is very, very smelly, and can be used only cooked, not grated. Try it sometime, though, to flavor soup in the same way that cabbage does.

PLEASE DON'T USE ALL THESE INGREDIENTS AT ONE TIME! Keep your soups simple, humble, and delicious. Only miso and seaweed need to be there every time, and burdock as often as possible.

As described in the previous chapter, miso is your protein and flavoring. Now that the rest of the soup is ready, here's what to do with the miso: use about one flat t per C of soup. Mash it with a fork, add a little hot liquid from the soup, mixing carefully to be sure there are no little salty lumps, add it to the soup, stir it in thoroughly, and serve. DON'T BOIL SOUP AFTER THE MISO IS ADDED — boiling destroys valuable enzymes in the miso.

Cooking grains: I'm going to drive skillful cooks wild, and say that for us amateurs the safest cooking method is to use a double boiler. The skillful ones use a pressure cooker for brown rice, and that drives *me* wild. It always ends up with a lot of rice stuck to the bottom of the cooker. They talk about how nutritious the scorched rice is, but there it is — *stuck.* And you're bound to waste some of it trying to get it out. Lima Ohsawa, in *The Art of Just Cooking,* recommends pressure cooking, of course, but then, bless her, she says (page 47) that it is "not necessary that grains always be cooked under pressure" (see Bibliography).

Rice may be baked — see recipe books. But not all are careful to specify a *covered* baking dish. They also don't mention that if grains around the edge of the dish begin to dry out you can drizzle a little boiling water on the dry places and cover again so they can steam and soften, rather than serving dental hazards for dinner.

Until you gain lots of confidence (and maybe acquire also a "flame minder" or "radiant plaque" (a perforated metal disk with a handle) or even just an asbestos mat to help prevent scorching) you may want to use my beginner's aid — a double boiler. You will also have lots less trouble with depressing boil-overs, because you don't have to watch the bubbling grains for very long. You can construct an inexpensive home-made boiler by mixing and matching large pans on the shelf at a cut-rate department store until you find a couple that fit together fairly well. Don't use aluminum for the top half of the boiler. Enamel pans are fine if you treat them gently so that they don't get chipped and cracked. Modern stainless steel is OK but I can't afford it. (I can't afford Corning Ware either, but it's very good except for three things: food sticks easily, you can't pour out of any of it without having a wet piece of paper towel handy to wipe the outside of the pan, and you couldn't make up a large-size double boiler from any of the pans I've seen. Use them for cooking other foods than grains.)

Grains need to be washed before cooking. First, start some water heating in the lower part of the boiler, if that's the method you're using. Then "sort through" larger grains such as rice, barley, and the like. We put a cupful at a time on a light-colored tray, or on shelf paper, and lightly brush the kernels across the surface, picking out very dark kernels or those that a bug chewed on first, weed seeds, pebbles, etc. You are, of course, working with back-to-nature food, so you have to clean up some of the results of the harvest. Don't forget to corral the kids and your temporarily sick person to do jobs like this. Wash a couple of cups of grains at a time by swirling them around in a large bowl of cool water, and pour them into a colander-sieve or strainer (small mesh for grains). Run cold tap water through the strainer for a few seconds. Two or three times of this process should suffice. (See below for seeds and beans.)

To continue with rice, put it in the top part of the double boiler and add water (see below for amount). We usually add just a tiny pinch of sea salt or solar salt per cup of rice; but don't really "season" it, in case you want to use it later with miso or tamari in soups or casseroles. To avoid stickiness you can add about a half-teaspoonful of sesame or corn oil for each 2 C of rice. Our rice turns out well if we use 3 C water per 2 C rice. Bring this to a boil, give it one graceful swirl with a large cooking spoon, and simmer covered for 15 minutes. By now the lower part of the boiler should be boiling hard. Don't peek into the bubbling rice kettle, but simply place it over the boiling water for 15 minutes. Turn off heat, allow to stand 20 minutes. Then pour it out into a very large bowl or small *clean* dishpan and gently "fluff it up." You can put it back into the kettle for storage.

Barley, soft white wheat, and other whole grains probably cook better if sorted, washed, and soaked overnight in a cool place. These grains *expand,* so you'd better cook just one cup in 4 or 5 parts of water. After simmering as for rice, or longer, cook at least an hour over boiling water. If any water remains on the grain, pour it off, or dip it off if it's thick, and store it for liquid in soup. Incidentally, if soaked overnight, barley, soft white wheat, and hard red winter wheat may be added in small quantities (for example, a 1-4 proportion) to rice before cooking. These things make for nice surprises — and for some reason they cook in the same length of time as the rice, although if cooked separately, it seems to me they have to cook longer.

You'll love the "faster" grains such as millet, oat flakes (oatmeal), wheat flakes, bulghur, corn meal, kasha (buckwheat groats), whole-wheat spaghetti and macaroni. Of these only millet needs a quick rinse. Usually I just put it in the strainer (it looks as if it would go right through, but it doesn't) and run cold tap water through it. All these cereals except the pasta may be roasted before cooking, if you like; many people think this improves the flavor, especially if the cereal is old. To cook, for millet and corn meal it seems best to me to use a 3-1 ratio with water; for the flakes, bulghur, and kasha, 2-1; for pasta — lots. Save any excess liquid. The flavors of millet and kasha are not compatible, by the way.

I may scandalize the skillful cooks by telling that I use boiling water from the tea kettle to start these "faster" grains. That makes them even faster, but that's not the real reason. We just like the flavor better. Millet needs to simmer about 30 minutes after returning to a boil, while the others require less time. "Cook to taste." If you're careful, and especially if you use a flame minder, you can get by without using a double boiler for these grains. It expedites your recipes to have one of the "fast" grains and one of the "slow" grains (in addition to rice) cooked and stored most of the time. Learn to use these fast grains cooked with some of the sweet vegetables — onions, carrots, parsnips, cabbage hearts, daikon if you can get it. This will give flavor to your breakfast cereal, for of course you must not use *any* of the accompaniments you have always counted on to go with cereal — no honey, milk or cream, butter or margarine, and no fruit for a while, at least. You'll be surprised how quickly you can learn to enjoy vegetables for breakfast!

Beans need to be sorted, rinsed, and, except for lentils, soaked overnight. Pinto beans need a lot of washing, as they're muddy (but tasty!) little critters.

Seeds: For economy, buy broken pieces of hulled sunflower seeds. You may want to give these a quick sorting. Then put them in a strainer and run cool tap water through them to remove dust. You can quick-rinse sesame seeds without sorting. Ditto for almonds. Drain these things thoroughly before roasting. (Sunflower seeds in large quantities can be laxative for some people; and pumpkin seeds if you can afford them make delicious crunchies to go with meals, but they are likely to be *very* laxative!)

Vegetables: Buy small ones whenever you can. The big ones lose some of their concentrated power. Abehsera says not to worry if vegetables are wilted — that only some of the liquid is gone. *Of course* we don't *peel* vegetables! Trim out only the worst blemishes. Wash them gently, and just before cooking if possible, for they don't especially like to be stored after being scrubbed. If you can ever find any vegetables with their top leaves, cook those, too. Cutting vegetables is a special art, for which you can study the macrobiotic cookbooks.

Re-warming, and **sauteeing:** If you cook and store grains in quantity, use a smaller double boiler to re-warm whatever you need for a meal. Or if you cook vegetables to add flavor to your breakfast grains, it is to be hoped that you can cook the vegetables fresh each time. Saute them if you like (they taste better and hold the color better) and then boil them quickly in a minimum of liquid. Let most of the liquid boil away and then add the cooked cereal, stirring gently to mix the flavor into the cereal. Continue the warming process over a flame minder or boiling water. If the cereal becomes too dry, drizzle just a little boiling water over it and continue to steam it until it's hot. About sauteeing — remember we're to have only 2 T of oil per day. So get the skillet warm first and then use only a tiny amount of oil, which should coat the skillet easily if it's warm (but not smoking!). Applying the oil to the skillet with a pastry brush is a good trick. Refer to your cookbooks for other information on sauteeing.

Bancha tea: I'll tell you about the all-important bancha (ku-kicha) tea and then we'll do something different. You already should have your tea roasted and stored, as per instructions above. To make tea, a glass coffee maker (with the coffee-making "hardware" removed) is best. (Other pans may have retained the flavor of previously cooked foods.) Use a rounded T of the twigs for each 3 or 4 cups (6-oz. cups). It's a good plan to get some fresh water (tap water or spring water, not distilled) rather hot in a separate tea kettle and pour it into the twigs and several cups of cold water which you have already put into the coffee maker. This lessens the risk of cracking the glass. Warm the tea over low heat for 10 minutes or so to get the tea and water used to each other, then turn the heat high, to bring it to a boil. It can boil over, so be careful. Turn the heat off and stir all the twigs down into the water. Add boiling water from the tea kettle up to the required level for the number of cups you're making. Then turn heat very low and steep the tea for about 15 minutes, without boiling or even simmering. The action inside the glass should be lazy like that of a lava light. Turn off the heat and allow to stand for 40-60 minutes to allow the twigs to settle. The longer it stands the better it tastes. It becomes an attractive reddish color, an aromatic, delicate-flavored beverage to sip and savor. If you made plenty, you can refrigerate it for three days at least, pouring out what you want to warm in a pan reserved for bancha tea only. The same tea can be kept warm for hours (as with the pilot light in a gas oven), or it can be often re-warmed. But please don't let it boil again, for you lose not only flavor but valuable enzymes. This tea, with 6 times as much calcium as milk, remember, plus 2½ times the Vitamin C of orange juice, but containing nothing harmful or stimulating, is a great aid to digestion. Even small children may drink it. By the way, it is very refreshing to sip cool — but never icy! (We should never use iced drinks, for reasons we mentioned early in this chapter.) Try never to drink fast, for our liquid, like our food, is better for us if we mix it with a little saliva.

If you have a large family, or often entertain and want to make tea for large groups, a 25-cup enamel ware coffee pot — the kind used for camping, in which one would put a bag of coffee and boil it (I think!) — is very practical. But don't use it for anything else except bancha tea. Of course, you don't *have* to use such tender-loving-care in making bancha tea, but if you want *supreme* quality, well, that's how to get it. We're going by the fact that we have never had anyone say he-she didn't like our tea. It seems to be immediately popular with guests.

Now that you have that primary information to build on, let's see what to do at various stages of macrobiotic development. *For our own protection, we must emphasize that these plans are guides in which we would have complete confidence if we were re-experiencing the sort of trials you readers may now be undergoing. We can neither prescribe nor advise, but can only report, with no desire to change our amateur rating.*

IN THE KITCHEN

Many proficient macrobiotic Cooks are here with you — all the Zen monks down through the ages (only the most outstanding were allowed in the monastery kitchen, says Michel Abehsera, who is also here), Cornelia and Herman Aihara, Lima Ohsawa, Iona Teeguarden, and Aveline Kushi herself, who welcomes you:

> There are many ways to study this Order of the Universe, yin and yang. Cooking is a particularly exciting and rewarding way. Your rice and onions, carrots and salt, your cutting knives and pots will prove to be your best teachers. And if you listen carefully to their silent lessons you will be able to develop your intuition and to make your family and yourself happy and beautiful.[1]

Easing your own emotional problems is very important, for the atmosphere in the kitchen should become one of serenity. This food is alive, after all, and it senses your tensions just as do living plants that Cleve Backster and others have experimented with. I used to talk to the rice. "You lovely little pearls are going to have to help me more than you do other people, because I'm 'way out of context here. You're going to have to do most of the magic of getting Jean well, no matter how unskillfully I work with you." (Brown rice grains *are* like little pearls, so that wasn't just idle flattery.) Well, the grains responded, straining at first from having to overcome my anxiety, but finally after a few months like light little dancers, whirling and laughing when I was rinsing them. And the beans responded, and the seaweeds stretched out their graceful but strong fronds to offer help. And I still have a healthy husband instead of an urn full of ashes.

But wonderful though these foods may be, they do demand that you be a co-worker. Help them and they help you and your family, as we said in Chapter 12.

We will lean heavily on Mari's consummate skill, the product of her heritage, intuition, knowledge, and experience. Mari is in our Chapters 1 and 2, and has her own case history included with the others in this book. We can begin with her recipes for the very seriously ill. These are highly specialized, and if your invalid is weak enough to need this treatment, you'll have to take a leave of absence from your job and hire help for maintenance duties around the house. Or, hire one of those young natural-foods cooks we suggested in the previous chapter, work with him or her for a week or two, and go back to your job leaving your Cook in charge at home. (Note the change from cook to Cook. A Cook is deserving of much gratitude and honor — especially after you show him-her the paragraph above about not licking fingers and cooking spoons!)

If someone in our family were dangerously ill enough to need to be fed through a tube, we'd first phone either Michio or Edward Esko to ask questions, then get help from an R.N. for a few days, and after that ask the latter's advice as the situation improved. We'd say nothing but very frequent positive and encouraging statements in the presence of the invalid, knowing that someone even in an apparent coma can hear (at least subconsciously) every word we say, and can sense much that we don't say. We would keep constant reminders in the conversation of reasons for getting well, and keep saying that we were using food that can work miracles, stressing the returning strength and the steady healing brought about by the food. We'd ask the East West Foundation where to find a macrobiotic friend proficient in shiatsu massage, and would have all members of the family, as well as the Cook, learn this technique as applied to our invalid. We think that if the latter has a strong determination to live, and a willingness to adjust, an adaptation of the same food could, in a couple of weeks perhaps, be administered by mouth.

Jean advises that even when critically ill your invalid is likely to be extremely distrustful — very suspicious of having to eat things he-she is afraid of not liking. You may have the problem of trying to overcome deep psychological resentment in the sick person. Here's where family reading of macrobiotic philosophy, suggested in the previous chapter, can gradually give you a knowledge to work from. Incidentally, everyone involved may also find it helpful to review the pronunciation hints about half-way through Chapter 12.

For all the following recipes we are assuming you have, as a prerequisite, read the previous chapter, and have sorted and/or toasted and stored the foods requiring such attention. Rinse other foods just before cooking.

Rice, of course, always means brown rice. Rice flour always means brown rice flour. w-w =whole-wheat. Spaghetti (often called noodles, remember) and macaroni are always w-w or soba (buckwheat). Salt is always solar salt or sea salt (see above). If we forget to specify the amount of tamari, add it to your own taste; but please train your taste to use moderate amounts.

As for oils, Mari uses only sesame oil, the most yang of oils, to impart a beneficial yang quality to her cooking. Since she is feeding healthy people now she doesn't *have* to be that careful; but people in poor health should use *only* sesame oil. At our restaurant our Cooks use corn oil for sauteeing and for gravies, sesame oil for pastry, salad dressings, wok cooking (corn oil here would bubble up too much). If the price of sesame goes *too* high, they have to regretfully substitute safflower oil, which Ken Burns says he finds as acceptable as corn oil so far as yin properties are concerned. Mari suggests combining corn oil with sesame or safflower, to keep the former from being so "heavy." But she drops the hint that daikon sauteed in corn oil has an especially delicious flavor.

Our recipes are all oriented toward the conditions we know here in the Midwest section of the United States. Wherever else you live you can adapt things to your own conditions, as you gradually learn more about macrobiotic principles. There's a world-wide list of macrobiotic centers in the Appendix to this book, so perhaps you can communicate with one in a climate similar to yours. Or subscribe to East West Foundation literature so that you will receive schedules of international seminars, which are becoming increasingly more popular. If you could travel to attend one of those, you would have hundreds of questions cleared up for you.

> A little note of interest: Macrobiotic food likes to be stirred *counter*clockwise in the northern hemisphere, clockwise in the southern.

A SUPPLY OF LIQUID FOOD FOR THE CRITICALLY ILL

(For several days, or up to one week. All this food should be refrigerated, then slightly warmed in small amounts for each feeding.)

1. Rinse 1 C brown rice, drain thoroughly. Roast in a large flat bak-

ing dish at 325° at least an hour, until golden brown and until some of it *pops*. Stir occasionally. Or, if you have time to stay with it, you can roast it in a heavy skillet on top of the stove, stirring almost constantly.

Cool the rice and put it in the blender with no liquid, on high setting. This makes about 1½ C of fine flour. In a large kettle stir this flour into 10 C cold water. Add 3 umeboshi plums, seeded, using also the beefsteak leaves (chiso), if any, in the jar. Add 2 T tamari (optional), and a 5-7 inch strip of dashi kombu (see seaweeds, above). Bring this mixture to a boil, uncovered, stirring occasionally. Simmer over very low heat for 2-3 hours, uncovered, stirring occasionally. (Later on, for feeding by mouth, you can cook it longer to make it thicker.)

Remove kombu. Run the mixture through the blender again, at the "liquefy" setting. If too thick for tube feeding, add 2 C cold water and bring to a boil again. Cool the mixture and squeeze it through cheesecloth, refrigerating the liquid.

2. Rinse 1 C azuki beans and soak overnight in 4-5 C water. Add a 3-inch strip of kombu and bring the beans to a boil, uncovered, in the soak water. Keep it simmering enough to bubble very lightly for four hours, or until the beans are very soft. Whenever more water is needed, use your skimmer to remove the scum that has formed on top of the bean juice, and add more cold water. For the last half-hour add a pinch of salt. When cool, run through the blender on "liquefy" setting, then strain the mixture and the cooking juice through cheesecloth.

3. *Butternut or acorn squash:* Wash and cut in cubes, cutting out the hard "ends." Place in kettle in about 1 inch of water, adding a few drops of tamari if desired. Simmer 30-45 minutes covered, adding cooked azuki beans the last half-hour if you wish (about 2 T for each squash). Cool, remove squash skins, blend the pulp (and beans) on "liquefy," and then strain through cheesecloth.

The feeding tube must be rinsed after each feeding with a small amount of spring or well water. After a few days, for one rinsing each day, you may use the nutritious water in which you have boiled kale.

"SOFT" DIET

When we begin to see signs of improvement that would make us think the liquid diet would soon be inadequate, we should again phone the East West Foundation or the nearest macrobiotic center to see how to go about changing to a macrobiotic "soft" diet. But it would probably be something like the following instructions. If your invalid is *not* critical, of course, the soft diet would be the one you could begin with instead of the liquid diet.

1. Cook rice extra soft, perhaps in a ratio of 1 C rice to 5 C water. Or, use rice already cooked for the rest of the family, add an equal amount of water, and boil gently till the water is used up. Or, use some miso soup for part of the liquid to add a little flavor; but in that case give your invalid another small serving of miso soup or miso broth during the day because what you boiled with the rice would have lost some nutritive value.

2. Cook beans extra soft, as per instructions in #2 of the LIQUID DIET, except, of course, don't puree them in the blender. Other beans will require longer cooking time than do azukis. Probably you should use very small servings of beans.

3. Vegetables should also be cooked very soft, using onions to bring out the flavor of other vegetables. In general, you could use the suggestions above for squash, or the vegetable recipes below, but with considerably *longer cooking*.

STRICT DIET

These recipes would be for convalescents who are "ambulant," but who must be on the fundamental macrobiotic program. The recipes are also for everyone else, and healthy people could have the "occasional" items a little more often. Check, too, recipes from (aa) on, for those which are labeled *Safe*. Some of these recipes you will find in the cookbooks we recommend, for because of their antiquity they are common property. But if you have them here, you can use them NOW, and won't have to wade around in the cookbooks looking for safe recipes to start with. Besides, Mari has made them more "understandable" for Americans and other non-Orientals. We hope you can locate an Oriental food store to find some of the more exotic-sounding items.

Recipes are printed in a format to save as much space as possible; but you will no doubt want to transfer them to your own recipe cards anyway, no matter how they are printed here.

MARI'S SUPREME VEGETABLES
(We hope a little of her magic touch
will be imparted to you!)

(a) Slice 4 large carrots thin, on a long diagonal; cut these slices into narrow strips. Thin-slice one medium-size or large onion from the top down; cut slices into strips if the onion will cooperate. Warm a heavy kettle or pan, spreading 1 T oil over the surface. Layer the vegetables — onions, then carrots. Sprinkle with 1 T or less of tamari. If the lid is close-fitting, water will not be necessary, but in any case use no more than ¼ C. Cover, bring to a boil, turn heat very low to simmer till carrots are tender. Do not stir for 30 minutes.

Or, use burdock (sliced as for carrots, not slivered as for soups), and carrots (fewer carrot slices than burdock). Burdock must be sauteed till it changes color before the rest of the cooking process is continued.

(b) *"Cantonese"-style vegetables:* Use amounts according to how much you want to make. (Remember that celery and snow peas are for occasional use, and should perhaps be omitted for a recuperating invalid. Substitute bits of chopped kale or other dark greens, sautéed after the onion.) Sauté chopped green onion till soft, then add other vegetables in this order, sauteeing each until it changes color: celery, snow peas, cabbage and/or Japanese cabbage, bean sprouts. Add tamari to taste. Do not overcook. If vegetables are too dry, add ¼ C water and cover while you soften 2 T kuzu in a little cold water. Add to vegetables and stir over low heat till liquid is clear and thick. Serve over rice or noodles.

(c) Nishime (a kind of "stew gone stylish"): Soak a long strip of a tender variety of kombu, rubbing it between your fingers to clean it. For a fancy touch, after it softens, tie pieces of gourd string tightly around the kombu, about two inches apart, and cut it between the knots. (If you can't find gourd string, use ordinary string but be careful not to eat it!) Boil kombu bows in 2 C water for 30 minutes. Save liquid. Slice one cake of tofu as thin as possible; brown it in a skillet in 1 T sesame or corn oil; cut it into 1-inch squares. For this sort of recipe, root vegetables are cut in chunks, alternating diagonal cuts so that the pieces look like "deer hoofs" (see recipe books). In a deep pan, place in layers: kombu bows, large pieces of onions, then burdock, carrots, or other root vegetables, then vegetables such as cubes of squash and, occasionally, whole green beans. For healthy people a few cubes of taro potato may sometimes be added. Tofu squares go on top. If you're in an exotic mood, and if you have konnyaku and lotus root, pieces of those would go in right after the kombu bows. (Broccoli, celery, and cauliflower do not fit in to this kind of combination.) Add the kombu stock, to which you have added a maximum of 1 t solar or sea salt and about 4 T tamari, plus enough water to cover about 3/4 of the depth of the vegetables. Cover the pan and bring to a boil; lower heat and simmer 30-45 minutes, or until carrots are almost tender, without stirring. Uncover and simmer until about one-fourth of the liquid remains. Leave in the pan until serving time, or until cool for storage. The remaining liquid is very flavorful for sauces, for mixing into unleavened breads, etc. Whenever you get clearance from your macrobiotic friends to use dashi iriko or chirimen iriko (little fishes), those should go into the bottom of the pan before any of the other layers. (People don't eat dashi iriko, usually, but save them for your dogs and cats! We do eat the tiny chirimen iriko, and they're *very* nutritious.) When the time comes that you can replace the little fishes occasionally (once or twice a month) with small pieces of sauteed chicken, you are *really* healthy!

(d) Ken Burns tells us how to prepare dandelion greens. They're bitter, but very beneficial! Use small servings as accents to a meal, or use a little in soups on days when you don't use burdock. Dig up the whole dandelion plant. Wash thoroughly. Sauté a large fine-chopped onion till translucent. Cut off dandelion roots, chop in small pieces, saute these and mix them with half the onion. Chop the leaves in small pieces, saute, mix with the remaining onion. Mix all ingredients together and add tamari to taste.

(e) *Boiled salad:* This may be recommended for your condition rather than raw vegetables. But its own goodness recommends it in any case! Use fine-chopped vegetables of the tossed-salad type, except, of course, for omitting off-limits vegetables. Put them in a pan, add half a pinch of salt and a little boiling water. Simmer covered 1 or 2 minutes, turn off heat and put some small pieces of wakame on top of the vegetables. After a few minutes pour off the water into some soup stock. Or, omit seaweed and sprinkle toasted seaweed on top of the salad when served. Or, use gomasio or umeboshi plum juice. For instance —

(f) *Gomasio:* Use about a 10-1 ratio of sesame seeds to solar or sea salt. Make only enough for about a week, used sparingly as a table condiment. Crush the roasted salt in a suribachi. Add the roasted seeds, hold the suribachi in your lap, and develop a light circular technique with the pestle, gently grinding 70 percent-80 percent of the seeds. Store in a glass jar. (A quick turn in the blender could be a second-best method, if you don't have a suribachi.)

Plum juice: Bring 1 or 2 umeboshi plums to a boil in a quart of

water. When they soften, fish them out and pop the seeds out.
Put seeds and pulp back into the water and simmer for up to an
hour. See macrobiotic cookbooks for details on gomasio and
plum juice.

(g) *Pressed salad:* Find a heavy rock and wash it — a size that will
be smaller than the top of one of your large crock-type bowls,
which should have an overglaze finish, please! Vegetables such
as these may be used, according to what you like: carrots, cabbage, lettuce, radishes, daikon, turnips, cauliflower. Thin-slice
the root vegetables and fine-chop the others. Put half of them in
the bowl, sprinkle with a *very* little salt; repeat with the remaining vegetables. Cover with a plate smaller in diameter than the
top of the bowl, and place the rock on top of the plate. Cover
with a cloth to keep out insects. As the plate sinks during the
next 3 days, pour off the liquid. A serving of pressed salad is
1 or 2 T. (Mari says that a *large* jar filled with water can also be
used as a weight, if you don't have a rock.)

(h) We'll ask Mari now about sprouting seeds and beans — alfalfa
seeds (for salads and sandwiches), wheat berries (see recipes),
mung beans (salads), and soybeans (see recipes). Wash these
little friends lightly and soak overnight. Drain off water. (Alfalfa
seeds may be strained through fine cheesecloth to avoid losing
them.) You can keep each kind of seeds or beans in a large glass
jar, gallon size if you can find them. Cover the would-be sprouts
with water, cover the top of the jar with cheesecloth (tie it on),
and store in a dark closet. Twice each day pour some water
down into the jar through the cheesecloth, swish it around to
rinse the sprouts, drain it off, and return the jar to the dark
place.

If you don't have any large glass jars, a flat Corning Ware pan
is good, covered with a double thickness of cotton cloth and then
with the pan lid, so that just a little air can be available for the
sprouts to breathe. This is dark enough without the additional
darkness of closet-storage. Or, you could use a deep earthen-
ware or china bowl (*over*glazed), with an opaque covering. After
the sprouts are nice and long and fresh they should be refrigerated, and used before they start to grow little hair-roots and
become little plants, for then their highly concentrated nutritive
elements become dispersed. If a green color is desired, expose
sprouts to the sunlight for a few minutes before serving.

We've mentioned before the benefits of training your family to
chew their food till it's creamy. But warn them also to "bite down
easily" on the first couple of chews. A tiny pebble may have been

missed in the sorting process, or grains may have dried out during baking, to become little tooth-breakers. Check the comments about baked rice, above, for the remedy (for the dried rice, not for a cracked tooth!). With these reminders about eating techniques, we can go back to a few samples of Mari's recipes for —

COMBINING GRAINS WITH OTHER FOODS

(i) *Rice cooked with vegetables:* Wash 3 C rice as described above. Put it in a large kettle and add ⅓ C fine-grated carrots and ⅓ C burdock, slivered thin. Add ½ C hiziki and 2 pieces of aburage cut into small pieces (see Recipe (s). Into 2 C water mix ¼ C tamari, pinch of solar or sea salt, 1 t sesame oil; pour this liquid into the kettle, mixing all ingredients gently. Add 4 more C water and cook as for ordinary rice (see above). Sometimes, if you are not too ill, you may add fresh garden peas at the point where you turn off the heat and let the rice steam. Very occasionally you could use frozen peas, for color.

(j) If you have to get something ready in a hurry, you can pan-fry cooked rice with a few grated or fine-chopped vegetables in a very small amount of oil, in a heavy cast-iron skillet if possible. First saute the chopped onion in the oil till the onion is translucent. If you happen to have cooked hiziki on hand you can add that next, then add other vegetables. Add rice, tamari to taste, and mix gently until all food is thoroughly heated.

(k) *Spring Rolls* (vegetables wrapped in a "blanket"): These seem very complicated at first, but they're well worth the trouble. Put 2 C w-w flour and ½ t salt in a bowl and stir in 1 C hot water to which 1 T oil has been added. Blend well, mix with fork, knead to "ear lobe" consistency, roll out very thin, cut in squares about 6 inches across, and roll the edges even thinner. Continue making squares until batter is used up. Then — chop fine: 4 stalks of scallions, one medium-size carrot, enough cabbage or Japanese cabbage to fill about ½ C, 1 stalk of celery (very little or none at all for recuperating invalids), 5 fresh water chestnuts. Saute lightly in that order in 2 T sesame oil or black sesame oil (more expensive, with stronger flavor). Stir in tamari to taste (up to 1 T). Mix 1 T arrowroot in a little cool water (try ¼ C). Stir into vegetables, thickening them enough to stick together but not using enough liquid to make a thin gravy. Allow to cool.

Lay one of the 6-inch square "blankets" on a cutting board in front of you. Scratch a light line across the middle. Imagine moving clockwise around the square, with 1 in front of you, 2 at the left end of the line, 3 at the top, 4 at the right end of the line. Place two T vegetable mix just below the line, folding edge #1 over the vegetables and pressing it lightly against the line. Fold over sides 2 and 4. Roll the bottom half, including the vegetables, upwards, so that 1 is about a half-inch below 3, allowing 3 to be folded down as a flap on an envelope. Dampen the edges of 3 and press closed against the envelope. While you are shaping the last few packets, preheat 3 inches of oil in a heavy skillet (see tampura, below). Lower the vegetable packets into the oil and deep-fry 1 or 2 minutes. Drain on a rack and then on paper towel. Fine gourmet eating! When you are healthy you can use bits of sauteed chicken in the vegetable mix.

Next we can offer a few combinations of

BEANS WITH OTHER FOODS

The basic method of cooking beans is given in the instructions for azukis in #2 of the recipes for the critically ill, except, of course, that we would not include the last step of liquefying in the blender. Some people like to pressure-cook beans, in which case the recipe books tell how much less water to use. Black beans won't work under pressure, as they bubble so much they clog the valve. All beans are likely to spit out of the pressure cooker, so you can't leave them alone very long. Lima Ohsawa says that pressure makes azukis taste bitter. Oven-baking is OK on a long, slow setting with a little more water than for kettle cooking. A crock-pot seems excellent. Mari uses a little more liquid than is suggested in some cookbooks, and we have some left over for soups and sauces. *Do not use kuzu for sauces, however, with any kind of beans or their juices, including lentils,* as the flavors do not go together.

(1) *Rice Balls:* These are all-important in macrobiotic life, for lunch boxes, for travel, for parties. Use cold salted water to wet your hands. Press rice into balls between your palms. Poke a hole in each ball and put in a sliver of umeboshi plum or a few drops of tamari and press it closed. Rice Balls will keep several days unrefrigerated because of the plum or tamari! Mix azuki beans with the rice if you like, although this will not stay fresh as long. Roll the balls in toasted sesame seeds. Or: toast nori over an open flame (just a few swishes back and forth) or in the oven and wrap the Rice Balls in nori. Sweet brown rice is especially good for Rice Balls because it holds together well. Sometimes poke little

surprises into the center of Rice Balls — bits of sauteed vegetables or toasted sunflower seeds, for instance. For *parties*, use
bits of cooked dried fruit, or something of your own invention.
Small rice balls without anything else added are delicious in
tempura (see below).

(m) *Red Rice:* Sort and rinse 1 C azuki beans. Soak overnight in 5
or 6 C water. Cook beans in this same water: bring to a boil uncovered and simmer uncovered 15-20 minutes, until the skins
are softened and *almost* ready to break. Pour off the liquid and
cool it. Using this liquid plus enough water to make 5½ C, soak
7-8 hours in a cool place 4 C sweet brown rice and 1 C brown
rice. Gently stir in the partially cooked beans, which have been
kept in a cool place; bring to a boil, covered, and simmer covered
about 45 minutes. Allow to stand 20 minutes. Gently "fluff it up"
before serving, sprinkled with gomasio if desired.

(n) *Carrots and kidney beans:* Cut 2 medium-size carrots into rec-
tangular slices about 1/8-inch thick. Put these and 1 C cooked
kidney beans in a large pan and add 3/4 C stock, to which you
have added 1½ t tamari. (See instructions for "Soup stock"
earlier in this chapter. If you don't have any put aside, you can
make it by boiling a 2-inch piece of kombu in 1¼ C water for 20-
30 minutes, covered.) When you have combined carrot slices,
kidney beans, stock, and tamari, bring to a boil covered and simmer covered till carrots are done but not overcooked. *Sauce:*
grind in a suribachi 1 block (about a 3-inch cube) tofu, 3-6 T
roasted sesame seeds, 1 t tamari. (In the absence of a suribachi
try a few seconds in the blender on low setting.) For *parties,* you
can mix 1½ T of pure maple syrup into the sauce. But save some
without syrup for anyone on the really strict diet.

(o) *Azuki beans and kanten:* Break 1 bar of kanten into small bits
and soak in ¼ C-½ C water. When soft, press out the water. Boil
the softened kanten in 1 C azuki juice till melted. (You need to
have planned ahead to have that azuki juice on hand!) Add ½ t
salt and up to 2 C azuki beans if you like. Boil again for a few
minutes, pour into a flat pan, and chill. If you are dieting to lose
weight, you should probably skip the beans, or add only a very
few. This may be served as a salad, on green lettuce leaves. As a
dessert for *parties,* use only a few beans, if any, and add ¼ C pure
maple syrup when you add the salt and/or beans. Or, you could
puree cooked squash and azukis to make about 1 C of puree, and
stir this and 2 T pure maple syrup into the hot kanten at the time
the salt is added. Then simmer again for a few minutes and chill
as above.

(p) *Mari's Golden Dream Pie:* This is so "safe" that you can have it from the very beginning! And you won't have to be macrobiotic very long before your taste buds get tuned up to imagine that the filling has a few marshmallows in it. A good recipe for pie crust is included with breads, so we'll give only the filling here (which of course may be used also as a pudding, stirring in a few toasted sunflower seeds, if you like, when the mixture is partially cool). You'll have trouble believing these ingredients, but just put your doubts aside and try it anyway. Saute one large onion, chopped very fine. Add 4-6 parsnips, sliced very thin, and one large acorn squash cut into 1-inch cubes. Saute these until the squash becomes a deeper color. Add 1¾ C hot water to which you have added a pinch of salt. Simmer uncovered till squash is tender. Pick out and discard whatever pieces of squash skin you can. Cool the vegetables and stir in 3 T w-w flour. (With this amount of filling, you'll need to use an electric mixer instead of a blender; mix ingredients thoroughly.) Pour the mixture into a pie shell and flute the edges. Bake at 425° for 15 minutes; reduce to 225° for 1¼ hours. Variations: Add 1 or 2 T raw carob powder with the flour. For *parties,* add 1 T honey, *or* 1 T pure maple syrup, *or* 2 T corn-barley malt syrup.

LESS STRICT!

If you are basically on the strict diet, but after a while are allowed more oil, for instance, or a small amount of sweetening, or fruit, you may find that you can use most of the recipes in this section. Probably pretty early in the game you'll be able to have tempura, and of course the Clear Soup you can have right away if you omit the little fishes.

(q) *Tempura:* Mari has hints to make this process completely successful, and tempura foods, properly prepared, are the ultimate in good eating. Probably once every two or three weeks is often enough to serve this type of food. Prepare the rest of the meal first, so that the tempura can have your complete attention just before serving. Keep food warm in the oven, where you can also put the tempura foods as soon as they drain. Do not break the little lumps in the batter. Do not make too much batter at one time, even if preparing a large quantity of tempura treats; make a moderate amount, use it up. and then make more batter. Do not over-coat the food with batter. Do not put more than one ingredient into the oil at a time, but dip each piece of food individually. Use about 3 inches of oil in a large skillet or wok; heat slowly to 350°. To test, drop in a bit of batter, which should sink to the bottom and rise again at about the same speed. One of the main secrets is to keep skimming flotsam and jetsam off the top of the oil. For cloudy oil, drop in an umeboshi plum and let it turn black before removing it.

Batter: 1 C w-w flour, ½ C corn flour (blend corn meal to make this), pinch of salt, cold water to make a medium-thin batter (try 1 C + 2 T). Use such foods as: small rice balls, 1 carrot cut in thin strips, dipping several strips in a little bunch; 1 parsnip prepared in the same way; 1 onion cut in thin slices; strips of burdock dipped in small bunches (m-m-m!); small thin slices of acorn squash; nori cut into 1½-inch pieces; parsley (cut off the stems, but save them to chop and drop into soups); broccoli flowers; green beans; occasionally, green peppers cut in strips; chrysanthemum leaves, if you've been to the Oriental store lately; any other "approved" vegetable that suits your fancy, but don't use too many at any one meal. Skim the oil clean and allow it to cool; if stored in a tightly covered glass jar with an umeboshi plum, it may be used over and over for several weeks.

Whenever oily food is served, the Japanese give each person a tablespoon or two of fine-grated daikon (if unavailable, use radishes or even turnips) to which a few drops (or up to 1 t) of tamari may be added. Dip some bites of tempura into the daikon "horseradish" to counteract the effects of the oil. Very often, as a prelude to a tempura meal, Mari will serve —

(r) *Clear Soup:* A basic soup stock is made of 6 C water and a 6-inch strip of kombu (plus ½ C bonita shavings if available; or, 8-10 dashi iriko (refer to Recipe (c). Bring to a boil and simmer 20 minutes. Allow to stand for 10 minutes and then strain. For Clear Soup add 2 T tamari and a maximum of 1 t solar or sea salt. Sometimes you may want to add chopped watercress and/or cooked carrot strips, or cooked w-w noodles (spaghetti). We dip pieces of tempura food, held with chopsticks, into the soup and eat them. Wow! Tempura warmed in the broiler a second day is just as good used this way as it was when freshly cooked.

(r-1) Mari sometimes makes Miso Soup by adding to the basic miso broth some very small cubes of tofu, pieces of wakame, and chopped scallions. See our basic recipe for Miso Soup earlier in this chapter, for the method of adding the miso.

(s) *Aburage:* Fried bean curd (tofu). Aburage is made of thick slices of tofu, pressed dry in paper towel and deep-fried. Pieces of aburage may be used in soups. It is also possible to make little "pock-ets" in aburage, stuff them with vegetable mix as for Spring Rolls (Recipe (k), or stuff with rice and vegetables as in Recipe (i), and warm them in the oven. This is best if the aburage is first boiled in basic soup stock. For parties, you can boil it in about 1 C of soup stock to which tamari and a very little maple syrup have been added.

(t) *Seitan:* Meat! The Japanese call this "vegetable meat," and it surely surpasses any kind of red meat you ever ate, if you can make it right. It's really called "kofu" (wheat gluten), I believe, up to the point where you slice it and simmer it in soup stock, after which it is called seitan. A complicated recipe — definitely a family project, or one for several macrobiotic friends, if you have been able to convert any or join any. People should take turns kneading this "meat loaf."

Mix 2½ C wheat gluten, 1½ C brown rice flour or sweet brown rice flour, 1½ C w-w pastry flour, 2½ C cold water. Knead 30 minutes, till smooth and elastic. Form an oblong loaf about 2 inches high. Place a rack in the bottom of a large kettle and add enough water to cover the loaf, then remove the loaf. Bring the water to a boil, lower the loaf into it, cover it with a cloth. Or, you can use a steamer such as a spaghetti steamer, bring the water to a boil, place the loaf in the upper pan and cover it with a cloth. Cover the kettle, bring water to a boil again and simmer 30 minutes, or until a metal skewer comes out clean. Drain off the water. Allow the loaf to cool and cut into two loaves.

In a skillet or deep-fry pan, heat 2 or 3 inches of oil, enough oil to cover one of the loaves. When the oil is hot enough to sizzle a bread crumb, grain of rice, or whatever, lower the loaf into it. Brown on both sides. Lift out the loaf, drain, and cool. Slice into ¼-inch slices. Repeat the process for the other loaf.

In a Corning Ware pan (probably 9 inches square) or a heavy (9-inch) skillet put 1 C basic soup stock (Recipe (r), adding 3 T tamari (1 t fine-grated ginger root is optional — see "Compres-ses," end of this chapter). Bring to a boil. Lay kofu slices from one of the half-loaves in the pan or skillet. The stock should cover the slices. If necessary, add a little boiling water, or more stock brought to a boil in another pan. Cover the 9-inch pan and return to a boil. Simmer about 30 minutes. Uncover and simmer, with the liquid making light bubbles, till the liquid evaporates or is absorbed. Repeat for the other loaf.

Seitan keeps very well, refrigerated or (not macrobiotically en-dorsed!) frozen. Once you have it, there are various ways to use it. A favorite is to cut the slices into small pieces and cook with vegetables. Cutlets are great! To make them, dip the seitan slices into thin batter (1 C pastry flour to 2/3 C water), coat with bread crumbs (see Breads, below) and deep-fry. Or, for a thick batter, without bread crumbs, use 1 C pastry flour, 1 C corn flour (simply run corn meal through the blender), and 2/3 C water. Often these are served with cabbage shredded *very* thin, garnished with parsley. Serve grated daikon also (end of Recipe (q), and don't eat too many cutlets! We're supposed to *go easy on oily foods,* remember; and also we should try to stay reasonably within the relationship of 15 percent ground grain to 85 percent whole grains. Seitan slices uncoated and lightly sauteed may be served with the following, delicious —

(u) *Mari-sauce:* Liquefy in the blender left-over pieces of seitan and left-over vegetables. Mix arrowroot with a little cool water (about 1 T arrowroot per C of blended liquid), stir it into the liquid, and bring the mixture to a boil, stirring till it thickens and bubbles slightly. Don't forget also the sauce in Recipe (o). These sauces can enhance many foods, but, again, *use in moderation.* Remember our best sauce is our own saliva, and thorough chewing!

(v) Mari could go on for volumes, but maybe we should let her take a rest after we get her recipe for a rice pudding loaf. For this you make rice flour of 2 C of brown rice, according to instructions in #1 of recipes for the critically ill. Then cook 1 C dried apples in 7 C water till apples are soft. Drain and reserve the liquid. Put the apples in the blender with another C water and blend well. Cook the brown rice flour in the reserved apple liquid for 30-40 minutes. Add the blended apples and mix well. Pour into a 9 x 11 baking dish or pan. Cover and place the dish in a pan containing 1 inch of hot water. Bake at 350° for one hour. When you are allowed to have a little soy powder (pretty yin stuff), you could sometimes stir ½ C into the dry rice flour.
The next day this pudding may be sliced and browned lightly in a skillet or under the broiler for a welcome addition to breakfast rice, or for a lunch-box treat!

Now we can go to our Harvest Moon Cooks for a few of their recipes for casseroles, sauces, breads, and desserts. These are typical of the dishes served in most natural-foods restaurants, with such recipes as are in the *Ten Talents* and *Deaf Smith* cookbooks adapted for macrobiotic use by the omission of herbs, spices, off-limits vegetables, etc., and the reduction of oils and sweeteners. Most of these recipes make about twelve *generous* servings.

(aa) *Lentil-Millet Burgers:* Mix 1 C cooked lentils and 4 C cooked millet (see "faster" grains, in the instructions for cooking grains, earlier in this chapter). Mix in 1 chopped onion, sauteed until translucent, 2 C bread crumbs (see Breads, below), 8 C cooked rice, tamari (try 3 T). Shape into medium-thin patties and bake on lightly-oiled cookie sheets, 350° for 30 minutes. Cover with aluminum foil the last 5 minutes to soften grains that may have dried out during baking. *Safe.*

(bb)   *Millet-Barley Burgers:* Mix 2 C cooked millet, 2 C cooked barley (you have to think a day ahead on this, to soak the barley overnight — see cooking grains, earlier in this chapter), 1½ C cooked oatmeal. Saute 3 large fine-chopped onions till translucent, and occasionally you could add and saute a fine-sliced stalk of celery. Add tamari (3 T or to taste, meaning *less*). Mix with other ingredients, form into patties, roll in bread crumbs (see Breads, below), bake on lightly-oiled cookie sheets, 350° for 30 minutes. *Safe.*

Make up your own variations for recipes like these "Burgers." They can also be baked in loaf form in a large flat baking dish — 350° for 30 minutes. About once a month, or for parties, you can use celery seeds or dried parsley, or less often, fine-chopped sauteed green pepper.

(cc)   *Vegeburgers:* When you have cooked garbanzos and cooked azukis (optional) on hand, you can grind or "blenderize" the garbanzos and mix in the azukis, 6 C of garbanzos to 1 C of azukis. Fine-chop 1 or 2 onions and saute until translucent, add about 3/4 C coarse-grated carrot and (occasionally) a little fine-chopped celery and saute a few minutes longer. Add tamari (maximum of 3 T). Mix all ingredients. If too dry to form patties, add bean stock; if too wet, add oat powder (or rice flour, or w-w flour). Shape into patties and bake on lightly-oiled cookie sheets, 350° for 30 minutes. Or, brown on both sides in a heavy skillet in a minimum of oil. Or, press into a lightly oiled cookie sheet, make narrow "separations" with a spatula so that the sheet is divided into 3 or 4 sections, to allow for better baking in the middle. Bake till lightly brown; cut in squares to serve. *Safe.*

(dd)   *Magic Pumpkin (or Squash!) Casserole:* Wash 4 acorn squash, cut into large cubes, sprinkle with a pinch of salt, steam until tender. Sauté 3 large onions till translucent, add and sauté 3 large coarse-grated carrots. In a large bowl, mix 10 C cooked rice, sautéed vegetables, 1 C toasted sunflower seeds, and a sprinkle of tamari. The seeds are optional, but very nice (see instructions for seeds earlier in this chapter). Place ingredients in a large flat baking dish, cover with bread crumbs sprinkled with a few seeds. Bake at 350° for 30 minutes. *Variation: Hiziki* may be added — to this and almost any other casserole. Wash hiziki in a large sieve, soak 10-15 minutes in water to cover. Drain off the water and discard it. Chop the hiziki and saute it over medium heat for 10 minutes, or until it no longer smells strong. Cool slightly, add water to cover it, and bring to a boil. Cover and simmer 30-40 minutes. Simmer uncovered till liquid evaporates. Experiment until you know the amount to add to your recipes, according to what you and your family will enjoy. *Safe.*

(ee) *Sunflower Casserole:* Heat 3 T oil in a large skillet. Stir in 4 C wheat flakes and 4 C oat flakes (oatmeal). Continue to heat and stir for 5 minutes. Add 5 C water, to which you have added a pinch of salt. Cover and simmer 20 minutes over low heat, stirring often. In another skillet saute in as little oil as possible: 2 fine-chopped onions till translucent, 1 fine-chopped stalk of celery (if you haven't served celery too often lately), ¼ C chopped parsley (or more if you like it), a little fine-chopped green pepper (very occasionally). Stir 3 T tamari into 1 C sunflower seeds. Then mix all ingredients together. Bake at 350° for 30 minutes, sprinkling a few seeds on the top during the last 5 minutes. *Safe.*

(ff) *Broccoli-Rice-Cheese:* Get well fast so that you can have this once in a while! Coarse-chop 2 or 3 bunches of broccoli and steam it until tender. Saute: 1 large onion till translucent, add and saute 1 large coarse-grated carrot. In a large bowl, mix 5 C cooked rice and ¼-pound grated cheese. Grate a few more T cheese for topping. (See Appendix for source of organic cheese.) Stir in the vegetables, place ingredients in a large flat baking dish, cover with bread crumbs (see Breads, below) and sprinkle with the grated cheese. Bake at 350° for 30 minutes. *Safe* only if you're allowed to have cheese.

(gg) *Macaroni in Vegetable Sauce:* Use 3 C cooked w-w elbow macaroni. Sauté 1 chopped small onion till translucent; add and saute 1 chopped carrot, 2 chopped kale leaves; add a pinch of salt while sauteeing. Put sauteed vegetables in blender with 2 C water and blend till smooth. Return mixture to skillet. In a cup or small saucer, thin 2 T tahini with several T of the vegetable mixture. Pour into the skillet. Dissolve 1 T kuzu in ¼ C cool water. Stir into the mixture in the skillet. Cook, stirring constantly, until the sauce is thick. Add tamari to taste. Combine macaroni and sauce and bake in a covered dish at 350° for 30 minutes. *Safe,* if you're allowed tahini.

(hh) *Pan-fried Noodles (Spaghetti!):* Use well-drained, cooked w-w or buckwheat noodles. Heat in a minimum of oil in a large heavy skillet or wok, stirring constantly, until they're no longer "limp." Sauté any ["approved"] green vegetables you like, until the color deepens. Serve over the noodles, sprinkling lightly with tamari or gomasio (Recipe (f). This is a "simplified version" of Recipe (b). *Safe.*

(ii) *Cabbage Rolls:* Steam large cabbage leaves until tender. Use 2 or 3 C cooked bulghur, depending on how many rolls you want to make. Follow the pattern in previous recipes for sauteeing vegetables. Add vegetables to bulghur, spoon the mix onto cabbage leaves and fold the leaves over to make enclosed rolls. Place the rolls in a baking dish and dip onion sauce over them (see below). Bake 20-30 minutes at 325°-350°, depending on the size of the rolls. *Safe.*

This type of cooking is limited only by your own imagination, which will stretch more and more as you keep working with this food. Many casseroles can be served with sauces, a few of which we will list next. Use your favorite sauces served *over* pasta dishes, as well as mixed in, as in Recipe (gg). But remind your family to be sparing with those sauces and not to *drown* the food in them, partly because, as we mentioned with Recipe (u), wet food is likely to be gulped and not chewed, and partly because, since the sauces have vegetable ingredients, they can play hob with the vegetable-grain balance. For variations, as soon as you turn off the heat under a sauce, sprinkle in some fine-chopped parsley, or kale coarse-blended for a few seconds; cover and allow to steam for a few minutes. Or, add toasted sesame seeds or sunflower seeds.

(jj) *Basic Sauce:* 1 C Clear Soup stock (Recipe (r). (For a quickie, use about 3 inches of wakame (as in "More seaweeds," earlier in this chapter). Give it a quick rinse, soak a few minutes (till soft) in 1¼ C water, bring almost to a boil, and lift it out to use in soup or salad. Add tamari, to taste, to the wakame stock. Dilute 1½ T arrowroot in a little cool water and add it to the cup of stock. Heat and stir until thick and clear. *Safe.*

Onion-vegetable Sauce: Cut 2 large onions in rings; saute in 1 t oil until lightly browned. Add 2 C hot water or vegetable stock (or pasta stock, or sometimes bean juice, etc.). Bring to a boil and add 2 T arrowroot softened in a little cool water. Tamari to taste. Heat and stir until thick and clear. *Safe.*

Onion-vegetable #2: Use 2 medium-size onions, 1 small carrot, occasionally a small stalk of celery, *or* daikon, *or* whatever your mood suggests. (I would like turnip, but probably I'd be in the minority.) Blend with 2 C water. In a skillet heat 1½ T oil, 2 C water, 4 T arrowroot softened in a little cool water. Continue heating, stirring till thick. Add the blended mix and cook slowly, stirring frequently till it bubbles slightly. *Safe.*

Bechamel: Fine-chop ½ onion and 2 scallions and saute in a minimum of oil until translucent. Use 2 C water. Use some of it to dilute 2 T rice flour (or toasted w-w or oat flour) and some of it to dilute 1 T tahini. Mix with remaining water, add ½ t solar or sea salt, and pour into the skillet with the onions. Bring to a boil, simmer 15 minutes, half-covered, stirring occasionally. *Safe,* if you're "cleared" for tahini.

Gravy: Use 3 times as much w-w flour as oil, 4 times as much water (or stock) as flour. Toast the flour in oil, add hot liquid, stirring constantly to avoid lumps, add tamari to taste, cook as for bechamel sauce. *Safe,* but use in moderation because of the oil.

The sauces included with the vegetables and grain recipes, above, may also be used with other foods.

Dessert Sauce: Cut dried apples and apricots into small pieces with kitchen scissors. Boil in a small amount of water, with a pinch of salt, until fruit is very soft, adding a little more water if necessary. Allow nearly all the water to boil away. Soften arrowroot (the amount will depend on how much fruit you have used) in a little cool water, add it to the fruit, heat and stir to thicken and clear. According to the amount you have made, add 1 or 2 T corn-barley malt syrup whenever you dare! Once in a while, sneak in a few chopped raisins before cooking, although they are very sugary. The cooked fruit could be put through the blender before thickening, if you would like it that way. (This is definitely for the occasional use of healthy people only!)

(kk) *Spreads:* Safe if you can have tahini, but even healthy people should use it somewhat sparingly. If you're still recuperating, spread it very thin and don't use it every day!

Garbanzo Spread: Grind in a food mill, or coarse-blend, 1 C cooked garbanzos. Add 2 T tahini softened in a little cool water. (Remember that tahini, if used in a recipe where it is not cooked, is one of those items requiring toasting according to instructions earlier in this chapter.) Add 1 T plus 1 t gomasio. Add one small fine-chopped onion sauteed in a little garlic powder (sneaky!). Mix well, adding tamari to taste.

Miso-Tahini Spread: Use 5 parts tahini to 1 part miso. Dilute miso in a little hot water. Add tahini and dilute further with cool water if necessary to mix the two together well and have the consistency you like.

Your own inventions: Use various combinations of leftover beans and vegetables, prepared as for garbanzo spread (but don't use that garlic powder very often!). One you could try would be the puréed squash-parsnip-onion combination (as for squash pie), plus roasted tahini diluted with water, plus a sprinkle of tamari. A few sunflower seeds may be added for interest.

Tahini-Apple Butter Spread: Once in a while you could make such a mix as this, with roasted tahini, of course. Apple butter should be purchased at a natural-foods store, so that you can get it unsweetened and non-chemicalized.

BREADS

(ll)   *Baking process for unleavened bread:* This takes special handling, and, in my amateurish opinion, it doesn't get it from the instructions in most macrobiotic cookbooks. I find it next to impossible to get the inside of the bread well done if a "normal"-size loaf is attempted. If you try a "normal" baking process you'll end up with a crust like kiln-fired clay, about 1/8-inch to 1/4-inch thick, with an interior like a wet mop. The maximum height of the unbaked loaf, I believe, should be 2½ inches, even if it's supposed to be "self-rising." Two inches would be better, in my opinion. I'd like to try the bread made by the Cooks who write the recipes in the books, for I have a feeling that in spite of what they say, a large loaf would have a soggy middle. Even the excellent Cooks at our Harvest Moon restaurant have a lot of trouble getting a good middle in a loaf of unleavened bread, although Gloria, our manager, is now making a very successful loaf (Recipe (mm), below).

So, I would bake a small, 2-inch-high loaf at 150° for one hour. This allows the warmth to penetrate to the interior of the loaf. Then I would turn the loaf over and, contrary to instructions in the books, *keep* the setting at 150° for another hour, covering it with foil or a lid if it begins to look too dry. Then try setting the temperature at 375° for another hour, removing the

cover for perhaps the last 15 minutes. Test the center by pok-
ing in a bamboo stick or a thin knife to see whether the tool
comes out clean. I would turn the loaf over again to cool.
Actually, I think mini-mini loaves are the most successful —
about 6 or 7 inches long and 1½ -2 inches in diameter. If you
have to make sandwiches you would either make them "can-
ape"-size or slice the little loaves the long way.

With sour-dough bread, Iona Teeguarden of *Freedom through
Cooking* suggests starting at 375° to "kill the smell." But after
about 15 minutes of that, I think the oven should be cooled
for a while and then the baking started again at 150° for one
hour, and continued as above.

Unleavened bread is always best if toasted — especially if you
get one of those "wet" loaves! And the best way to toast it is in a
small electric oven-broiler appliance. I find mine indispensable for
toasting (since unleavened bread is likely to have funny shapes, and
flat breads are too thick for regular toasters), and for warming many
of our other foods. If you object to abusing the ecology by buying
still another electrical gadget to drain our energy supplies, you
could use the broiler on your stove.

Back to baking techniques: even the batter breads ("flat
bread") will be more successful if the slow-oven process is
followed. Smooth the batter onto a lightly oiled cookie sheet,
making it less than ½ -inch thick. After the first hour — or
whenever the hot batter becomes manageable, cut it into large
squares and turn it over, just as for loaf bread, and cover with
foil. (You can use those large sheets of foil several times.) Complete the baking process as above, and turn over again to cool.
Toast to serve.

All these breads (as well as all other macrobiotic foods!) have
a better flavor the second day and thereafter.

Be sure these natural flours are always thoroughly cooked.
Otherwise, you may have to chew raw rice for a few days to clear out
intestinal parasites. Additionally, remember the approximate 15
percent-85 percent ground-grain-to-whole-grain ratio mentioned
under "Beneficial" at the beginning of this chapter.

Healthy people may eat yeasted bread, provided it's at least
second-day and well-toasted. There are many recipes for this kind
of bread in your macrobiotic cookbooks; or you can now usually
buy loaves of excellent bread in natural-foods stores. (If buying any-

where else, read the ingredients!) Dependable unleavened bread is
also sometimes available in natural-foods stores. So maybe all you'll
have to bake, to have variety, will be "flat" or batter breads. We'll
give you one example of an unleavened loaf bread and a couple of
examples of flat breads. Eating these is good exercise — a small bite
will give you a mouthful by the time you chew it enough to swallow.
And it gives you more flavor all the time!

(mm) *Unleavened Rice Bread:* In a large bowl, rub together between
your palms 4 C w-w flour and 4 C cooked rice. If the rice is
slightly sour, all the better! Or sour spaghetti is also good. The
bread will taste slightly cheesy. Add a scant t solar or sea salt,
¼ C sesame seeds, 2 T oil, and enough water to knead. Knead
at least 5 minutes, but the longer the better. Place in a lightly
oiled bowl, coat the top of the loaf with a little oil, cover with a
towel, and leave 6 hours or overnight in a warm place. Knead
again, adding more flour to again make a dough consistency.
Shape into loaves, according to instructions in (ll), and set
aside for one more hour. Make horizontal slits in the top of the
loaves and bake according to (ll). *Safe.*

Gloria's Wheatless Flat Bread: Toast 2 C rolled oats and 1 C
sesame seeds (see "More Toasting," earlier in this chapter). In
a large bowl, combine 2 C rye flour, 1 C rice flour, 1 C corn
meal, 2 t salt, and add ¼ C corn oil. Mix well, and then mix in
the toasted ingredients. Add enough warm water to make
dough, and knead for 7 minutes. Spread the dough evenly onto
a lightly oiled cookie sheet, smoothing it with oiled hands and
rubber spatula. Bake according to (ll); cool on linen cloth. *Safe.*

Moon Squares: (so-called because our Cooks at the Harvest
Moon experimented for some time to perfect them. Veralu,
Ruth, Rick, Teresa, Barbara, Cheryl, and others, as they came
and went, all contributed.) Blend 1 C dried apples cut in small
pieces, 3/4 C sunflower seeds, and water to cover. In a large
bowl mix 3 C w-w pastry flour, 3 T arrowroot, ¼ C corn meal,
1 t salt, 3 T oil. Add ¼ C sunflower seeds, and occasionally
sneak in a few raisins. Add the blended mix, spread the batter
onto an oiled cookie sheet, and proceed as for the Flat Bread,
above. Or, *for a safe version,* use onions and carrots and/or
parsnips and/or squash, chopped and sauteed so that you have
about 3 C sauteed vegetables, blended with 2½ C water. Or,
blend *any* leftover vegetables. These vegetable blends would
replace the blended mix in the Apple Moon Squares — and of
course you'd never put raisins in Vegetable Moon Squares.

Waffles: Comes now this Jean Kohler with his baker's hat on,
such a tall hat that it's a good thing it's only imaginary! You

should see the flair with which he dips out into a large bowl or pitcher those 2 heaping cups of w-w pastry flour and 1 heaping cup of buckwheat flour! They are rather easy-going measurements, but you'd better not have even one extra grain in that 1 t salt, or one extra drop in the 1/3 C of sesame oil. Stir in 4 C water, humming contentedly, and then add about one more C water, till the consistency is just the RIGHT degree of runny. Since there's no leavening, the batter has to be thin. Actually, it's better if it stands at room temperature for 4 hours or overnight; the second day you may have to add a little more water. When the waffle iron is preheated and lightly oiled, you pour a *thin* coating of batter, with just the right p-f-f-ss-ss sound, pouring slowly in a circular motion — counterclockwise, please, in harmony with the Universe — to coat the griddle evenly. The waffles should come out brown and crisp, and taste a little bit like the cone for an ice cream cone (tsk, tsk!). In warm weather w-w flour should replace the buckwheat. We eat these plain, crisping them again lightly in the toaster after the first day, but you might once in a while coat them with a very little apple butter from a natural-foods store. They can be a help in lunch boxes (see below). *Safe.*

Pancakes: You can use the same batter as for waffles. Place a heavy skillet on low heat; when warm, lightly coat the surface with an oiled pastry brush. Preheat the skillet, testing with a drop of batter; but don't let the skillet get so hot it smokes. Ladle the batter into the skillet to form very thin pancakes. When bubbles appear, turn pancakes over. Because they have no leavening, these pancakes must be cooked very slowly and turned often so that the inside will cook before the outside scorches. Serve as for waffles; or you might use a thin coating of one of the sauce recipes. Toast the next day in the broiler — another lunch-box possibility. *Safe.*

Gloria's Tortillas: In a large bowl thoroughly mix 1¼ C corn meal, 2½ C w-w flour, ¼ C sesame seeds, 1 t salt. Add warm water to make a dough and knead for 2 minutes. Oil a breadboard and rolling pin with corn oil, roll up balls of dough in your hands, flatten them with the rolling pin into thin circles, and cook them on a lightly oiled griddle or skillet, a few seconds at a time on each side, turning frequently till they brown. Same uses as for waffles. Or, wrap them around cooked beans and serve as a main dish. *Safe.*

Moonsavers: (We call them this because we cut them with a doughnut cutter and hope they save people from chemicalized snacks.) Mix together 3/4 C corn meal, 3/4 C w-w flour, 1 C w-w pastry flour, ½ C sesame seeds, and 1½ t salt. Stir in ¼ C corn oil and mix until the ingredients form into beads. Add very warm, but not hot, water to make dough. Roll out about 1/8-inch thick on floured surface. Cut into desired shapes, with a doughnut cutter or whatever else you wish. Bake at 375° for 30 minutes. For variety, part of the water could be replaced with flavoring from cooked vegetables (Recipe (c), or with a little corn-barley malt syrup; or invent your own variations.

Prowl through the macrobiotic cookbooks for other snacks to add interest to meals — various crackers, and karinto (don't miss this one as soon as you can have tempura!).

(nn) *Macrobiotic Pizza:* For crust: Mix 2 C w-w flour or pastry flour, ½ C sesame seeds, ½ t salt, 2 T corn oil, and enough water to make dough. Knead 3 minutes. Roll out on floured board. Place on oiled and floured pizza pan and trim the edges. (You can also use ordinary pie pan.) Bake at 425° for 5-7 minutes. *Filling:* A great variety of combinations or vegetables, grains, and sauces. For example: Mix ¼ C tahini with ½ C cool water and 1 T tamari. 2 T gravy, as in (jj) above, could be added if you have it on hand. Add 2 T arrowroot and mix in well. Add 1 C fine-chopped sauteed vegetables of your choice, plus 1 to 2 C cooked rice, or less rice and some cooked bulghur; or 1 to 2 C cooked millet; or 1 C rice and 1 C millet; or cooked macaroni or cooked chopped spaghetti. Spread filler on crust, top with bread crumbs and seeds if desired, and bake at 425° for another 5 to 7 minutes. Sprinkle with sprouts (Recipe (h) to serve, if you like. *Safe,* if you can have tahimi; if not, use a sauce that is on your list. When you're really well you can sprinkle a little organic grated cheese around on the top before baking.

Pie Crust (one double crust — 9 inch): Mix 3 C w-w pastry flour, ½ t salt, ½ C sesame seeds (optional, but *good*). Cut in ¼ C corn oil. Add water to dough consistency and knead 3 minutes, or, as they always say, "to the consistency of your ear lobe." Press out on wax paper, cover with wax paper, and roll out between the papers to pie-crust thickness (or "thin-ness"). *Safe,* but don't eat too much because of being attentive to the percentage of oil and the percentage of ground grain in your food balance. For a delicious *Safe* filling to brighten your macrobiotic strict diet, refer to Mari's Recipe (p).

Oatmeal Crust: Pan roast 2 C of oatmeal until it gives off a nut-like aroma; pan roast ½ C corn meal. Mix the toasted cereal into 1/3 C corn-barley malt syrup to which you have added a scant t salt. Add enough warm water to make a consistency to press into a pie pan. Bake after adding a filling of your choice.

DESSERTS

(oo) *Fruit Pie:* For parties, or for you sometimes after you're "out of the woods": Put 2 C dried apples in a pan with 2 T raisins, pinch of salt, and a small amount of water. Simmer till partially softened. Cool, place in pie shell, sprinkle with 1 or 2 T roasted carob powder and 4 T arrowroot. Cover with top crust and flute the edges, making slits in the top crust; or, make a lattice top. Bake at 350° for 40-50 minutes until lightly brown; in Pyrex use a 325° oven setting.

Gloria's Peaches 'n' Cream Pie: Soak 1½ C dried peaches in salt water for about 10 minutes (a scant t salt to 2 C water). Drain and rinse. Cook in 4 C water and ½ t salt for 20 minutes. Puree in blender, put back in pan, and add 3/4 C arrowroot softened in a little cool water. Cook over medium heat, stirring constantly until thick. Allow to cool and pour into the pie shell of your choice. Bake at 300° for 40 minutes. You could also make an Apple Cream Pie or an Apricot Cream Pie.

Carob Pie: Blend till smooth 1 C almonds and 1 quart water. Add ¼ C corn-barley malt syrup. Mix ½ C arrowroot, ¼ C roasted carob powder, ½ t salt. Slowly add the almond liquid to dry ingredients. Mix well and cook over medium heat, stirring until thick. Cool and pour into pie shell; refrigerate to set. Makes one deep 10-inch pie. A very yin dessert — go easy!

(pp) *Rice Pudding:* Mix ¼ C pure maple syrup or ⅓ C corn-barley malt syrup, ⅔ C oat powder, 1 T arrowroot, ½ t salt, 2½ C water. Cook over medium heat 10-15 minutes, stirring often. When mixture thickens, add 4 C cooked rice and ¼ C coarse-blended raisins.

(qq) *Kanten desserts* (also called agar-agar): We promised weight-losers some ideas for using this seaweed which has no calories but is high in minerals. A basic way to cook the kanten is to break one bar in 1½ C water and soak 10 minutes. Bring to a boil, stir to dissolve, add a pinch of salt and 1½ C apple juice, which I hope you're allowed to have if used in this manner. Simmer the mixture 10 minutes. If you can have fruits in season, arrange small pieces of fruit on the bottom of a flat dish and pour the kanten mix over it. Chill for about 2 hours. Or, if you've been given the go-ahead to use dried fruit, cut it in small pieces and cook it with the kanten. Or, in place of apple juice use juices in which sweet vegetables were cooked, such as we suggested reserving in Recipe (c). Puree cooked, sweet vegetables and add to the hot kanten. Or, in place of fruit, use fine-grated carrots and a little fine-shredded cabbage.

(rr) *Kanten Whip* (an ice cream substitute): Break up 1 bar of
kanten and soak the pieces 10 minutes in 1 quart of apple
juice, adding "2 pinches" of salt. Simmer 10 minutes, or until
kanten is dissolved. Chill a couple of hours, until kanten is set.
Whip in the blender till frothy. Keep chilled to serve, and if it
jells again, whip it again. Try also 1 C pureed cooked dried
apples and/or apricots, mixed with hot kanten (1 bar cooked
in 2 C water), chilled and then whipped. These are for hot
weather only, of course, and are obviously not for the strict
diet.

Soy Ice Cream: Most people don't seem to mind the slightly
"grainy" consistency of the soy powder. Mix 1 C soy powder,
2 C water, 2 T oil, ¼ t salt, ¼ -½ C pure maple syrup, 1 t slip-
pery elm. Add 1 C roasted carob powder; or, use chopped
dried, cooked fruit for flavoring, blended if you prefer. Follow
the manufacturer's instructions for your ice-cream freezer.
Four times the above measurements will be the amount for a
5-quart freezer. (Soy powder is very, very yin, so please govern
your servings accordingly!)

COOKIES

Cookies without soda or any other leavening agent will have to be
baked slower and longer than you might expect. They should be thin
in order to bake all the way through and turned over a time or two to
help them bake evenly. For special occasions you can add a few
raisins to almost any of them, so we'll not repeat that in every recipe.

Wheat Berry: Whoever invented these should have a macrobiotic
medal, for they are both *Safe* and sweet without sweeteners! (There
is a slightly bitter "aftertaste," but that's a minor disadvantage for
those who will be allowed very few desserts for a few weeks; and it's
not the *harmful* aftertaste of chemical sweeteners.) Use 3 C wheat
berry sprouts (Recipe (h) blended at medium speed in enough water
to cover, making a thick paste. Add w-w pastry flour with ½ t salt to
make a stiff cookie batter. Lightly oil a cookie sheet and your palms.
Flatten balls of batter with your hands to form medium thin cookies.
Bake at 350° for about 25 minutes, till lightly browned on both sides.
Gloria's skill has made these a popular item at our restaurant. Mari
uses more water, to make a consistency to drop from a teaspoon onto
the cookie sheet, baking at 300° till brown and crisp.

Pumpkin (or butternut squash or acorn squash): Saute 1 small fine-
chopped onion till translucent, add thin-sliced parsnips and pumpkin

or squash cut in 1-inch cubes (enough that you will have about 2 C of vegetables). Saute till the squash or pumpkin color deepens. Add a little hot water and simmer till squash is tender. Cool and beat the mixture till creamy. Mix ¼ C sesame oil and ¼ C corn-barley malt syrup (or 3 T pure maple syrup) and add to the pumpkin mixture. Sift 4 C w-w pastry flour, 2 T raw carob powder, and ½ t salt. Mix the dry ingredients with the pumpkin mixture. 1 C sunflower seeds would be optional but delicious. Press into flat cookies on a lightly oiled sheet. Try 300° till lightly browned. *Safe* IF you omit the syrup, in which case you could mix 4 T arrowroot with the dry ingredients.

Oatmeal: Cut dried apples in small pieces to make ½ C. Blend for a few seconds in 3/4 C water; stir in ¼ C oil and 3 T corn-barley malt syrup or 2 T pure maple syrup. Mix 5 C rolled oats, 1½ C w-w pastry flour, ½ C sunflower seeds, ½ C bulghur *or* corn meal, 2 t arrowroot. Stir the apple mixture into the dry mixture. With dampened hands form small balls and press into flat cookies on a lightly oiled cookie sheet. 300° till lightly browned. For a plainer version, try mixing 1½ C rolled oats, ¼ t salt, 1 T oil, 3/4 C water, ½ C apple juice, and 3 T sunflower seeds.

Carob: Mix 1¼ C water, 2 t oil, ¼ C corn-barley malt syrup. Mix 4 C w-w pastry flour, 1½ C roasted carob powder, ½ C sunflower seeds, water to make dough consistency. Mix all ingredients together, form small balls and press into flat cookies on a lightly oiled cookie sheet. Bake at 300°, but they're so dark you can't tell whether they've "browned." Try 35-40 minutes.

Carrot Brownies: Mix ½ C water, or sometimes apple juice, ¼ C corn-barley malt syrup or 3 T pure maple syrup, 2 T oil. Mix 2 C w-w pastry flour, 2 T raw or roasted carob powder, 2 T arrowroot, ½ t salt. Mix ingredients together and add 1 C grated carrots. Spread thin in an oiled baking dish. 350° for 45 minutes.

Almond Gems (for parties): Mix 1 C sesame oil and ½ C pure maple syrup or corn-barley malt syrup. Add a mix of 2 C w-w pastry flour, ½ t salt, and 1½ C toasted, coarse-ground almonds. Shape into walnut-size balls (leave them that way — don't flatten!) and bake on a lightly oiled cookie sheet at 350° for about 20 minutes or until lightly brown.

Carob Sparkles (for parties): Toast 2 C soy powder mixed with 3/4 C sunflower seeds. Mix 3/4 C roasted carob powder and 1 C corn-barley malt syrup. Mix all ingredients together, make small balls 1 inch or less in diameter; roll in toasted sesame seeds.

These examples should give you enough to go on till you can get acquainted with some macrobiotic cookbooks. The key word

with all of them is *"omit."* Learn carefully the list of harmful foods
and leave them out of your versions of the recipes. You can learn to
dream up substitutes for some things, such as 1 t raw carob powder
(also yin, however, so don't overdo it) in place of cinnamon, arrowroot in place of egg, umeboshi plum juice (Recipe (f), in place of
vinegar or wine or grated lemon peel, *nothing* in place of mint and
other heady herbs and spices! There are infinite ideas that you *can*
use, however, in these books. In addition to recipes, you'll find lists
of yin and yang foods, nutriments in various foods, protein compari-
sons, sketchy menus, and an affectionate respect for the food, char-
acterized by Iona Teeguarden's humility in saying her book was
written not *by* herself but *through* Iona Teeguarden.

Beverages in Macrobiotic Land can be quickly dealt with. Mostly it's
bancha tea, unless you want to count the two cups of soup that most
people can have each day. As we mentioned before, all those teas in
the Muramoto *Healing Ourselves* are for specialized use and should
not be experimented with unless you check it out with macrobiotic
friends. In a moment we'll mention a couple that are OK to use sometimes. For an occasional change from bancha tea you could drink
cereal grain coffee (see recipe books), or "tea" made from roasted
grains; but they're not in the same league with bancha tea. If you are
healthy, you can have fruit juices on special occasions in hot weather,
and beer once in a while. This is all on a different level from the custom of constant guzzling which has become a national and international habit! After you get used to the new way you're just not
thirsty.

Foods for lunch boxes: If yeasted bread (at least second-day, and
toasted, remember) is allowed, you can make sandwiches with the
various spreads in Recipe (kk), or with seitan (ah-h-h!) (Recipe (t).
Don't forget to use alfalfa or mung bean sprouts (Recipe (h) on sandwiches, or in salads with chopped lettuce, radishes, carrots, or whatever, wrapped in plastic paper. Sometimes include a little "Pressed"
salad (Recipe (g). Leftover casseroles wrapped in foil are very helpful,
especially if you can find some other method of warming them besides in a microwave oven. (Prop the foil packet up on a work-lamp
for a while, maybe?) Rice Balls (Recipe (1) are a *must,* of course.

A thermos of Clear Soup (r) could be either a prelude or a postlude
to the meal, but is not drunk *with* the food, remember. If the soup is
to precede the meal, then a little bancha tea in another (glass-lined)
thermos could be used as a chaser. Now if you have to use unleavened
breads your sandwiches may look kinda funny, but will be delicious.
Your rice bread (mm) may hold together better if you slice the pieces
in half after toasting when you make the sandwich. Or you can use

toasted leftover waffles, but don't toast them too much or the edges will get so hard you can't bite through. If your vegetable Moon Squares are thick enough, you can slice them through the middle and toast the insides a little in the broiler. And Gloria's Tortillas should work very well. You'll no doubt have to open up all unleavened sandwiches and eat them open-faced, or you won't be able to bite through the bread. Better pack an extra napkin. You can let everyone else in your outfit do the gossiping while you chew. But you'll have the *heartiest* lunch of all! (The unleavened breads are all part of Recipe (mm).)

Menus: Macrobiotic recipe books will give you a small insight into variations for location and season. Someday I want to try a few weeks (and maybe then lots longer!) of the kind of routine Mari had in her student days in Japan. That was like this:

Breakfast: Miso Soup (maybe with tofu, green onions, and wakame; or, with aburage, Spanish onions, and wakame; or, with daikon, green onions and wakame). Rice with nori crumbled over it. Charcoal-dried small fish. Pressed salad. Natto with soy sauce and chopped green onions. (Natto is not in our recipes, as few Westerners would relish it: very (phew!) fermented soybeans, very nutritious if you can get near enough to get used to it. It seems they would eat Natto for a few days and then omit it for a few days.)

Lunch: Clear Soup, sometimes. A noodle dish with vegetables (perhaps in tempura) on top. Rice Balls, and perhaps a "sushi" dish. (If I understand it right, "sushi" means various combinations of rice and vegetables in sweet-sour flavoring.) Occasionally they would have some fruit, in season, no doubt.

Supper: Clear Soup, sometimes with tempura vegetables, but not if they had tempura for lunch. Steamed fish. Vegetables prepared, perhaps, as in the "Nishime" recipe (c). Rice with tamari, or Red Rice with sesame seeds. Pressed salad. A possible dessert (?!) might be sweetened azuki beans.

Miso Soup *is* the very best way to begin the day, to pull yourself back together again after the yin night. Use hacho miso in the winter, and probably kome miso (Chapter 12) in the summer. Hopefully, you've made Miso Soup the day before so that all you have to do for breakfast is warm it.

Breakfast also calls for a bowl of rice, of course. As for ourselves, we have this almost one hundred percent of the time, usually with toasted wakame crumbled over it. Other ways to vary rice are suggested under "Cooking grains," earlier in this chapter. Barley, soft white wheat, hard red winter wheat, and millet, for example, may be either added to or cooked with brown rice. Sometimes you could boil sunflower seeds for a few minutes in just a little water and add them to rice while it's warming. (This combination reminds me of mashed potato flavor. Macrobiotic practice would consider it more acceptable to use *toasted* sunflower or sesame seeds.) Leftover vegetables are very good mixed with cooked rice for variety. Maybe once a week you can cook chopped dried apples and/or apricots, and a very few raisins, boiling them in a little water till it is almost evaporated, and mix the fruit with cooked rice. Leftover casserole is often very good for breakfast. Millet is an excellent breakfast grain, cooked with fine-chopped green onions and a few lentils for flavor. When cold, it may be sliced, sauteed, and served with a thin coating of a sauce from the above recipes (jj). We always warm small pieces of unleavened bread to eat with our rice. Then we have a little bancha tea if we want it.

Lunch is often small servings of casserole with sauce or gravy, and rice with gomasio (f) or vegetable sauce, even if the main ingredient in the casserole is rice. We have lettuce, a little raw cabbage, or any other [approved] raw vegetable we happen to want. We eat these unadorned, but you could use gomasio, or plum juice (f), or an approved dressing from macrobiotic cookbooks. We might have a little rice-bread toast. One or two cookies from the above recipes, plus a little bancha tea, would complete the meal.

Supper might go something like this: Miso Soup made with kale, bits of tofu, and onions, in the basic stock of course. "Cantonese" vegetables (Recipe (b), served over rice. We might have "seconds" on rice, with a couple of tablespoons of azukis on top. Carrots prepared as in Recipe (a). Small serving of leftover three-grain casserole (make up your own recipe for this). "Pumpkin" cookies made with squash. Bancha tea. OR: Clear Soup with noodles in it. Tempura vegetables served with rice, and we might put a little kuzu sauce on the rice. Azuki bean kanten (Recipe (o). Squash pie (Recipe (p). A few sips of bancha tea. OR: Clear Soup with leftover tempura. "Nishime"-type vegetables as in Recipe (c), which might sometimes include bits of seitan (t) instead of tofu cubes. Boiled kale mixed with toasted sesame seeds; or, sometimes sauteed and simmered green beans mixed with toasted sesame seeds ground slightly in a suribachi, plus a little tamari, served cool. Waffle square. A little bancha tea.

All the foods used in the macrobiotic way of eating are actively beneficial to health. To make this idea more graphic for you, when you are thinking grateful thoughts for your meals, we can give a few examples of the way Oriental medicine assigns foods rather than drugs to bring about specific improvements:

Lung troubles: at least once a day a side dish of root vegetables such as carrots, burdock, daikon, etc. Control liquids, drinking only when thirsty.

Kidney and bladder: beans often, very moderate intake of salt (sometimes temporarily eliminated entirely).

Heart trouble: use round vegetables like cabbage, and whole round grains, avoiding crushed grain or flour products.

Liver and gall bladder: plenty of leafy green vegetables. Oil — sesame and corn only — in moderate amounts.

Spleen, pancreas, stomach: no animal foods; use cooked round vegetables and grains, and some beans and seeds, every day.

Intestines and sex organs: Miso Soup (which contains seaweed, salt, and bacteria from the fermented miso, all in liquid form) every day, for these organs correspond to the moist, dark, warm environment of the ancient primordial ocean (see genetic diseases, end of Chapter 8).

Mr. Kushi has devised a generalized list of foods helpful in the recovery from yin cancer and from yang cancer (see Chapter 8). (If you have a cancer which is not definitely in either the yin or the yang category, you should check with a macrobiotic center (in our Appendix) for aid in devising a middle-of-the-road diet.) In any case, of course, chewing each bite 100-200 times is essential.

Cancer from yin cause; Grains — 50 percent-70 percent of total intake // Gomasio — 1 part salt to 8 to 10 parts of sesame seeds // Miso Soup or tamari broth — rather strong // Vegetables — longer cooking (10-14 minutes), slightly salty // Beans — azuki, garbanzo, lentils // Seaweed — longer cooking, stronger taste. Hiziki is recommended // Beverage — strong bancha tea or grain coffee; sometimes Mu tea (see macrobiotic cookbooks) // Salad — none, or occasionally (preferably boiled for 3 minutes) // No fruit or nuts // Oil — sesame only, and as little as possible // Animal or dairy food — none, except very small quantity of fish, preferably little fishes cooked in soup.

Cancer from yang cause: Grains — 40 percent-50 percent of total intake // Gomasio — 1 part salt to 10 to 14 parts of sesame seeds // Miso Soup or tamari broth — rather weak // Vegetables — shorter cooking (2-10 minutes), almost no salt // Beans — variety of beans // Seaweed — shorter cooking time, not too strong in flavor. Wakame, nori, dulse are good // Beverage — weak bancha tea or grain coffee; NO Mu tea//salad — up to 10 percent of the day's food. Frequently use boiled salad, adding chopped vegetables to boiling water for 2 or 3 minutes, with tamari if desired; or saute 2 or 3 minutes, adding a pinch of salt // Fruit — occasionally, if there is a craving for it. Use dried or cooked local fruits, or a very small quantity of fresh local fruits in season. No fruit juice. A few nuts, preferably almonds, are allowable // Oil — sesame or corn oil may be used sparingly in cooking. No raw oil // No animal or dairy food.

Kuzu is often used as a food to relieve various digestive symptoms. It may seem expensive, but not if you compare it with commercial nostrums. It should be kept on hand as a friendly helper. Grown in Japan, it is a root some 3 or 4 feet long, and therefore is very yang and soothing. It is sold in a starch-like form. Use about one tablespoon per cup of hot liquid (water, kombu stock, etc.), but soften the kuzu first in a little cool water. Some cooked rice may be added to the mixture, if desired. Simmer a few minutes, stirring till the mixture thickens and clears, adding tamari to taste. It is best to take it an hour before meals, especially before breakfast. Having a slight resemblance to chicken broth, it is a pleasant treat you can use occassionally if you're "starving" late at night, yet know you shouldn't eat anything for three hours before retiring. (Don't tell Boston we suggested sneaking in this little snack!) *Postscript:* We've learned that those awful vines that seem to be choking out acres of forest vegetation in many southern and mid-southern states are *kuzu* vines! Someone should form a company to excavate the roots and thus eliminate many of the vines. The company could prosper and the price of kuzu might begin to compare with that of arrowroot.

Umeshoban tea (listed in *Healing Ourselves* on page 88 as "Plum-Soy-Ginger-Bancha Drink") is good to relieve chilling. Bring a cup of bancha tea to a boil (forget about retaining enzymes in this case!), add half an umeboshi plum, 5 drops of juice from grated ginger, and 1 t of tamari. In spite of the praise the Muramoto book expresses for this drink, it is too yang to be used very often.

Compresses are *external* uses of foods! You can't believe the benefit from compresses of this type until you see it happen. We can give instructions for a couple of the most common ones, so that you'll have them easily available in case macrobiotic friends suggest their use before you can get any books to help. (Mr. Kushi's *Book of Macrobiotics,* incidentally, includes some good pages (129-134) on this topic.)

Ginger compress: Buy the large "fat" roots often available in groceries (not the small, hard "un-grate-able" ones from drug stores). If you don't find them, ask the grocer to try to order a supply. Meanwhile, you *can* use the powdered ginger. Tie the ginger (2 heaping table-spoons grated, per 1 quart of water, or about 2 teaspoons powdered) in cheesecloth and drop it into boiling water. After that keep the water hot, but not boiling. Press on the cheesecloth with the back of a tablespoon until the water turns slightly yellow. Fold a terry cloth hand towel the long way, twist it a little, and dip the middle of it into hot water, holding the two ends so that you can handle it without burning your hands. Twist out the water enough that it doesn't drip, and apply to the afflicted area. The patient should be ready to lift it several times for a second or two till the skin gets used to the heat; but it should be as hot as he or she can withstand. Dip the cloth three times in ten minutes, covering the patient to avoid chilling while you "re-dip." The skin should turn very pink. For people with very bad circulation a half-hour of application may be necessary. If there is any water left, it may be used again, for up to 24 hours.

Taro potato compress (also called "albi," and by Puerto Ricans "yuca"): See early in this chapter for places to buy; in cities you may find these potatoes at Oriental stores or Puerto Rican stores. Buy young, small, light-colored ones if possible (which may be called "jinenjo"). If you just can't find taro potatoes, you may be able to find albi powder at the above stores or some natural-foods stores or some drug stores. (Or, see Variation, below.) Mix grated potato with 5 percent-10 percent grated ginger, then mix in ordinary white flour, which is "pastier" than w-w flour. Use from 1/5 to nearly 1/2 flour, depending on how wet the grated potato is; you should have a spread-able paste, ¼-inch to ½-inch thick. Wrap the mixture in cheesecloth and shape it large enough to cover the afflicted area. Use first a ginger compress to warm the area thoroughly; then apply the taro plaster. Cover with muslin (pieces of old sheets are good for this). In some areas the plaster will have to be held on with tape; in others, with wide bands of cloth pinned around the area, such as a wide sash of the muslin pinned around the upper or lower abdomen, etc. Leave on, usually, 4 hours or overnight.

Variation with common potato of the grocery-store variety, if nothing else is available: coarse-blend potato and an equal amount of some kind of greens — weeds, or in winter any *dark* greens available as food from the grocery. Then add the other ingredients as for the taro potato compress. This variation is likely to be messy and somewhat smelly, so wear old bedclothes or else you will be trying to take out stains with ecology-poisoning bleaches. These applications are often continued for 2 to 4 weeks, but check your case with your macro-biotic center or the East West Foundation. You'll be amazed at the inflammation these plasters will pull out!

Thus is food used for physical improvement, internal and external, maximum benefits resulting from external applications only if the diet is what is should be. Then, of course, with *physical* betterment comes greater *mental* clarity. Aveline Kushi revealed the *spiritual* element which develops, in time, to become the intuition she mentioned as we entered the kitchen. Of this, Michio Kushi says, "That faculty of pure intuition, the highest form of thinking, is nothing but infinity itself, our true nature, which never dies."

Note for Chapter 13

[1]Aveline Kushi, *How to Cook with Miso* (Tokyo, Japan: Japan Publications, Inc., 1978).

CHAPTER 14

Case Histories (Second Hand)

Most of the stories we summarize in this chapter began before our time, macrobiotically speaking, and since (by ordering the East West Foundation Case Histories listed in the Bibliography) you can read them as their protagonists have written them, we'll give only very brief sketches. The first one, however, not included among the Case Histories, is unique, and is so fascinating that we'll tell that one somewhat in detail.

ISABEL AND ROBERT LANDES, et al

The Landes' live in Yellow Springs, Ohio. (But see the "Postscript" at the end of their story.) In 1972 Isabel had been nursing their second child for about fourteen months when she developed a severe case of viral pneumonia. There was also a "generalized rash," which one doctor's report considered to be a possible result of food supplements. Her diet had been Adele Davis's; yogurt, liver, brewer's yeast, wheat germ, molasses, much fresh and dried fruit, salads and super-protein. She naturally felt disillusioned with health-food routines, and especially when to her other weakness were added cystitis (with which she had had problems in the past) and a vaginal yeast infection. She traveled from specialist to specialist and finally by chance in Saratoga Springs, N.Y., met a girl who told her about macrobiotics. At the friend's suggestion, Isabel visited Mr. Kushi in Boston and began eating macrobiotically. Within three days she felt better, and in three weeks the cystitis and yeast infection had disappeared. Except for an occasional "small deviation," she still eats macrobiotically, and she credits Mr. Kushi with "giving me the courage to change myself."

Isabel didn't stop with healing herself. She has done much to instruct others in macrobiotic cooking, one night each week and one morning each week in her home. In August of 1975 she began a gourmet "International Food Center" in Yellow Springs.

223

Meanwhile, husband Bob had been skirting around the edges of macrobiotics, not feeling any need for a special diet because of being sure that he was in perfect health. In spite of being impressed with Isabel's recovery, he just never quite "made it" to get into the program for himself. Besides, his work kept him away from home for varying periods of time, so that it would have been difficult to get the food. His profession was training and racing horses. But when he was thirty-nine, severe arrhythmic heart beats developed, and atrial fibrillations catapulted him into the cardiac intensive care unit of the Springfield, Ohio, Community Hospital. His heart would stop and then would start beating wildly, 180-200 times a minute. He recovered enough to leave the hospital; but after that, more than a year of medication, and consultations with specialists and general practitioners, helped not one bit. They all said his heart could never be normal again. He had very limited energy for his work, and he said his "whole personality underwent rapid changes."

Finally, in late April of 1975, he visited Michio Kushi. After six weeks of following a fairly restricted macrobiotic diet most of his symptoms disappeared. Within six to eight months he was jogging three or four miles a day and working full days. Eighteen months later he spoke of feeling ten years younger than he did before his trip to Boston. "I thank God that I have a beautiful wife who cooks me wonderful meals. Without her it would have been very difficult for me." Aside from times when he was thinking about Isabel, his heart — which doctors had predicted could never be normal — was again beating normally, at age 42. By late 1976 he was driving in races again, something he had thought he would never be able to do.

As if all that were not amazing enough, listen to this: Bob and Isabel found out that Michio was going to visit the Ball State campus in Muncie in January of 1976, and they asked him whether he might stop in Yellow Springs for a couple of days on the way. This was arranged, and on short notice they got 500 people to turn out for a Kushi lecture. (How could they do *that,* when we worked like beavers for several months and had half that many?!) Bob drove Michio from Yellow Springs to Muncie, so we had the pleasure of meeting and visiting with him. And what he told us left us gasping! Early in his acquaintance with macrobiotics he had begun to figure that if it worked so well for people, it ought to work also for horses! They would be perfect "students," he reasoned, because they were dependent on the food they were given and would not have the choice of going off on a binge as people often do.

He was taking care of a twelve-year-old former champion

pacer, Good Knight Lobell, now arthritic and unable to race. The horse was in pain, with large calcium deposits in his ankles and knees, and had a vicious disposition. His monetary value had dropped from $25,000 to $200. Bob took away all sweet feed, which, he says, for horses as well as humans is absolute poison, since, just as for people, it drains minerals from the system and gives a horse artificial "highs" with subsequent "lows." The water intake was controlled, and the horse had free access to salt — but sea salt rather than commercial salt. Bob adjusted Lobell's food by trial and error until the horse tamed down considerably. Moreover, he took Lobell to Florida, having learned from a horse magazine that there was a veterinarian there who could administer acupuncture, a treatment now becoming somewhat widely used by veterinarians. After three weeks of treatments this horse who could barely walk when Bob started his therapy won three races in a row at Pompano Beach Park! This was in the winter of 1974. The purse for the third race — a claiming race — was about $700-$800, and Lobell was "claimed away" from Bob for $2000. Sadly enough, the new trainer laughed at the diet-acupuncture therapy, and within two weeks Lobell was again unable to race.

Another lame horse, a trotter with terrible ankles, was in Bob's care later on and returned to good condition with a macrobiotic diet, acupuncture, and swimming-pool training instead of trotting. Bob then worked him out for ten days and he won the first race he entered, besting his own previous record. The owner quit business, sold the horse, and Bob didn't hear any more about him.

Bob said he was planning to continue his experiments on a larger scale. Jean asked about cooking some foods for horses, since cooking is an important principle in macrobiotic beliefs. The reply was that actually it's not uncommon to give horses cooked grain as a treat after a race. He's going to try using oats and corn (the more yin grains) in the summer, cooked buckwheat and seaweed in winter. And he's going to see what soy meal will do for horses.

Macrobiotic all the way, the Landes family feed their dog the same diet they eat, for if his majesty reverts to commercial food those mournful basset-hound eyes become very bloodshot.

So how's that for a story! We've considered it a privilege to be acquainted with Isabel and Bob, and we're happy to have this opportunity to introduce them to you.

Postscript: A letter from the Landes' in March of 1978 contained the big surprise that they had enjoyed a winter in Florida and were planning to move there — to Lake Worth — in September! Isabel captured the essence of the adaptation of macrobiotic food when she wrote, "We learn a lot about macrobiotics in this warm clime. Oranges and grapefruit are disaster for the teeth. Rice must be tamed with barley, oats, or corn — and 50 percent grains still seems a good rule." For example, she used a combination of 25 percent barley and 75 percent medium-grain rice, cooked without salt. She would wash the grain (say, 3 cups) and mix it with an equal amount of water. She pressure-cooked it, putting a few inches of water in the bottom of the cooker and then pouring in the grain-water mix, cooking it about 45 minutes.

She describes a good hot-weather condiment: 1 C roasted sesame seeds, 1 heaping T roasted wakame powder or kombu powder, ground in a suribachi till seeds are nicely crushed. (It sounds as if this would be less yang than gomasio with sea or solar salt, and therefore preferable in hot, yang weather.)

Isabel advises that fruit, even in warm climates, "should be eaten in small quantities, preferably cooked, not every day, and not by everybody!" She considers it better to keep cool by using boiled vegetables, a little less salt, more yin cooking, "or a long swim in the ocean. As always, individual goals and differences must be considered, but the best advice still seems to be to eat less, chew more and 'pray without ceasing.'"

(Our discussions concerning foods in relation to climate and location are in the early part of Chapter 9 and at the beginning of Chapter 13.)

Incidentally, getting back to pets for a moment, we've known other people who fed their dogs macrobiotic food. Our friend Mari tells us that Japanese people, who eat *very* little meat, give their dogs some fish scraps, plus the grains, beans, vegetables, seaweed, etc., that people eat. (In recent years, of course, commercial dog food is infiltrating Japan, preservatives, artificial coloring, dead vitamins, and all the rest of it.) Ida Honorof (you met her in Chapter 6) was telling us that when her daughter Faye was a teenager she had a dog who became very sick with distemper. After $200-worth of shots and other medication the veterinarian finally said that she might as well accept the inevitable and take the animal home to die. Once home, the dog lost control of every bodily function and collapsed on the kitchen floor in a very unpleasant mess. Its eyes rolled upward till only the whites showed, and Ida was sure they had a dead dog to dispose of. But Faye phoned brother Don, who hurried over and cooked some brown rice and a whole carp, which he boiled until even the bones were soft. The dog did rally enough to eat a little. They then fed the dog macrobiotically and it recovered completely except that the hind quarters never quite regained their original strength. After four years Faye had to leave home to go to college, so she gave the dog to a friend who continued the program for a while but who eventually became lax in keeping up with the dietary care. The dog became ill again but this time, sad to relate, had no one to come to its rescue.

So of macrobiotics and laboratory mice and men — and women and children and horses and dogs. There are gradual gains, but macrobiotics is still not exactly a "household word"!

We have three main purposes in giving synopses of some of the cases published by the East West Foundation. One is to show the variety of ailments thwarted by macrobiotics; the other two we'll point out later.

The first case has so much variety that we'll include a little more than an outline.

"PAUL AND BELLE KATZEN are alive and well and still living in Miami Beach" — on Bay Drive, to be more specific, where we phoned in March of 1977 to ask permission to include their story. That phone call was a stimulating experience, for they are very vital and enthusiastic people. When their story appeared in the EWF Case Histories (Summer, 1975) their ages were 68 and 69, and their physical symptoms had been these:

Belle: "a constant battle with fighting blackouts," shortness of breath, pains in chest, arms, jaw, and teeth. Three hospitalizations in 14 months had led to diagnosis and ineffective treatment, first for heart trouble, then for hiatal hernia, then for severe middle-ear disturbance. Eye problems developed, with less than one-fourth vision and danger of detached retina in the left eye; there was a similar threat for the right eye. Each day's routine included 15 pills.

Paul: paroxysmal heart attacks which according to the doctor were "nothing to be alarmed about," plus an arthritic condition in the neck, left knee, and toes, which the doctor said he would "just have to live with," plus constant headaches.

Then they heard about Michio Kushi, through friends in Pennsylvania whose son had studied with Michio in Boston and whose mother had cured migraine headaches through macrobiotics. They traveled to Boston, so that Belle could tell Michio her several complaints. As sometimes happens in the case of the partner who accompanies the "sick" person, Michio spotted more serious trouble for Paul than for Belle, and he told her privately that Paul's heart was in very bad shape. So they *both* began eating macrobiotically, and stopped all medication. After three days on the diet, Paul had a severe headache, but took no aspirin. And he hasn't had a headache since. On the fifth day all arthritic pains disappeared. After two macrobiotic months a "new" arthritic pain developed in his right knee, then disappeared in about a week. No arthritic discomforts have ever returned.

Paul had previously tried to increase his life insurance to comply with a requirement in the firm where he worked. However, the application was turned down because of a poor electrocardiogram. Some time "after Boston" his firm merged with a large national firm where he would also be a partner, but a complete medical checkup was required. He quoted his doctor as saying, after the examination, "Paul, I'm very pleased to report to you that your cardiogram shows absolutely normal. If you want to, you can get a million dollars' worth of insurance."

Now Belle, whose trip to Boston had unexpectedly brought about Paul's recovery, was checked by her opthalmologist five months after that trip, and improvement in the left eye was evident. Another year, another checkup — no cataract, no glaucoma, and two more lines read on the chart! Seven months after Boston her internist had found her blood pressure, blood count, cholesterol level, and general condition improved. A year after that, all was normal! Belle remarked that she was sure the hernia was gone. The doctor smiled indulgently and drew a diagram showing how the hernia could not be cured without surgery. But to please her he ordered a GI series of tests. Amazed, he announced that neither he nor his assistant could find any trace of a hernia. "Tell your Japanese friend to come to Pittsburgh and set up a center here!"

Naturally, Belle is very happy about the whole thing. She ended her account in the EWF history by asking, "Let me put it this way. How does one say, 'Thank you,' for getting another chance to live?"

Another very interesting person we'd like to tell you about is DR. RUTH S. SHAFFER, an osteopathic physician from Ardmore, Pennsylvania (Valley View Road). Dr. Shaffer spoke at the important EWF Seminar on Nutrition and Cancer we mentioned in Chapter 6, and she proved to have an entertaining style of presenting some significant information.

In 1948, at the age of only 38, she had a malignant tumor removed from the left breast. A resultant severe burn from X-ray therapy affected her left shoulder and arm. Nevertheless, she was in good health until June of 1973, when she began experiencing shortness of breath which she tried to tell herself was because of too many cigarettes. By September she was so lacking in energy that she "could barely walk thirty feet," but still she continued her practice, planning to ignore the cancer she strongly suspected in her left lung. Her food included fruit, milk, meat, butter, heavy cream, coffee, and rich desserts brought to her by her patients.

One patient who noticed she was not feeling well suggested Laetrile when she told him she was sure she had cancer. Deciding on the Laetrile route, Ruth went to the hospital for tests to confirm that there was indeed inoperable cancer. After three weeks of Laetrile treatment in Mexico, she brought back a supply to use at home. But in May of 1975 a liver scan showed the cancer had spread to that area. She was finally forced to discontinue her practice.

Then in July a student at the Philadelphia College of Osteopathic Medicine told her about Michio Kushi. After six strict macrobiotic months she had an X-ray which showed possible but not confirmed liver cancer, and a "cloudy" left lung. By May of 1976 tests showed the liver normal! The lung was still cloudy, and because of scar tissue she did not have full use of the lung, but she felt well and had lots of energy.

That much we knew from an EWF Case History Report. But in her talk at the Seminar, Dr. Shaffer recounted that when she was in Mexico she had made friends with eight other people who were trying Laetrile and she kept in touch with them. She who had rejected Laetrile in favor of the macrobiotic way had returned to her osteopathic practice, and was giving a speech crediting macrobiotics with much of her good fortune. The other eight were all dead.

The following are sketchy outlines of case histories typical of many now being compiled by the East West Foundation. Of course theirs are presented much more in detail, and make very interesting reading. Dates of birth are shown in parentheses.

MONA SCHWARTZ (8/11/35), c/o East West Foundation Center, P.O. Box 330892, 3043 Grand Avenue, Coconut Grove, Florida, 33133. Ideopathic edema, low-grade fever, high white blood cell count, kidney infection, thyroid condition. Tests included a lymph-node biopsy and a liver biopsy; leukemia was suspected. Treated by specialists for years, at a cost of thousands of dollars. Had fluid in the lungs and developed pneumonia. Was taking ten water pills daily, plus other medication: Potassium supplements, vitamins, drugs for thyroid trouble as well as for a kidney infection. Then began taking vibramycin, the strongest antibiotic (the last-resort drug). In April of 1974 she heard about macrobiotics and began following those principles and practices. There was a month by month improvement: the swelling went down, and in the summer of 1975 there was a normal red and white blood cell count for the first time in fifteen years. A snapshot shows a very trim and youthful figure. Mona is now a partner in the Miami branch of the East West Foundation at the above address.

EDWARD ESKO (10/16/1950), Boylston Street, Brookline, Massachusetts, 02146. Constant allergies, especially in the "hay fever" season. He had periodic severe attacks, with a particularly bad reaction to cats. When he was twenty, he discovered macrobiotics and realized that the allergies were caused by the quality of his blood, determined by what he had been eating rather than by external factors. After two days of macrobiotic food, he felt no discomfort when a cat slept on his bed! Other symptoms disappeared one by one.

Edward and his wife Wendy are members of the East West Foundation staff, so there have been references to them elsewhere in this book. We have found it necessary to have frequent contact with them for advice and information, in a relationship which for us has led to a feeling of warmth and friendship which we have found most pleasant. *Postscript:* Eskos infiltrate U.S. capital! See Appendix: WASHINGTON, D.C., for new EWF National Center.

WENDY ESKO (11/26/49), same as above. Anemia, sluggish mentality, pains in back, headaches, severe pains in right wrist and arm. Her food had included meat and much sugar, particularly in six to twelve bottles of carbonated drinks each day, especially during the five years after she was sixteen. She took "nerve" pills for headaches, and also had sharp pains in the kidney region during these years. In 1970 she began using drugs in order to be accepted by her friends, and consumed large quantities of candy, beer, wine, and meat. She became quite overweight, unable to concentrate or to remember anything she read. During this time she also had a very unpleasant scaling and itching condition in her ears. Severe pains developed in her right wrist and arm, for which casts, cortisone shots, and surgery for a pinched nerve were ineffective. In 1972 she learned of macrobiotics, and in time this new way of life brought complete relief from all her symptoms. In 1974 Wendy and Edward Esko became the parents of a very healthy Eric, and Wendy de-

scribes both the pregnancy and the natural birth as experiences
entirely free of problems. Then in 1976 Eric was joined by a baby
brother, again with no difficulties for mother or baby.

AUDREY ISAKSON (5/28/48), near Kennebunkport, Maine,
04046. Too frequent menstrual cycles, early in 1977; by mid-summer
as often as every week and a half. Complexion blemishes, constant
dull lower back ache. In July she began checking her symptoms
with doctors. While they were awaiting further developments in her
condition, she happened to visit a friend who was enrolled in the
East West Foundation's Intensive Macrobiotic Course at Amherst
College in Massachusetts (Summer, 1977), and she attended a Michio
Kushi lecture on — "of all things — the treatment of female disorders." Audrey had been already "softened up" by learning something about macrobiotics in the spring and had been making some
incomplete attempts at using a proper diet. After hearing Michio's
lecture she spent more time at Amherst and became aware that she
could heal herself by diet, but still lacked the conviction that diet
could be *more* effective than medical treatment. She did, however,
begin eating a larger percentage of macrobiotic food.

In early September the doctor diagnosed a growth (a dermoid
tumor the size of an orange!) on her right ovary. Because of the possibility of cancer, the recommendation was for surgery within a
month. She told the doctor she would consider it — and then had to
buck the typical advice from family and friends who begged her to
follow the medical route. But Audrey decided to try macrobiotics
first. A visit with Edward Esko, executive secretary of the East West
Foundation in Boston, provided still more detailed knowledge about
the macrobiotic way. She began using a strict food program, plus
daikon baths for a week, and taro plasters (see our Chapter 13)
over the tumor for two or three weeks. Edward said she should see
her doctor again in six weeks. In spite of increased pressure from
family and friends, she steered her own course, and says she became
"quite proficient at making taro plasters that stayed put and didn't
leave little bits of taro everywhere." (That's no small accomplish-
ment!) Luckily, she did receive "considerable support, especially in
'imaging' the healing process, from the friend who introduced her to
macrobiotics." (Compare with our previous examples of Simonton
techniques, Silva Mind Control courses, and other such devices.)
Audrey gives her own account of the results of her regimen:

> Slowly my skin began to clear and the back pain
> subsided. I knew changes were taking place, but the

"proof of the pudding" would be my upcoming appointment with the doctor.

My visit to the doctor that day seemed interminable. Because of one delay or another, it was several hours before she could examine me. To her amazement and to my delight, she could find no evidence of the tumor which had been so large just six weeks before. My ovary had returned to its normal size. I asked if perhaps her initial diagnosis could have been in error. She said no, she was certain I had a dermoid tumor. Not only was she sure of this diagnosis, but one of her associates who examined me at the time of her diagnosis was also sure. How could it be that the tumor had disappeared? She had never heard of or experienced such a reversal. She had no explanation. I told her a bit about macrobiotics. She said she wasn't a believer in that sort of thing, but that whatever I had been doing seemed to have worked. I asked again if she had any alternative explanation for what had occurred. She said she had none. But she did say that on the basis of the recent change in my condition it certainly wouldn't be necessary for me to undergo any surgical procedure.

I returned home and reported the results to those friends who had encouraged me to have surgery. They were pleased, amazed, delighted, but I assure you none of them was more delighted than I was. I knew that I had found a way of providing for my own health and well-being: macrobiotics.

To complete the process of improvement, by early 1978 the menstrual cycles had become regulated (in macrobiotic harmony) in accordance with lunar cycles.

KEN BURNS (11/1/34), Warren Street, Brookline, Massachusetts, 02146. Drugs. For two or three years Ken had been following a "life of drugs," which by the spring of 1966 had led to complete depression: mental, physical, and spiritual pain. Internal pressure made him feel he was being pulled to pieces; a deep burning sensation he had felt for years on his right side was intensified. He "felt eighty years old and wanted to 'curl up and die.'" A friend who had heard about a strange diet and who had just returned from a trip to New York to get some information about it, stopped at Ken's room in Detroit, saw that he was in even worse condition than usual, and silently handed him a book and walked away. The book was George Ohsawa's *Zen Macrobiotics* (see Bibliography). It had a powerful impact on Ken right where he needed help. He and his partner Ann

— of Armenian and Syrian descent and therefore comfortable in the presence of grains and vegetables — decided to try macrobiotics.

The following winter Michio Kushi came to Detroit to lecture. Ken and Ann were so much impressed that the following spring they moved to Boston "seeking guidance and encouragement. And we found it. How we found it! Seen from the long-view, our lives since becoming macrobiotic have taken on the soft glow of a fairy tale."

They lived in Vancouver for a while teaching the macrobiotic way, then in Seattle, for the same purpose, and finally back in Boston to be associated with the East West Foundation.

> In the four years since we have returned our lives have improved in every way — financially, emotionally, intellectually and spiritually. ... I don't mean to imply that since macrobiotics life has been a bed of roses. ... The real student of yin and yang is sometimes a very lonely person. We can never again blame anyone or anything for our condition. Our life is exactly what we have made it and if we are not happy with our product we are completely free to create any other kind of life.

In the previous chapter we referred to Ken's expertise in natural agriculture and his advice to us on using natural foods. A number of other times we have phoned him for help on related matters and are always impressed with the extent of his knowledge. In the constant chain of seminars sponsored by the EWF, Ken lectures on natural agriculture and the use of wild plants, as well as on acupressure massage. He also wields a colorful pen or typewriter, whichever, as you will see if you order the EWF Case Histories (see Bibliography).

SHERMAN GOLDMAN (2/3/37), University Road, Brookline, Massachusetts, 02146. Large duodenal ulcer. Sherman stated that he had always been melancholy, and that for six years prior to 1970 he had been gradually declining in every vital function except gaining weight. In January of 1970, X-rays located his ulcer, for which the medication had to be continually increased, and the pain sometimes required sedatives. Colds, hay fever or other allergies, and intermittent colitis had always been a part of his life. He tried a vegetarian diet and began getting relief from pain in only a few days, attaining complete relief in two weeks.

He met a macrobiotic friend, read Ohsawa, and was attracted by the philosophy and the way of life. On macrobiotic food, he soon began to lose weight, and became "peaceful," with a feeling of "physical and mental buoyancy." He took a job doing hard manual labor in a New York warehouse. Lulled by his feeling of good health, he began eating coffee and doughnuts every day. After a couple of weeks the ulcer returned suddenly and viciously, causing intense pain. Surgery was required to stop internal hemorrhaging, and part of his duodenum and lower stomach were removed.

In 1972 he went to Boston to study macrobiotics properly and has been encouraged by steady improvement since then. He now has energy and the ability to concentrate, and is not bothered by any of the other symptoms mentioned above. This Harvard graduate in philosophy, who has had additional study in Greek and Latin at Stanford, and who is the editor of the *East West Journal,* finds macrobiotics intellectually and philosophically stimulating, as well as physically healing.

When Jean was in Boston to speak at a weekend seminar in September of 1976, he spent a pleasant hour with Sherman preparing the interview which appeared in the March '77 *Journal.*

OLIVIA OREDSON (8/7/47), c/o East West Foundation, 359 Boylston Street, Boston, 02116. During first 21 years was plagued by frequent colds and other respiratory and sinus disorders, for which she took all the usual medications. Unhappy, sometimes desperately so, slightly overweight and sluggish, experiencing menstrual irregularity, visual difficulty, and long-term energy drain from mild mononucleosis. Experimented briefly with drugs, with terrifying results, and then used birth control pills for over a year.

She acquired a somewhat better sense of direction by dropping out of college to do secretarial work. In 1969, through friends, she discovered macrobiotics. After one meal at their cooking class she cleared out all her old food at home and began cooking macrobiotically. "Since then, my life has changed dramatically," for within a few weeks the unhappiness, the colds, the headaches disappeared, and within three years the menstrual cycles became normal. Her mental and emotional state both became clear. Moving from her native Minnesota to Boston, she worked in the many areas of activity of the East West Foundation. She notices that when she does not eat properly some of her old problems begin to send out warnings, but by being careful again about macrobiotic balance, she can very soon bring things back under control. Her main goal now seems to be to help disseminate the knowledge all over the world that everyone can own "this key to a healthy and happy life."

PATRICIA M. GOODWIN (11/10/51), Brooks Street, Boston, 02128. Since late teens, bothered by serious, swollen, painful varicose veins and by arthritis (later diagnosed as a tendency toward rheumatoid arthritis), both ailments considered inherited and impossible to cure. Rejected prescribed pain killers after only a couple of weeks' trial.

A close friend began working at the Seventh Inn Restaurant (an endeavor of the East West Foundation) and persuaded Patricia to work there, where after a few weeks she began sampling the food. In 1975, when she wanted to marry a "macrobiotic man" (no, not *bionic!*), she became macrobiotic in a hurry, and with his help and patience learned to cook this way. One day, after a few months, she ate cheese and wine. Right away she experienced pain in her back, making her realize that for some time she had forgotten all about the constant arthritic pain she used to have to live with. As time went on, although she still had dull pain or discomfort occasionally as a result of weather or of "off-limits" food, there was no more sharp or persistent pain, and she began to understand that with consistent proper food she would become entirely free of arthritis. And the varicose veins by early 1978 had almost disappeared, with only the largest still not completely reduced, but with no pain or difficulty in walking.

Her former "anger at the world" which had brought jibes from her roommates, dissolved, and she was "happily in love" with the man she soon married. Depression and hopelessness disappeared, along with 15 unneeded pounds of weight. She became a much more out-going person and now had "no fear of the future...in a world I know will only get better."

BILL TIMS (Christmas Day! 1949) Myriad allergies while growing up. Overweight, listless, recognizing an emptiness that even a good relationship with his parents failed to satisfy, nor did school nor did church.

As a university student, he "partook of" and "encountered with" whatever fad was current — anti-war demonstrations, drugs (which he calls "social toys"), yoga and meditation groups (new "social games"). Then somewhere he came across a "ragged copy" of Georges Ohsawa's *Book of Judgment,* and it had a "stunning" impact (see Bibliography). Friends told him of a man named Michio Kushi, a former student of Ohsawa who was teaching macrobiotics in Boston. That was all Bill needed to know to quit his job, drop out of school, and move to Boston to study. In two months he had lost thirty pounds, and in six months the allergies were "under complete control." The inner emptiness became replaced during the next four years with an "intense aliveness," a feeling that he was "radiating at the roots," and a deep appreciation for parents and friends and Kushi and Ohsawa. *Postscript:* Fall, 1978, with wife Carol, moved from Atlanta, Georgia, EWF Center to Boston to serve in Esko's place in EWF "home office."

ALAN KENNEY, M.D. (1/20/47), Moncton, New Brunswick, Canada. Dr. Kenney was unaware that his health had become eroded and endangered, even though he had undergone the usual intensive training to earn a B.Sc. at McGill University in Montreal and his M.D. degree at Dalhousie University in Halifax, Nova Scotia. This, plus the usual self-neglect experienced by young doctors getting a start as general practitioners, allowed for the typical rapid consumption of cafeteria food, as well as of cheeseburgers, eggs, french fries, and citrus fruits. Then he chanced onto macrobiotics and tried the strange (and at first tasteless) food, unaware of even the names of some of the "substances" he was eating. In spite of "strong intellectual skepticism," the program brought rapid benefits. As early as the third day he noticed that his sleep became deeper, shorter, and satisfying, undisturbed by nightmares; and he awakened in a positive mental state. Encouraged by this relief to continue eating this way, he further noticed that a number of unpleasant physical irritations began disappearing, and his entire skin texture was being altered. "In a larger sense, there was an incredible release from an unmistakable feeling of dying and deep decay — changes proceeding from inside. Soon, my mental state was revolutionized..."

Dr. Kenney's more serious symptoms had included one compared by Mr. Kushi to a condition "similar to multiple sclerosis:" with "fluctuating weakness" and weakening of the legs, hands, and facial muscles, reduction of bladder function and capacity, intervals of staring into space during conversation, prolonged and irresistible daytime sleeping, and general lack of initiative. But after some months of a fairly strict macrobiotic regime, he developed "an increased sense of body and mental lightness," the stamina, "if needed," to run six miles a day without fatigue, a lowering of blood pressure from 140/90 to 110/70, and a loss of 25 pounds of excess weight. In addition, he improved unpleasant kidney and intestinal weaknesses.

Before going abroad for further study, Dr. Kenney, during about two years of his own practice, "utilized macrobiotics as much as possible, and drugs as little as possible." The many advantages he observed led Dr. Kenney to declare, "Macrobiotics is and continues to be the fundamental discovery of my life, and I feel its study and application have saved my life. This is a totally subjective, non-scientific claim, but it has been my experience. However, it must be constantly emphasized that the unexpected healing of any serious disease is a multilevular process involving multiple unknown factors, favorably interacting with natural diet, stress reduction, personal and family growth processes, and a widening philosophy of life. Nonetheless, I am among a great many who have become very grateful to Michio Kushi for his teaching and example. Thank you."

We said we'd tell you later of our other purposes in writing this chapter, besides that of demonstrating the variety of troubles we know the macrobiotic way has solved or nearly solved. If you'll check the Goldman, Oredson, and Goodwin accounts, you'll notice they have one element in common: all three people found they had a recurrence of trouble if they jumped the macrobiotic track. This fact is borne out also in the Landes story with horses and dogs. It also happened in the Ivan Samuelson account and in the sequel to the story of one of your friendly authors, namely, Jean. The success that people have with the macrobiotic way, as well as the relapses they have when they disregard universal "regulations," indicate to us that the macrobiotic plan is what our bodies really need. Then the last four stories — Oredson, Goodwin, Tims and Kenney — strongly emphasize the improvement which macrobiotics can bring in mental and emotional conditions.

Now there's one more friend who belongs in this chapter. We consider all these people to be stars in one field of life's drama. They all deserve acclaim for conquering their own problems, then for re-enacting their experiences for others to absorb. But we believe they'll all agree with us that the feature star of the group is one EUGENE WILLIAMS. Gene's story was in the *Reader's Digest* of October, 1975, compellingly written by Allen Rankin.

Gene's mother Katie, is living in Walton, Indiana, to care for her semi-invalid mother, and we met her when she was one of the out-of-town registrants for the cooking classes Mrs. Kushi held during her January '76 visit to Ball State in Muncie. Katie is a live wire who learns everything interesting that crosses her path and then goes out looking for more. She found it *vitally* interesting that a hopeful theory was introduced to her after she heard the discouraging prediction at the Arthritic Clinic at George Washington University that nothing could be done for the arthritis from which she had been suffering. Gene told her about macrobiotics, and she attended a Michio Kushi psychology seminar. She states that she "dissolved" her arthritic trouble. "Macrobiotics has done it for me. When I slip and eat sugar or meat, I get the stiffness and pains again."

Katie became an accomplished macrobiotic cook. All guests at her home are served macrobiotic food, and we'll wager that's a favorable, flavorable promotion for that way of eating. Applying macrobiotic principles in caring for her mother, she has brought about considerable improvement in that lady's health, especially in relief from arthritis, high blood pressure, and heart problems.

Once in a while Katie will be in or near Muncie and will come to our Harvest Moon for a meal. On May 19, 1977, she phoned from Walton to say that she would like to bring a friend to the Moon for lunch and could get there in a couple of hours. The "friend" she brought was her son! So Gene Williams has eaten with us at the Harvest Moon! You can keep your "George-Washington-Slept-Here" signs. We could put up one saying, "Gene Williams Ate Here." We're sure he's a much more delightful, out-going personality than the other G.W. was. You'll be properly impressed when you hear his story.

It was one of those incidents where one second things are O.K. and the next the world has come to an end. On Thanksgiving Eve in 1966, just before a somersault in a wrestling practice session, Gene Williams was a football hero and co-captain of the lacrosse team at St. Albans School in Washington, D.C. He was popular as a bass fiddle player in a combo, and had won recognition at his school as an artist. As he executed the somersault he heard his neck pop, and suddenly instead of an athlete he was a *quadriplegic, paralyzed from the neck down.*

When he was able to think again, he determined to play this game with all possible winning maneuvers. Very gradually, painfully, repetitiously, he learned to re-activate arm muscles that almost weren't there and use them to re-enter active life. He learned to balance himself to sit up in a wheelchair, and over a long period of time reduced from more than three hours to thirty minutes the time it took to dress himself. His parents gave him a new car, with hand controls but no other special equipment. He could fold his wheelchair, pull it into the car, and drive off. With many regrets, he had to substitute drums for bass, piano, and guitar, but he applied the same stubborn struggle that had taught him to sit up and dress and feed himself. The apartment his parents had wisely remodeled for him in part of their Georgetown home began to jump with music.

In June of 1968, Gene graduated from St. Albans near the top of his class and entered Harvard in the fall to major in musicology. Incredibly, he became a member of a successful jazz-rock group, as well as a disc jockey on a Harvard radio station. In the summer of his sophomore year he and his car and his wheelchair made a trip West, and in the two following summers, to Mexico!

The B.A. from Harvard was earned by 1973. When Allen Rankin interviewed him Gene was living independently in a rented house in Boston, a member of a wild but successful jazz trio. And he was painting again. He declared that, more than from allopathic medicine, he had benefited from massage, exercise, macrobiotics, meditation and prayer, and the support of his parents, of a favorite physiotherapist, Janet, and other quadriplegics.

We're glad, of course, that macrobiotics had a part in Gene's comeback. For about a year and a half he lived in one of the East West Foundation student houses near Boston, and because of the quality of the food was able to forgo all medication. He also attended all Michio Kushi lectures in order to thoroughly absorb macrobiotic principles, and made a careful study of acupressure massage. In time he acquired enough of the essence of macrobiotics to work out his own adaptation in order to achieve a balance for his own needs, adding herbs, more sprouts, a higher percentage of raw foods, some juices, but no salt.

This man has carried out a new dream of his by doing demonstration teaching for the rehabilitation section of Massachusetts General Hospital in Boston. He was talent director for a Public Broadcasting System series shown in the spring of 1978 on the subject of handicapped children, entitled "Feeling Free," produced by the Workshop on Children's Awareness through a grant from the U.S. Bureau of Education.

You don't have to be with Gene Williams very long to feel as if your life has been improved in some mysterious way. The feeling stays with you like the ruminations after reading a fine novel or hearing a penetrating symphonic theme. If this be charisma, more of us should be blessed with it.

CHAPTER 15

Case Histories (First Hand)

We'd like to ask you to join us now in getting acquainted with some of the people for whom Muncie was the source of information about macrobiotics. They have all had success in making improvements in their health; they are typical of many, many others whose problems were not so serious. There have been still others who were getting along well but who drifted off course from the "universal way" and are still keeping company with their illnesses. There were some who, to our sorrow, did not learn about this way until after they were unable to retain food. And there have been one or two for whom we had hope in spite of an advanced stage of their disease, but who didn't make it. If Dr. Hutschnecker is right in his *Will to Live,* that was the way they wanted it to be, even though their desire to put aside this life was not apparent to us or perhaps not even to their families. (See our Chapter 4, second paragraph.)

As you can see when you read each of the personal histories, the process of *healing* by diet makes it apparent that it must have been *wrong* diet which was mainly responsible for the onset of the illnesses. The eating of too much rich food may have been an attempt to counteract feelings of stress by coddling the stomach, the stress, it seems, being commonly considered as the main cause of the illness. But the accepted food-group nutrition itself, we now believe, was both inadequate and damaging, playing hob with all the natural body functions. In our own case, macrobiotic eating would probably have allowed us to withstand the feeling of stress until things calmed down enough that we could get on top of our self-imposed over-crowded schedule (maybe after retirement?).

Because it seemed obvious that poor food was the main cause of sickness, we did not feel it relevant to pry into the long-range background of each of our friends as we compiled their offerings designed to help you. What is important with most of them is not so much the correctible past as the promising future — the future which for some of them probably would soon have been non-existent, on this level, without our macrobiotic discoveries. We now tend to believe that for a majority of people "mind-control" techniques would need to be accompanied by proper food, and even that, as "post-graduate" macrobiotic disciples believe, the prolonged use of proper food automatically brings about the mind control.

This chapter of our book, then, contains case histories of cures other than our own, to show that our experience was not an isolated one. These little stories grew out of our own, so that we know *how* they happened — a fact which we hope will prove convincing for others who are ill. We hope we can be forgiven for a bit of sentimentalism in our descriptions of these friends, for we naturally admire their courage and self-discipline — which often were more rigid than our own!

Names of doctors and hospitals have usually been withheld because our friends wanted to avoid any possibility of embarrassing their doctors. But if a member of the medical profession wishes to verify the authenticity of any of our claims, these names can be provided.

MARI SAMUELSON — AND IVAN AND GEORGE

We introduced Mari and Ivan to you in Chapter 1, but there have been significant additions to their story since then. Our lives are so closely woven together that we have practically become a family of four.

We were already eating dinner at Mari's several times a week before Jean found out about his cancer, for, while she was an excellent cook, it seemed uninteresting to fix substantial meals just for herself and five-year-old Ivan. She needed a bigger audience than that, and we two Kohlers were ardent fans, very willing to applaud her artistry. When we phoned her from Boston after visiting Michio she was shocked to hear that we were eating brown rice, miso soup, and azuki beans, and drinking bancha tea. "Poor man's tea!" she snorted. And the other things — heaven forbid! Those were from her childhood, willingly, eagerly, forgotten. They now brought back memories of an army-officer father who would not let the children speak at meals for fear of spraying germs in the food, or turn their heads for fear of having a hair fall in the food. Her mother cooked many reminiscences of ancient traditional foods, although of course she had never heard of macrobiotics. She did not say to the children, "Eat this — the flavor is delicious." But, "Eat this — good for your skin." Or, "Good for your hair." Your stomach. Your eyes. Your circulation. Meals were not exactly carefree occasions! How could Mari go back to *that* association with food, having enjoyed the preparation and consumption of rich American foods and desserts for many years? With a background of fine training in music, specializing in voice and piano, she had first learned to cook from her Scandinavian in-laws, after their son brought her as his new bride to their home in Tacoma, Washington.

In the sixth year of their marriage, her husband, as the aftermath of a bad fall on the ice, discovered that he was a brittle diabetic. Then Mari learned to prepare a diabetic diet, and keep it exact, but varied and interesting. While she and both Georges — husband and first son (now grown and married) — all ate this diet, she still enjoyed concocting the scrumptious desserts and main dishes for parties where other people were involved. Until her divorce, cooking meals presented no problems.

For months after we got back from Boston, Mari would fix the "peasant" food for us when we ate there, but continued to cook many American items for herself and Ivan. What's more, Ivan drank quantities of carbonated drinks, and every day he drowned in milk and sugar several servings of junk cereal which he would have wheedled his mother into buying for the "prizes" in the boxes even if he hadn't enjoyed gorging on the contents. Typically American, he frequently ate hamburgers, hot dogs, and french fries buried somewhere under all that catsup.

But Mari's inventiveness in cuisine kept popping up like a cork in water, and almost involuntarily she made those macrobiotic dishes more and more delicious, finally attaining gourmet status. And this, friends, is one of your legacies from this book — an association with, and guidance from, one of the world's best cooks, the incomparable Mari, in learning to prepare food that is entirely safe for you, beautifully simple in structure (if not always simple in preparation!), and capable of making you slap your sides in satisfaction as if every meal was a Thanksgiving dinner (which, of course, it is if your attitude is properly and gratefully macrobiotic).

Mari had inherited a very strong constitution, fortified by the good food she had had in her childhood (albeit no one knew better than to eat sugar and drink too much liquid). But she did have rheumatic fever as a young woman; and her main ailment after we knew her was that she contracted poison ivy very easily, suffering from a lengthy and agonizing siege every summer. She — and especially Ivan — both had kidney problems, and small tumors in various places. And Ivan had frequent respiratory ailments, including attacks of asthma, plus chronic attacks that resembled epilepsy. One of these, after a "long, hard day" at King's Island in August of 1972, was so terrifying that we thought he was dying. Late that night we followed the ambulance siren and flashing emergency lights from our motel to a hospital near Cincinnati. But he bounced back, and although tests showed a condition similar to epilepsy we were able to return home in a couple of days.

In spite of dilantin prescribed by Ivan's doctor, the blackouts kept recurring about once a month, always at school, frightening teachers and classmates. After an especially bad one in January we decided to have a chiropractor examine him. This proved to be a lucky decision, for his spine showed evidence of a damaging injury when he was a small child, recalling to Mari a sudden stop in the car which had thrown his forehead very sharply against the dashboard. Chiropractic treatments helped immeasurably, so that although we gradually reduced and finally eliminated the dilantin, there were no more blackouts to disrupt classroom routine.

Ivan had a way of disrupting things otherwise, being always hyperactive and often rebellious, along with his real nature which was very intelligent, unusually sympathetic and concerned, irrepressibly cheerful, and ingenuously charming. Like his mother, he had an amazingly strong constitution and was gracefully well-coordinated in spite of his recurrent illnesses.

During a three-month tour of her homeland in the summer of 1975, Mari took Ivan to an eminent orthopedic surgeon who gave him several treatments and confirmed the fact that we had followed the correct course in regard to the blackouts.

Then the Kushi's came to Muncie, in January of '76. A glance at Mari's forehead told Mr. Kushi that kidney stones were forming, and he knew that she could be relieved also of the poison ivy sensitivity by eating properly. Ivan was on the verge of becoming a real mess, healthwise, so he was also zapped onto the strict diet. Of course, tumors began dissolving, constant trotting to the bathroom soon became unnecessary, asthma soon amounted to only occasional headaches and sniffles. Ivan still misses school more than he should, not because he is sick but because he doesn't feel quite up to par. These lapses usually follow visits away from home, during which he naturally eats unhealthful food. His desk no longer has to be within swatting distance of the teacher's desk. And at home he no longer talks incessantly and domineeringly, or climbs all over his chair at meals like a monkey on a trapeze. Of course some of this would have come about with natural maturing, aided by Uncle Jean's collar-grabbing restraint. But with the soothing influence of good food, the learning of considerable self-control has come about without withdrawal or inner repression, so far as we can tell. Ivan is still all Ivan, strong in personality and ability, but now a partner instead of an adversary. He's going to be a skillful athlete and an uncommonly good pianist, with obsessions toward engineering, literature, geography, science, and theater. Macrobiotics, chiropractics, Uncle Jean, and Mari's magic cuisine and patient teaching, have combined to rob juvenile delinquency of a potential victim.

The summer of '76 Mari worked like a buzz saw in the yard, kneeling right down in the weeds and bugs with nary a rash or a bite more than a "normal" person might have. She also went swimming, did vigorous exercising at an Elaine Powers studio, and acquired a fashion-model figure.

Friendship with psychic people mentioned in Chapter 2 convinced us that Mari had exceptional healing power in her hands, but it frightened her a little to try to use it, so the ability lay somewhat in limbo except for an unscientific version of acupressure massage, the actual study of which was curtailed by many other duties. Certain it was — and is — that she has a very reliable intuition in all matters related to healing. Occasionally she helps someone who is critically ill, showing the family massage techniques and very specialized cooking. And she is forever helping people who come to her with questions about cooking for a family invalid.

Fittingly enough, she went to Boston for the whole week of the seminar study on Nutrition and Cancer (Chapter 6 and Sequel to Chapter 9), taking part in *everything,* to the point of actual exhaustion. Her intuition can now be combined with the best knowledge. Among other things in Boston, Mari translated all week for Hideo Ohmori, the eminent guest lecturer from Japan, and that association with him had side effects that benefited us in most unexpected and fortunate ways. These you read about in the Sequel to Chapter 9. Now our tremendous Mari is all set to be a significant force as a source person for macrobiotic know-how in the Midwest. People are clamoring — understandably — to study with her the art of re-creative cooking. As a blueprint for good health, there's no better way to go.

This would be an appropriate place to mention George Samuelson's use of macrobiotics to combat the diabetes we spoke of above. As we said in Chapter 1, he and Mari were divorced when Ivan was four. Remarried and living in a town near Muncie, George was having an extremely difficult time regulating the intake of insulin with his prescribed diet, and although his doctor suggested several variations to use with the 48 daily units (sometimes even 50-60 units) of insulin, nothing seemed to solve the imbalance. Moreover, he had so much arthritic pain in his shoulders, elbows, and knees that even cortisone was of no avail. All his problems motivated him to see Michio during the Ball State visit. Inspired to follow the macrobiotic diet, as a number of others were after the contact with Michio, George found he could soon begin reducing the amount of insulin he required, as well as reducing his waistline. The first month of macrobiotics allowed him to cut the insulin dosage from 48 units to 24, and his weight from 170 pounds to 150. Within a few months the insulin was down to 16 units.

Since he and his wife both work, finding time to prepare macrobiotic food was of course difficult, but yet he remained almost completely strict in holding to his diet. Later on, he decided to add some meat to counteract a feeling of weakness. He believes that inexperienced diabetics should remain with grains for their carbohydrates, but should have the guidance of a professional dietician to help adjust the balance of carbohydrates to insulin. He knows well how to measure carbohydrates for himself and make the necessary adjustments. (Compare with Michio's statements on insulin dosage in the fourth paragraph of Chapter 5.)

In time, George found that he could hold the diabetes at bay on a 30-unit insulin level, besides holding his weight at a steady 150 pounds, a balance which he is finding quite satisfactory.

Postscript: As we make a final up-dating in June of 1978, we can report that Mari has for some months been working a few hours a week at a local "health spa," where she is much in demand because of her perceptive ability in helping people with exercises, devising special ones for individual needs. (Her college training in Japan had included a "minor" in physical education, along with the "major" in music — and the P.E. training has since been highly refined by her macrobiotic study!) At the spa, people also are docile about accepting her firm, but gentle, scolding to keep them in line on their individual dietary programs, into which she has incorporated as many macrobiotic principles as the "traffic will bear"!

THE FAMILY RUSSELL

We became acquainted with the Russells late in the fall of 1974 when they contacted us after finding out about Jean's recovery. Ingrid was following a recent interest in natural foods, and the family heard about Jean when they ate at our natural-foods restaurant. We learned that Ingrid was a native of Germany and had come to this country when she and John Russell were married in 1956. Their sons, Jerome and James, were born in 1957 and 1960. The more we were with the Russells, the more we recognized the unusually idyllic quality of their marriage.

We soon learned also that Ingrid had grown up in a comfortably well-off family, eating the typical German diet of heavy sauces, meats and sausages, many sweets and plenty of whipped cream. And then, World War II exploded when Ingrid was in her mid-teens, resulting in the loss of her brother, her father, and her home within one year! But even during the meager times following the war, she managed to continue eating sweets, a small haven that gave momentary escape from all the hardship she had experienced. In 1954 she began having severe pain deep in her hip joints which made walking, even standing, a periodic hardship, especially after being seated for any length of time. Hydrotherapy and a series of novocaine injections did bring relief. Then early in 1960 her right thumb became painfully swollen; but cortisone injections seemed to take care of the problem. Three years later this same symptom recurred, and the same therapy was even more effective.

Only recently we learned that during much of this time she suffered also from stomach disorders and insomnia, her anxieties being further intensified by the severe illness (arterial sclerosis) of her mother, still living in Germany. Soon after her mother's death, in November of 1970, Ingrid's right knee became swollen and extremely painful, so that she had to remain either in bed or in a wheel chair. There was painful weakness in other joints as well, especially in hands and arms. Medications and periodic drainage of fluid from the knee were not helpful. Yet she refused exploratory surgery on the knee (luckily!), and then doctors in England, where the family lived for a time, and also in this country told her she would have to learn to live with — rheumatoid arthritis! Cortisone relief was now only temporary, and she was warned against using it excessively. Increasingly severe stomach trouble ruled out the use of aspirin, and substitutes were ineffective. Because of swelling in her ankles and lower legs Lasix was prescribed to help eliminate excess fluids. "Unfortunately," Ingrid told us, "no effort was made to try to find a better way to make my kidneys function normally — like looking for the cause of the swelling, or the cause of my arthritis or stomach disorders, or the cause of shattered nerves. After many, many examinations it was recognized that I was troubled, tense, and suffering acute insomnia, but that was 'due to my personality.'" New prescriptions were offered — among them Doridin, Librium, and Valium — but her system continued to deteriorate, and deeper depression set in.

Worried about being a burden for her family, Ingrid began to think that there must be a more natural method of healing than to be steeped in drugs. It was about this time, then, that the Russells and Kohlers got together. The former were easily and eagerly convinced that the direction Jean was following sounded like a possible natural method that Ingrid had been hoping for, so they arranged an appointment with Michio Kushi and flew to Boston. It proved to be an exciting experience for Ingrid. "I'm so thankful I still had enough insight and will power left to realize the importance of that balanced, simple, but fantastic diet! My appointment with Mr. Kushi was one of the most touching and revealing experiences of my life. Meeting him, listening to and observing him, one couldn't help but develop immediate confidence and respect."

After three macrobiotic years, she added up the score: no more pain and swelling in the joints, and the little nodules on many of the joints of the fingers and toes had all but dissolved. Her strength had returned — she was doing intelligent exercising (sometimes with suggestions from Mari, by the way), and was starting to play tennis again. There was normal kidney function and deep sleep for the first time in years.

> All without prescriptions — only through a change to the macrobiotic diet! I could go on and on...! It is almost unbelievable to realize that I will continue to improve in the future as my system repairs itself.
>
> Looking back, I'm especially disappointed with myself for adhering so blindly to the seemingly simplistic, but only palliative, dependence that our society has placed on synthetic medicines. The obvious solution to most of our ills — if not to all of them — rests in nutrition. Why has it

taken our society so long to recognize that nutrition should be a major core of medical education? Proper nutrition ought to be a part of our daily existence! It's beyond my comprehension, now. It seems obvious now how poor my eating habits had always been — with that addiction to sweets from early childhood, to say nothing of all the other harmful food. Besides all that, I became a heavy coffee drinker! What with the combination of that kind of "diet," the severe trauma of war, and the endless stream of drugs my system was subjected to, it's no wonder I was not sound of body or spirit!

As might be expected from a husband like John, he was completely supportive. In the script for a local radio interview promoting a macrobiotic workshop, he extolled the beneficial results their new program had produced for their family during the first few months they practiced it.

It wasn't entirely smooth going, by any means. Ingrid had discouraging problems with various types of discharges. Kidney irritation. Tumors that had to dissolve. Swelling in her face, periodically so severe that she could hardly open her eyes for the first few hours in the morning. But with rigid self-discipline, with helpful telephone conversations with, and occasional visits to, Michio, she gradually learned to cope with what seemed to be disheartening setbacks and recognize them as essential discharge. Through it all she had John's constant encouragement, and they both seemed never to doubt that their work would lead to the success they now have achieved.

We have watched Ingrid commit herself with amazing dedication and skill. There was no "stewing around" — if you can forgive the pun — with the new cooking experience. Questions were asked, macrobiotic cookbooks were purchased, the pantry was restocked, and literally overnight fresh and exciting meals were appearing on her dinner table. Without pressure, she gently nudged their sons into macrobiotic territory by keeping the menus varied and interesting. The joy of discovery and the results from the new way of life have stimulated her to help others. She has found time to visit sick friends, taking tasty morsels from her natural kitchen. She has introduced macrobiotic specialties to friends at her dinner parties, some of them in connection with John's social obligations as chairman of the landscape architecture department at Ball State University. And she has unobtrusively persuaded others of the value of macrobiotics, assisting them in redirecting their way of life. She feels this is only the beginning!

Postscript: In April of 1978 we happened to be visiting with Ingrid at the Harvest Moon, and she remarked that the last place she had noticed any pain (now completely gone) was an occasional minor twinge in the right knee — the place where the arthritis began years ago and where she would naturally have expected it to make its final exit.

Arthritis sufferers, are you listening??

THE HOLDERREADS — LAURETTA AND LEE

Lee and Lauretta Holderread are an attractive young couple who have two nice-looking, well-behaved daughters, ages seven and thirteen. Lee is an agent for Farm Bureau Insurance Company and Lauretta teaches at a county high school — the kind of a teacher about whom the kids say, "She's *OK,*" when parents ask at the end of the first day of school. And the kind of teacher who engenders a sudden interest in the fathers of the kids to attend Parent-Teachers meetings that year.

The Holderreads ate at our restaurant rather frequently, so we knew them casually, but didn't know till they made an appointment with Michio Kushi in April of 1976 that Lauretta had multiple sclerosis. In the fall of 1971 she had begun to notice a kind of numb sensation on her left side. Her left leg became numb, then began causing pain when she walked; and finally she began to feel weak all over. Her doctor said only that she should wait to find out whether it was a temporary condition. But by Christmas she was in too much pain to walk from one end of a shopping mall to the other, and grocery shopping wore her out completely.

Still neither her doctor nor a neurologist could find the trouble. The numbness became chronic. For three years it was mostly in her hands and feet: something was always numb or tingling or weak. All this time she continued teaching, but after three-and-a-half years her right arm became so numb that she had no control in it. Teaching, and especially writing on the blackboard, became increasingly difficult. A couple of months later a very painful intestinal symptom developed, changing day by day from constipation to diarrhea. The intestinal pain became more severe, and drugs were no help. She was sent to an internist, underwent a hysterectomy, and thought she had found the answer, for immediately afterwards she felt better than she had for 18 months. But four weeks later, after she went back to teaching, all the pain, all the intestinal spasms closed in again.

In connection with the Michio Kushi visit to Ball State in January of 1976, Lee heard on the radio that macrobiotic information could be picked up at our restaurant. After reading it, Lauretta began eating macrobiotically, and in April went to Boston for a visit with Michio. By the time school was out she felt much better, and by mid-summer was a lot stronger, minus pain and intestinal spasms.

"Now, now," friends (?) said when she told them she was getting well. "You know m.s. has remissions like that. Your diet couldn't have *that* much influence!"

With an unusual daring which belied her soft-spoken manner, Lauretta deliberately ate, in addition to her macrobiotic food, a lot of ice cream, which Michio had said would be the worst thing she could eat! By fall she was having pain again. Returning to the diet again for two months, she became pain-free. Still adventuresome, she tested herself and the diet again at Thanksgiving and Christmas parties, bringing back the pain and the intestinal difficulty. She went with Lee for a wood-cutting outing, which she had enjoyed without any reaction the previous summer. But this time it made her so weak she had to stay in bed for several days.

Since then she has been pretty careful about her eating, and is feeling better all the time. She still is using ginger compresses twice weekly on her back and abdomen (see end of Chapter 13). She can swim a half-mile with ease, whereas before she became macrobiotic, four lengths at a YMCA pool did her in, and she would be sick the rest of the night. She comments on how much her tastes in food have changed. When she feels hungry while they're doing their laundry at a laundromat, she tells Lee she can hardly wait to get home to a bowl of rice cream. A few months earlier she would have said *ice* cream!

Her doctors seem receptive to her program, her surgeon saying that the diet makes sense, that sugar can certainly cause intestinal spasms.

So here's Lauretta — joining the others in this chapter and the previous one who have voluntarily played the role of guinea pig to show multiple sclerosis patients, arthritis, diabetes, and cancer patients, and all of you who don't want to contract such diseases, that this food offers us the power of control over our bodies, to make them well or keep them well.

TEREZIA MATYAS

One night in August of 1974 we had a phone call from Chicago. The anxious long-distance voice was that of Charles Matyas, a life insurance salesman who is a brother-in-law of Dr. Francois D'Albert, president of the Chicago Conservatory College. Francois, a superior artist as a violinist, had come down from Chicago to teach at Ball State when local faculty members were on leave, and he and Jean had enjoyed a very cordial relationship working on a number of successful recitals they performed together. As a matter of fact, one of those recitals was the night before Jean went into the Indianapolis hospital for tests to find the cause of his symptomatic itching. We mentioned in Chapter 1 that our family doctor had allowed a few days' extension so that this recital could be performed, but wouldn't let Jean finish the last few days of teaching for that term. While he became angry with us later for not following the medical route on treatment, the doctor was right about the need for urgency — it could easily have turned out that that was Jean's last recital! With characteristic Hungarian emotional intensity, Francois was crushed by Jean's illness and overjoyed by the cure, which he related to all his Chicago friends and relatives. So Charles Matyas knew all the details, little dreaming he would ever need to use them!

But the telegram he had received on August 5 read thus (translated): "Our dear mother is in very bad shape. If you want to see her please hurry home immediately." It was from his brother.

Charles had not seen his mother — Terezia — for eighteen years, but of course he knew all about her surgery in 1969 for intestinal cancer, at which time twenty inches of the colon were removed and a colostomy bag was required. His sister Erzsebet had been for more than twenty years the chief laboratory technician in the same hospital where the surgery was performed. Their father had died of cancer in 1973 — and now their mother was in danger! The telegram had been prompted by the report from a complete examination for Terezia on August 1, showing that the cancer was again in the intestines, had spread to the stomach, but was mainly in the uterine area, which was a mass of cancer, inoperable, and causing constant bleeding. Doctors predicted death in about a month.

Instead of going home, Charles wired his sister asking her to take their mother to her home so that he could talk to her by phone and could send food which had cured cancer of the pancreas for a friend of Francois named Jean Kohler. Terezia had been transferred to a sanatorium for terminally ill patients. Erzsebet wrote that there were many cancer patients there receiving drug treatments, but no cures were reported. "Looking at the problem through medical eyes, I do not think that a brown rice diet will help at all." Nonetheless she yielded to Charles' request and in September took Terezia home with her. So elated was Terezia to hear Charles' voice that she would probably have agreed to eat dog food. We wish we could have heard that conversation!

Erzsebet kept a careful record of her mother's progress from September 22, three days after the first shipment of rice and bancha tea arrived from Charles. We have the latter's translation of Erzsebet's almost daily account, as her mother's condition alternately improved and wavered; but even when things were not going well, Terezia needed only an occasional dose of narcotics for pain. By September 28 she felt good — in fact she had four consecutive very comfortable days — and she began walking! She took medication only once for an "ear noise." Some bad days were followed by a time with no problems at all, from October 4-24, when she started eating vegetables and miso soup, for by then further information about the diet had arrived from Charles.

The entry on November 14 records that Terezia walked three miles to the hospital for a complete check up, which, to the bewilderment of the doctors who had predicted her death within a month after the August 1 examination, *revealed NO trace of cancer*. Charles' translation says, "Cancer had fragmented to zero," stating that that might have been the cause of an intermittent discharge of cancer cells she had had from the uterus. The log notes that from mid-November on there was pain only rarely and there was no further discharge. A December 24 entry tells that Terezia, having enjoyed six weeks of feeling well, returned to her own home.

There were a couple of brief times after that when she had a few bad days, but by summer she was "feeling great," or the Hungarian equivalent thereof, and was happily working in her garden growing vegetables and flowers. She lost weight, and seldom had to rest during the day.

Congratulations, Terezia!

But July a year later brought us a shocking phone call from Charles. He said that at the end of that last good summer his mother had gradually started slipping away from macrobiotics. How often these things happen! Sometimes well-meaning friends bring in tempting delicacies, or convince the dieter that the weight loss is too extreme. Terezia had begun cooking for her family, and their type of food was at her fingertips, so that eating it was too easy and irresistible. Charles said she ate no meat or milk so far as he could tell, but did use too much oil and fish, along with other deviations. Terezia could not be blamed for returning to her former eating habits. She was very much alone as a macrobiotic person. There was no Michio to phone when doubts arose, and there was no one to warn her that although the cancer was gone, eating worldly foods could bring on other difficulties, especially for one who had already experienced some sort of serious ailment.

So on December 9 of '75 the log entries begin again, but this time they are not good. Terezia spent three days in the hospital to check hemorrhaging from the uterus, and had to have a blood transfusion. Apparently all was well again until February 19 ('76), when there was a five-day session in the hospital. Then March 13 to May 27 was spent in the sanatorium, with Erzsebet doing all the lab tests. June 26 saw Terezia back in the hospital for three days with a high fever; she was given a blood transfusion. She went home for one day only but then went back to the hospital because of swelling in her ankles. Doctors at the hospital, assuming cancer, gave her a cobalt treatment, which helped her condition not at all, for the swelling remained. Erzsebet protested, declaring that the symptoms seemed to indicate kidney infection; but the doctors disregarded her arguments and gave another cobalt treatment. Furious, Erzsebet asked that they give no more treatments without her permission. Overriding her wishes completely, they then tried intravenous chemotherapy.

That night Terezia died.

"They killed my mother!" Charles said bitterly, echoing the expression Erzsebet had used in her telegram telling him the sad news. A letter a few days later voiced the same sentiments: "They killed her...they treated her for cancer, which did not exist any more."

We were terribly saddened by this news, of course, for we had been feeling very close to Terezia since learning of her recovery, a feeling heightened by the exuberant native joy of the Matyas family. We would have been devastated by a sense of failure but for an O. Henry twist to the story which unfolded as Charles regained his composure and continued the conversation.

Erzsebet had seen the records of Terezia's last two hospital visits, but when she went to the files to get them to make copies to send to Charles *they were nowhere to be found!* She could locate a record of only one blood test. No one would admit to any knowledge of what had happened to the other records.

Charles had experienced similar frustration when he had tried to get permission from the Hungarian government to have Michio Kushi give some lectures for doctors while he was making a European tour. He also wanted to have his mother visit with Michio, of course. The fruit of that effort was a telegram from government authorities on June 7, 1975: they could not receive Mr. Kushi.

As Charles told us still more, we began to realize that even in death Terezia had made a significant contribution to medical history. For Erzsebet had also seen the report of the autopsy. But when she went to get a copy of that she was told that it had been classified as information to be released only to the courts or to legal authorities! For her own purposes she would never need a copy: imbedded in her memory from her one reading of it were the statements that *Terezia's last illness had been the result of a severe kidney infection which the autopsy revealed — that there was no trace of cancer — BUT THAT THERE WAS SCARRED TISSUE WHERE THE CANCER HAD BEEN.*

Rest in peace, Terezia Matyas.

GLORIA AND DAN

What a wedding that was! They had cleared a small grove down the hill by the stream on Sam's farm, and the water was flowing by just right and the birds were singing and the sun made long cylinders of light down through the high trees. The wind blew Gloria's long black hair and her skirt and the white, orange-trimmed tunics she had made for them both in the style of her Mexican Indian ancestry. They wore flowers in their hair. Families and friends gathered there, Sam read some unpretentious thoughts, and Paul sang to the accompaniment of his guitar. Afterwards, up the hill by the big farmhouse, the wind joined in the festivities and whirled around with all the decorations and paper plates.

Sam — hard worker, farmer, minister, college instructor of business administration — owned Mazda Natural Foods Store, which Dan managed in the wintertime. During the rest of the year he helped Sam on the farm. Gloria was manager at our Harvest Moon restaurant, where her dark beauty and her culinary talents were exceptional assets. Devoted to the continuation of the "Moon" in spite of the threat of its constant poverty, she calmly but resolutely tried one idea after another to "make it go," each time learning to be more practical and coming a little closer to what seemed to be a workable plan. Her study and application of yoga and astrology to every situation provided her with a perspective which prevented her falling apart from the unavoidable frustrations of this job. She was deeply appreciative of the spirituality and the power of natural foods, and began to realize during the lectures of Mr. and Mrs. Kushi at Ball State in January of 1976 that natural food was elevated to its most valuable use and balance by macrobiotics. So she began restricting the honey, peanut butter, fruits, and juices which had always been an important part of her food (but which, because of her tropical heritage, probably didn't harm her as much as they would damage natives of temperate climates).

Dan, unobtrusively intellectual but possessed of much common sense, had some American Indian in his blood, and he, too, ate simply and admitted no "junk" foods, although even after he learned of macrobiotics he didn't feel he wanted to be *that* strict. Gloria assisted Mrs. Kushi with her cooking classes during her three-day visit here, and Gloria and Dan both had an interview with Mr. Kushi, for there was a baby on the way and they wanted to learn how macrobiotic principles applied to pregnancy.

It would take a union like this to produce a very special, nearly macrobiotic baby. Ricky found the name for him (Ricky, our artist and artist-chef, who had been with the Moon since shortly after other owners started it in 1972, and on whom we depended — although we were considerably more than twice his age — for all sorts of advice and guidance on how to run the place). He found the name on a record jacket in a list of names, with their meanings, from various languages. AhKin (Ah-keen), meaning Sun, is apparently a Mayan name. And so on August 8 of 1976, the Sun, figuratively speaking, entered the House of the Moon. He was Sun, and son, to Gloria and Dan — and to all of us associated with the Harvest Moon.

AhKin *was* different. From the very first he seemed like a person and a personality. He looked out on the world with a mixture of alert inquisitiveness and understanding. The word that kept coming to me to describe him was "peaceful." Oh, I don't mean he didn't assert himself with vigor when it was time for Mother to hold him close for meals or when other services due him were not forthcoming soon enough. But on the other hand there was never any resentment of his lot in having to begin life on this planet as a baby. He accepted it, yet never lost his dignity with any of his many "mamas and daddies" on our Moonship.

AhKin was small but very strong and active and consistently healthy. (Macrobiotic friends assured us that whenever he decided the time was right, he would catch up on his growing.) He had none of the common physical complications of babyhood and so could turn his entire attention to remaining healthy and happy. Showing very early in life (at only 6 weeks) a propensity for sharing his mother's love of learning, he accompanied her and Ricky, with Susie and Chris, two more of our valued staff members, to Boston for several days of East West Foundation workshops. All our representatives were insatiable in their desire to learn all they could about the macrobiotic way of life.

In one way AhKin was a "test-tube baby": whenever Gloria went to a party and ate even small servings of party food, it showed up very soon in AhKin's complexion and disposition! Only at times like this would he have a facial rash or a temporarily "cranky" mood. Thus he was a sensitive indicator proving that foods we should seldom eat really *do* have a harmful effect on us. The occasional indulgence is soon absorbed and dealt with, but over a long period of time, stored almost unnoticed in tissues conditioned to and hardened by constant abuse, the insidious buildup eventually may erupt in serious disease.

We have for seven months resisted holding this baby, for until we wrote this much of his story, we wanted to remain totally detached from this Leo child, in order to give a fair and unbiased report saying that his charm is irresistible, that his eyes are a bright and sparkling dark brown, that his smile, while it is also directed toward others, is most especially for both of *us,* that he is, in every way we can impartially observe, an outstanding person in the true sense of the word, that one day you will be hearing of AhKin Walter — and you can say then that you remember that his renown was predicted by two observers who viewed his superior qualities from an absolutely unprejudiced vantage point.

TAILS OF TWO CITIES

We say that this chapter is made up of stories of "Muncie-influenced" cases. The others in the chapter are tales of individuals, mostly, and their families; but this one has a cast of hundreds, with a potential of becoming thousands — we might call it a tale of tails. We're speaking of the mouse experiment begun at Ball State University in February of 1976 (see Chapter 4). You remember we said it would take many months to complete. But because of a couple of setbacks more time will be required than was first envisioned. Setback One occurred when a student who was cleaning the cages inadvertently mixed up the groups of mice. Oh no, oh no! Begin again almost from the introduction. The other setback resulted from an airplane trip.

The principal investigator in the experiment is Dr. Peter Nash, medical microbiologist at Ball State until the fall of 1977, at which time he changed to the biology department at Mankato University in Minnesota, which welcomed the continuation of the mouse experiment. But the mice didn't welcome that plane trip — they didn't like it *at all.* They were so upset they'd hardly speak even to each other for several months; so the breeding program was severely handicapped for a while. But in spite of these frustrations, Dr. Nash is beginning to see signs in the project that are hopeful for macrobiotics.

We know of one other extensive experiment involving mice and a simple, primitive type of diet, described on pages 4 and 5 in Dr. K. Morishita's book *The Hidden Truth of Cancer* (see our Bibliography). The mice on the primitive diet were completely free of disease, while those on East Indian and English diets had many ailments, including impairment of the nervous system resulting in aggressive behavior. That experiment, carried out by the chief physician at the Nutritional Institute of India, showed significant results proving that diet determined the state of health, but we didn't like it because they killed all those mice for autopsies. By contrast, in Dr. Nash's work, the emphasis is on getting the mice well, or on preventing illness in the first place. And the control groups are given food that is commonly considered healthful for animals. Feeding them that way is no less responsible than giving our children the accepted food-group diets that many of us grew up on.

Since the report from Dr. Nash is expressed in scientific style, (with its typical reservation, obviously!), we'd better enter the report here as he gave it to us, to prevent distortion which might result from our lack of knowledge if we were to attempt any condensation or "editing." You will see quite a number of similarities to the government recommendations described in our Chapter 6.

The increase in knowledge in the field of diet and nutrition on the effect of tumor production in humans makes it important to try to understand direct interactions so that changes in diet can be made to prevent and cure these diseases. Dietary habits have been shown to correlate with the incidences of certain forms of cancer. In particular, stomach, colon and breast cancers have been linked to nutritional changes. The complete epidemiologic and laboratory data are needed to pin point the importance of diet as a factor in the causation of various forms of cancer.

The use of human patients for direct experimentation on the effect of diets on tumor production has created two major problems for current research. Patients with tumors usually produce only one tumor or one group of tumors at a time, making it difficult to repeat experiments. In addition, most tumors develop at an undetectable rate, so that by the time they are detected it may be too late to study the effects of diets.

The study of tumorgenesis in animals has continuously offered new approaches to the study of human cancers. Although not ideal for human study, animal systems have been developed as models which can overcome at least part of these problems. Mouse strains which develop non-induced tumors have been shown to provide for a good system to study diet factors on tumorgenesis.

The research reported here was a preliminary study to observe the effect of diet on two strains of laboratory mice, i.e., non-induced tumor strain (A strain) and non-tumored strain (Balb strain), both from my colony at Ball State University. Observations were carried out on the animals to study weight changes, breeding changes, blood paremeter changes and tumor development.

The animals were divided into six groups of 3 to 5 animals. Two groups of Balb and two groups of A strain mice were fed a special experimental diet: 50%-60% grain, 20%-25% cooked vegetables, 10% raw vegetables, 10% beans, and mixed with miso broth. This diet was made as needed 2-3 times a week. Two groups of mice, one of A and one of Balb strain, were used as controls. They were fed a Purina Laboratory Chow for mice, containing 23% crude protein, 4.5% crude fat, 6.0% fiber, 8.0% ash and 2.5% added minerals. All animals were given water ad libra. Specimens of blood were collected, animals were weighed monthly and births and tumor development were recorded.

In general, we observed that the experimental animals gained weight at a slower rate than the control animals and did not appear to get as fat. The blood parameters stayed normal, with the A strains having a lower hematocrit* of 45% as compared to the Balb strain, which has a reading of 55%. As tumors developed on the A strain the hematocrit readings dropped drastically. Birth rates appeared to be normal, but more information is needed because of the low number of females which were allowed to mate. The tumors appeared at a slower rate and were fewer in number in the experimental group.

The data collected for this experiment appear to support work reported by others. As the caloric intake is restricted there appears to be a decreased incidence of non-induced tumors of the breast. It might be noted that the special diet has less unsaturated fats and no preservatives or animal fats. The Purina Chow contains both animal fats and preservative BHA. Samlaska at Mankato State University (Personal Communication) has recently demonstrated that linoleic acid, an unsaturated free fatty acid, inhibits immune responses to human breast carcinoma cells. The possibility exists that the change in diet allows for less immune repression and for fewer tumors to develop. The animals seem to be able to survive on the special diet with little or no animal fat. The rest of the parameters seem to remain "normal." As has been demonstrated by others, the animals are less fat, and the lower the body weight the lower the incidences of specific tumors.

The preliminary results reported here from this study appear to indicate that this mouse system can be used to study the effect of diet on tumor production. The mouse metabolism has been shown by others to be similar to the caloric use by humans. The lack of fats in the diet may affect the immune response and might even stimulate the responses. The A strain of mice is an inbred strain that shows genetic defects with a high incidence of breast and other tumors. Further research is needed with these

---

*An evaluation provided by a hematocrit machine showing the percentage of red blood cells to a given volume of plasma (if we got it straight!)]

mice on the possible effect of diet on the histocompatibility leucocyte antigens (HLA) and their effect on tumor
prevention or treatment.

Thank you very much, Dr. Nash!

(An uncertain glossary: histocompatibility = tissue compati-
bility; leucocyte = white blood corpuscle; antigen = a protein or
carbohydrate substance to which antibodies in the blood stream react. Can you add that up? We can kind of get the idea!)

Even if we miss the full impact of the punch line, we think the
progress report is promising. Dr. Nash said that after his colony
builds up to 100 mice — and it was nearing that in August of 1978 —
people of scientific knowledge will begin to believe that his reports
are worth listening to.

HEATHER EINSEL

This is the story of Heather. We learned of her illness through
mutual friends, Maxine and Al Nussbaum, who live here in Muncie.
Heather's family had lived in Muncie some years ago, and we knew
her father as organist and music director at a local church, but we
were not acquainted with the rest of the family. When Heather was
seven they moved to West Hartford, Connecticut, where Richard
has another prestigious position as organist and minister of music
at one of the community's largest churches. But they kept contact
with the Nussbaums.

Maxine and Al had been interested in Jean's recovery from
cancer and in case histories we knew about which dealt especially
with cataracts and Parkinson's disease, for Al was having difficulty
with both. He began working on a do-it-yourself try at macrobiotics
from information he got at our restaurant, and then decided to go to
Boston for an interview with Michio Kushi, stopping en route for an
overnight visit with the Einsels.

The result of that visit was written into a beautiful story by
Heather's mother, Grace, who generously shared it with us. We sin-
cerely hope that Grace will be able to find a magazine that will accept this story, for it should be told in detail in her own version,
which we do not have space for here. She titles it "Life Begins on a
Diet," and opens the story by saying, "February of '75 was a bleak
month. Our daughter, Heather, was now seventeen. Epilepsy had

struck her at the age of five and since that time her medication had had to be increased to a heavy dosage just to control the illness." From the very beginning the illness greatly impaired her progress at school, and she suffered constant pain which became so much a part of her that she assumed that all other people were in pain. Deeply frustrated because of being forced by her handicap into special education classes, Heather became more and more antagonistic at school and at home, until, after Heather's sister Lynne went away to college, the home situation reached crisis proportions. The two girls had always been especially close to each other and to the parents — even more so since Ricky, the only boy in the family, had been *killed by lightning* five years earlier!

Consultations with a psychiatrist provided no help whatsoever for Heather, and then Al came for that brief visit. Here he was, going to Boston for a check up for cataracts and Parkinson's disease — not with a physician but with an Oriental philosopher! Yet somehow his description of macrobiotics reached a long-suppressed hope in Grace's inner being, and she asked Al to make an appointment for Heather.

There were many apprehensions and misgivings for husband Dick and herself, especially when Al politely but firmly refused the food they had bought for snacks and when he ate only rice and bancha tea for breakfast! Even Grace was "not enthused" about the "weird" macrobiotic diet. "I always felt I tried to give my family balanced meals, and I tried to buy the best available. After forty years of thinking milk, orange juice and meat were essential for proper body development, the prospect of a diet free of these things did not seem to make sense."

But Al phoned from Boston that he had made the appointment, although Mr. Kushi cautioned against false hopes. Al urged that Heather begin eating macrobiotically during the three-week interim before the appointment. So began Grace's "mental freedom and kitchen imprisonment," to paraphrase her description. Surprisingly, Heather was docile about trying the food, and Grace decided to follow the diet herself.

Forty meals later, having cooked and cleaned pots and pans for macrobiotics as well as serving regular food for Dick and for Lynne's houseguests, Grace's weariness was counteracted by the fact that Heather had stopped snoring at night, a problem since childhood in spite of the conventional removal of tonsils and adenoids. Her speech also improved! And she stopped the exaggerated blinking which had always occurred in strong sunlight.

By March 26, when they went to see Mr. Kushi, Grace "was at an all-time high level of enthusiasm," although Heather balked at seeing still another "doctor," especially an Oriental! Grace's only regret after the interview was that she had not taped the "glorious moments" with Michio Kushi. *No brain damage* — imagine that! Heather was to follow the diet strictly for another five months, and then relax it slightly for another five months. After four weeks she was to begin a gradual reduction of medicine, periodically dropping one more of the eleven daily pills. The two worst foods for her would be fruit and excessive liquid. Fruit, if any, would be only a few dried apples or raisins, and liquid would be bancha tea or water adequate to satisfy thirst.

For about a month things moved along smoothly, but then Heather contracted a severe case of flu. She had already lost fifteen pounds, and the flu weakened her to the point where Grace's enthusiasm turned to doubt and then to agonizing fear, a fear that was deepened because her brother had given her some of the major periodical articles attacking macrobiotics. Luckily, however, they were visiting Grace's mother and sister, both of whom were so much impressed with Heather's general improvement that they encouraged Grace to stay with her program.

After seventeen days Heather returned to school and to the opposition of the school nurse, who phoned Grace to protest that she was "slowly killing" her own daughter! Still, Grace stayed right on course.

In June there was another trip to Boston, with Dick included as a new convert. Mr. Kushi was pleased with Heather's progress, but said there was still too much water in her system and that more time and patience would be required. Gradual but continuous improvement began to bring joyous remarks about the changes in Heather. She began smiling! Cooperating! And taking less medication.

But then in July, to the great disappointment of family and friends, and mostly of Heather, she had an epileptic seizure. Because of that the family canceled vacation plans in order to keep things calm for Heather, and mustered the courage to continue reducing medication, until on August 8 all pills were stopped. The enslavement was ended.

"It still seems to be nothing short of miraculous. All our family and friends seem totally amazed and of course share our joy, for they, too, see a whole new person emerging." Reminiscent of the moment in *Amahl and the Night Visitors* when Amahl impulsively extends his handmade crutch to the Wise Men to take to the Christ-

Child as a gift — and realizes he can walk — must have been the moment when Grace asked Heather, "Well, how was school today?" and heard the reply, "It was beautiful, Mama, just beautiful!"

Meanwhile, Grace's mother had gone macrobiotic and was reporting "remarkable success in her fight against arthritis."

Still there were to be setbacks. On August 26, Michio said Heather would have only two more seizures. These occurred on November 1 and November 30. Unfortunately, too, the winter brought another debilitating attack of flu; but this time the big difference was that teachers and even the school nurse were now approving the regimen Heather had been following. For months she had been successful academically as well as personally.

And what of Maxine and Al? Well, Al was very faithful to his diet, and Maxine followed it to a considerable extent. In March of 1977 Al told us that the eye with the cataract had had no further deterioration, and the other eye had not developed a cataract. Maxine had diligently applied ginger compresses every night to Al's head, back of the neck, and eyes. To this routine, and to the food, Al attributed the fact that the Parkinson's disease was held in check even though his medication had been reduced to half dosage. He wanted very much to improve on this improvement, of course, and was hoping someday to have time enough away from his work to experiment with using no medication. During 1977 he had one two-week and one three-week trial without medication, neither time long enough for a real test. When he works, because of the need to move around freely, and to drive a car, he has to stay with the partial medication. Mari helped a great deal by using shiatsu massage and teaching the technique to Maxine; but again it's hard to find time to be consistent with such routines. Al enjoys doing part of the cooking, and Mari is going to plan some menus to be sure the balance is as accurate as possible for his needs. Time is the main hurdle: if you're an invalid you can devote your full attention to getting well, but if you're well enough to run a business, you have problems finding chances to complete the getting-well process.

Postscript: Early in March of 1976 when we talked to Grace Einsel by phone, she was happily musing about the *two thousand* pills Heather had *not* taken since August 8, and about the continued success in every other way. Her story had spoken of gratitude to Mr. Kushi "for his guidance and wisdom," for being "an inspiration to all who are fortunate enough to meet him." The family is grateful for "having been shown that nature does provide cures as well as illnesses. Macrobiotics has freed us from the bondage of medication, from the bondage of tensions and frustrations, from hopelessness to a new sense of joy."

We had another telephone visit with Grace — and even with Heroine Heather! — in early April of 1978. All news continued to be very favorable.

Grace's "Life Begins" story of Heather was printed in the Spring, 1978, issue of East West Foundation *Case Histories*. While we still hope to see it someday in a national publication, you would have a more *worthwhile* publication on hand if you ordered the EWF *Histories* (see Bibliography). In it, Heather has done an excellent job of giving her own appraisal, and Grace has added new deeply expressive comments.

A long, long distance was traversed in a short time between Grace's, "Institutional care had been recommended by the medical profession, a step we couldn't even consider," and Heather's, "I feel really great. ... My pediatrician checked me in June [1977] and said I was in fine shape."

We feel very lucky to have people like these as our friends, and we are glad that you can now know them as your friends, too. We hope their favorable experiences with macrobiotics may give you inspiration and encouragement.

Epilogue

In summary, I should like to state first that my wife and I are not attempting to display any medical expertise whatsoever. A musician-teacher and a housewife are hardly qualified to encroach on the field of medicine. So we are keeping a wide and humble distance between us and any intention of advising, diagnosing, or prescribing. We are only re-telling and informing according to our acquired information as we interpret it.

One of our main hopes is that our case histories (most of them about people we know) are convincing enough proof for sick and well people alike that they may come to realize the value of the macrobiotic approach — that sick people will thus be willing to test it against their illness and that those who are in good health will adapt at least a large percentage of the principles to ensure a life-time free of disease.

Families, in our opinion, could go a long way toward good health simply by veering in the direction of the macrobiotic harbor — by serving meat less often, finally to the point of using fish and fowl only and those in small amounts such as to flavor casseroles, by cutting back drastically on the amounts of cheese (using organic cheese if at all possible), replacing egg dishes with fish (not fried), serving the harmful vegetables as infrequently as possible, gradually drying up the fruit supply till it is indeed mostly dried fruits that grow locally, and introducing bancha tea more and more often to replace the copious present-day intake of damaging beverages (including milk, fruit juices, and vegetable juices!).

We hope also that this book and its readers will call to the attention of the medical profession the effectiveness of the macro-biotic diet. We want the latter to give it the critical judgment of working out a system of control-group testing, which is the only system that is convincing for scientifically-minded people. A few doctors are now considering the possibility of trying to develop such a program in conjunction with the East West Foundation in Boston.

There are those who will feel that we have committed a disservice in writing our book *before* medical verification can clear this method which has sometimes been called a "dangerous fad diet." But we are so certain that our claims are valid, for people who study attentively and follow instructions carefully, that we do not feel we should wait for the years of research required for control-group proof, during which time thousands of people would suffer and die instead of finding help they may be yearning for. Until such time as the medical profession becomes interested enough to make its own investigation, the only proof we have to offer are the medical records of our case history people, which can be made available to any qualified physician. Only the records of Terezia Matyas, closed off by the Iron Curtain, cannot be verified at the present time.

The question naturally arises: What about the failures? Does everyone following the macrobiotic program have nothing but success? Unfortunately, no. And unfortunately, since the background of macrobiotics has been philosophical rather than medical, records have not been kept to allow for any sort of check on percentages. (The East West Foundation is moving toward correcting this deficiency.) However, we have personally known about many successful cases beyond those we have space for in this book; and the EWF staff, of course, know of hundreds of people world-wide who have gained significant relief or have been restored to good health through macrobiotics.

Where there has not been improvement (usually in cases doctors have declared hopeless) the reasons are very often apparent: (1) perhaps long-term vacillation and procrastination in beginning the program, or (2) lack of thorough study and attention to detail if it *is* begun. There are too many people like one friend, whom we knew by correspondence only, who had pancreatic cancer and was very enthusiastic about the improvement she was making. But a few months later we were shocked to receive from her a "macrobiotic" recipe she had "invented" for spaghetti sauce. It contained *herbs, spices, tomatoes, mushrooms* — as if she had completely forgotten the restricted list or had never read it at all! She was one of those who did not survive.

Some people are not strict enough because of lack of will power (look who's talking!), or because they keep on having doubts that the program will really work. (In a few cases people do themselves harm by being *overly* strict; but usually other macrobiotic friends will notice such rigidity as this before it becomes serious.)

(3) The lack of a will to live probably causes many failures, and this is very hard to counteract, for usually there is a home situation the patient wants (subconsciously perhaps) to get away from. Even if the will to live is basically present, a home situation can be a near impossibility simply from the standpoint of logistics, as with the

young man who had a rare and fatal form of lupus erythematosus. He had realized some temporary improvement from medication but could tell he was starting to go downhill again. He and his wife came to talk with us one evening, and then worked out a very good program for themselves and their family of small children. In a few months he went from being too weak to turn off a water faucet to being able to work dawn to dusk six days a week at his construction job and then participate in winter sports in sub-zero cold on Sundays. But then, since he no longer felt ill, the food program seemed too arduous to maintain. It *is* difficult when there are several small children, to have so much food to prepare in advance, and special lunch boxes to pack instead of "picking up a quick snack" somewhere. After nearly a year the young father told us that he was amazed at the effectiveness of the diet, but felt that it was just too much trouble for long-range use. He had continued it on an irregular basis for several months and was surprised and gratified that he saw no signs of returning symptoms. This impressed him. We can only hope that if he does begin to slip backwards again he will again take advantage of macrobiotics, this time, perhaps, getting outside help to make things easier at home.

There are also those sad instances where people learn about macrobiotics only after they can no longer consistently retain food. But even in such cases as this, where families have solicitously helped the invalid to eat whatever could be retained, they reported relief from pain and sometimes much less need for sedatives.

As a matter of fact, under all types of circumstances in our experience, the macrobiotic way has measured up astonishingly well, as we hope we have shown by this account of our life and observations since August of 1973. *In every case we know of there has been at least as much, and usually considerably more, benefit from macrobiotics than would have been expected from orthodox methods.* We'd like also to call attention to the improvement in other illnesses besides cancer, although doctors we have talked to about these are very impatient with the ideas because they say these diseases ebb and flow for too many other reasons. But we think, and so do the friends who have had the illnesses, that the macrobiotic improvement is more definite than the commonly-accepted "remissions." And some of the more daring ones have made their symptoms reappear and disappear again in direct relationship to the food they eat! Thus YOU don't need to risk this sort of experimentation: others have already done it for you.

Most people on the diet will find that they will have to adhere to it rather strictly for a number of years at least, and perhaps, with occasional modifications, for the rest of their lives. But as we have pointed out before, even if harmful food is still tempting, one finds it less so because of knowing the havoc it can cause. And anyway, there are so many *safe* macrobiotic substitutes!

A reminder on discharging! This can go on for months in the form of symptoms of varying degrees of annoyance. It can seem as if some nuisance — such as bladder irritation, pain in the joints, diarrhea — will never end. But then suddenly it does run its course, and, as Ingrid Russell described it, another page is turned backwards and you're rid of one more stored-up potential illness that could have become really severe. Sometimes the discoveries are pleasant, such as realizing that the "flaking off" at the sides of your nose hasn't been there for ages, or noticing that your fingernails and lips have become, and are remaining, a healthy pink.

A final subject I feel I must mention before closing is one that we would never have thought of if we had not gone through the experience of talking to many people about our diet. I'm referring to the matter of religion. We are astounded when someone says, "I can't follow that diet because I'm a Christian." Our reaction is to wonder what in the world that has to do with it! The same people would be unlikely to say they can't go to a doctor because they are Christian, nor do they say that because they're Christian they can't "go on" a diet to lose weight.

We encourage everyone who has religious convictions to use them in every way that may be helpful. Maybe it was unseen forces in your religion, whatever religion it may be, that allowed you to find out about macrobiotics in the first place. And having guided you there it can be your partner in giving you the courage not to wander off the macrobiotic track. But don't expect it to do the job alone! Rather, it can *help* you stay involved, as farmers must be involved in growing their crops. World-wide, no matter what their nationality or religion, they can't just sit back and pray for a good yield till after they've assumed their share of the partnership and the necessary hard work.

Followers of Eastern religions may find the healthful elements of macrobiotic grains and vegetables more credible than do Westerners. However, if your background is Christian or Hebrew, the Biblical story of Daniel (1:11-16) should be persuasive for you, recounting as it does Daniel's confidence in a diet of pulse, rather than in the meat and wine offered by King Nebuchadnezzar in a test of superiority against a group of the king's people. Pulse is a porridge made of meal, vegetables, and the seeds of leguminous plants such as peas, beans, and lentils. Daniel asked for ten days of this food for himself and his friends, at the end of which time they appeared so well that they were allowed to continue. (Compare with the ten days macrobiotics claims as necessary to begin showing improvement!) Then at the end of three years, the king found Daniel and friends "in all matters of wisdom and understanding...ten times better than all the magicians and astrologers that were in all his realm." (Compare this with the macrobiotic theory that mental and spiritual faculties are heightened by proper food.)

It has been our intention to advance rather than retard the cause of good health for many people. As you have recognized in reading our book, we had a lot of help along the way. We're sure you feel well acquainted with Mari. We could never have finished the book without her expertise and artistry, nor without a similar high quality and understanding in the cooperation of our staff at our Harvest Moon Restaurant. Then, in clarifying our uncertainties, supplying us with information, and generally facilitating the organization of our material the assistance from the staff at the East West Foundation in Boston has been immeasurable. We list the names of our Moon and EWF helpers, with deepest gratitude, at the beginning of the Appendix.

We hope our readers will find our book continuously useful. Obviously each reader will have to form an individual opinion as to the direction he or she wants to take in maintaining or regaining good health. Whatever means you choose, I hope you have the kind of good fortune that came my way when I needed it!

We know it's a nearly impossible dream, but just in case many in this generation, and most people in the next generation, were to embrace the way of macrobiotics, it would be as if the human race had finally returned home after a long and arduous journey.

Appendix

(including occasional bits of gossip)

As mentioned in the Epilogue, we would like to bestow accolades on full-time staff members who worked at our Harvest Moon Restaurant during the last few months this book was in "intensive care": Gloria Alva Walter, our manager; Teresa Avila, Shari Flanders, Susan Groves, Veralu King, Ruth Grobey Herr, Molly Reeves, Barbara Torchio, and our ever-dedicated publicity agent, Freda Zegman. Then we include those who "lifted off" from the Moon to important natural foods situations in other locations: Rick Roy Ratican, Betsey Kiel and Peter Murray, Dan and Alison Plummer, Chris Smith, Susie Sufana and Barbara Parrott Williams, who with her husband Robby created their own fine restaurant and bakery in Atlanta, Indiana — "Our Daily Bread." Our gratitude is continuous to Paul Justad, a young business administration major who has made a special project of finding ways to correct the rocky financial orbit of the Moon, and to Dan Walter, manager at Mazda Natural Foods, who is even more invaluable to us than the store itself!

During this same period, the following friends, being at one time or another on the staff of the East West Foundation in Boston, were indispensable in easing many of our problems: Edward Esko, vice-president; Stephen Uprichard, vice-president; Ken Burns, Wendy Esko, Jack Garvy, Sherman Goldman (editor of the excellent *East West Journal),* Tim Goodwin, Rod House, Lenny Jacobs, Ann Stevens LaFlair, Olivia Oredson, Mona Schwartz, Bill Tims, Teresa Turner, Tamra Uprichard, Phil Janetta. You will recognize some of these names as belonging to people who have been "graduated" to start in far-flung locations the East West Centers we list below. And you will also remember some of them from the Case Histories in Chapter 14. The dedication of these and hundreds of other friends in working to enlarge the scope of the EWF stems from the macrobiotic relief they received in overcoming various illnesses and miseries which were ruining their lives.

MACROBIOTIC CENTERS

East West Foundation: federally approved, non-profit, educational and cultural institution, 359 Boylston Street, Boston 02116,

APPENDIX   271

phone (617) 536-3360. The Foundation is qualified also in Maryland, Pennsylvania, Florida, and Washington, D.C. At many of the Centers listed here there is a great deal of activity, providing a constant bustle of workshops, seminars, cooking classes, instruction in shiatsu (acupressure) massage, and other promotions. At all of them you can find a lot of information about macrobiotic food, cooking, and philosophy, offered with all-encompassing understanding and friendship. But before you count on visiting a Center, make a phone call, for before the rough draft of this page is finished there will already be changes! Many restaurants, as we well know, are especially uncertain as to their status from one week to the next. *(We will save space in the list by not repeating "East West Center," nor the name of the state, in each address.)*

ARIZONA: Bob Salazar, 620 W Howe St., Tempe 85281. (602) 966-9076.
CALIFORNIA: David Hinckle, 204 Baywater, Burlingame 94010. (415) 347-2058 /// John Fountain, c/o Erewhon, 8454 Steller Dr., Culver City 95436. (213) 836-7726 /// Patrick McCarty and Merideth James, 1137 G St., Eureka 95501. (707) 445-2290 /// Joseph Arseguel, P.O. Box 37, Forestville 95436. (707) 887-2828 /// Roy and Marijke Steevensz, East West Center for Macrobiotic Studies, 1756 N Sierra Bonita Av., Los Angeles 90046. (213) 876-9153 /// Inaka Restaurant, 131 S LaBrea Av., Los Angeles 90036. (213) 932-9895 /// Mrs. Gooch's Natural Food Store, Los Angeles — not an EWF Center, but one of the most outstanding stores anywhere. By the time you read this there will be at least two stores (see Chapter 10, and addresses near the end of the Appendix). /// Jacques and Yvette DeLangre, 160 Wycliff Way, Magalia 95954. (916) 873-0294 (see Bibliography for their *essential* books on massage!) /// George Ohsawa Macrobiotic Foundation (G.O.M.F.), 1544 Oak St., Oroville 95965. (916) 533-7702. Established in 1971 by Herman and Cornelia Aihara for the purpose of disseminating the teachings of macrobiotic scholars as well as those of other persuasions, the Foundation accomplishes its purpose through workshops and publications: books, pamphlets, and a high-quality monthly magazine, *The Macrobiotic,* plus sponsorship of a retreat-type summer camp for natural, self-sufficient living. The Aiharas, early leaders in this way of life, are now internationally famous among macrobiotic people through their books and their extensive travels to give instruction at seminars all over the world. (A choice bit: on some cookbooks, you will see the spelling *Cornelia;* but we have it straight from a member of their staff that she now prefers *Cornelia-San* — one *l,* and the suffix which would compare with our Deep South "Miss Cornelia." Friends and students also say "Herman-san," for which we know no equivalent. "Uncle" Herman,

maybe?) /// Smith's Sandwich Shuttle — at least that's what we're calling it until Chris makes his own decision on a name for his unique, innovative enterprise, taken over from a friend in June, 1978. Chris was one of our Harvest Moon staff members, and his new business consists of selling *macrobiotic* sandwiches (chapati for bread, and tofu, sprouts, vegetables, etc., for stuffing) to retail outlets. (Not yet an East West Center in 1978, but something this clever *should* be!) 639 W 16th St., Richmond 94801. (415) 237-6832 /// Good Karma Cafe, 501 Dolores St., San Francisco 94110. (415) 621-4112 ///

COLORADO: Frank and Marion Calpeno, 1013 Venus Dr., Colorado Springs 80906. (303) 475-2554 /// Lynn Pitt-Taylor, 3881 S Sherman, Englewood 80110. (303) 761-3846 ///

FLORIDA: Sanford Pukel and Mona Schwartz, P.O. Box 330892, 3043 Grand Av., Coconut Grove 33133. (305) 446-0120. Mona: (305) 446-0548 /// Oakfeed Restaurant, 3008 Grand Av., Coconut Grove 33133. (305) 448-0076 /// Su-shin Restaurant, 3339 Virginia Av., Coconut Grove 33133 ///

GEORGIA: Unity Natural Food Market, 2915 Peachtree Road, NE, Atlanta 30305. (404) 261-0110 ///

ILLINOIS: John and Charlotte Palumbo, 2525 W Gunnison St., Chicago 60625. (312) 561-8023 /// Plowshare Natural Food Restaurant (and store), 6155 N Broadway, Chicago 60660. (312) 761-0500 /// Larry Pagni, For Goodness Sake! Natural Food Centre, Plaza de las Flores, 1608 E Algonquin Rd., Schaumburg 60195. (312) 397-7292 ///

INDIANA: Gary and Judith Viehe, 259 Washington Av., Evansville 47713. (812) 425-0777 /// Harvest Moon Natural Foods Restaurant, 207 N Dill St., Muncie 47303. (317) 289-8194, c/o Mr. and Mrs. Jean Kohler 2900 Torquay Rd., Muncie 47304. (317) 282-0761 /// See below for Mazda Natural Foods (grocery) and Our Daily Bread (restaurant and bakery) — not East West Centers, however) ///

KANSAS: Jim Sleeper, Box 44, Alden 67512. (316) 534-3685 ///

MAINE: Larry Landau, Box 525 A, Kennebunkport 04046. (207) 967-4070 ///

MARYLAND: Murray and Pam Snyder, 6209 Park Heights Av., Baltimore 21215. (301) 358-5143 ///

MASSACHUSETTS: Main offices in Boston, as listed under MACRO-BIOTIC CENTERS, above. William Tims, director, having trained as manager of the important Center in Atlanta, Georgia /// Sanae Restaurant, 272A Newbury St., Boston 02115. (617) 247-8434 /// Seventh Inn Restaurant, 67 Providence St., Boston 02116. (617) 261-3965 /// Jim and Janet Sadler, 5 King Av., Florence 01060. (413) 586-4592 /// Joseph and Diane Avoli, 32 Burncoat St., Worcester 01605. (617) 852-8816 ///

MICHIGAN: Carlos Meeuws, 3800 Dexter Rd., Ann Arbor 48103. (313) 662-6135 /// Michael Potter, c/o Eden Foods, 4601 Platt Rd., Ann

Arbor 48104. (313) 973-9400 /// Don Wycoff, Good Earth Foods (an *excellent* restaurant!), 546 Portage Rd., Kalamazoo 49006. (616) 343-3622 ///

MINNESOTA: Tom and Jean Hurrle, 1447 Durand Ct., Rochester 55901. (507) 289-2997 /// Russell and Linda Desmarais, 993 Portland Av., St. Paul 55104. (612) 226-7472 ///

MISSOURI: Bill Worden and Dale Deraps, Rte. 3, Box 114, Bowling Green 63334. (314) 669-2222 ///

NEW MEXICO: Bill Rosenburg, 408 Salazar Pl., Santa Fe 87501. (505) 988-1695 ///

NEW YORK: Shizuko Yamamoto, 40 E 12th St., Penthouse B, New York 10003. (212) 674-8490. Teaching in New York, and traveling widely, Ms. Yamamoto is highly esteemed for her instruction in the art of shiatsu massage! /// Cauldron Restaurant, 306 E 6th St., New York 10003. (212) 473-9543 /// East West Cookery, 105 E 9th St., New York 10003. (212) 260-1994 /// Sou-En Restaurant, 2444 Broadway, New York 10024. (212) 787-1110 /// Gary and Sharon Goldberg, 589 Washington Av., Albany 12206. (518) 465-4124 /// Michael and Melanie Melia, 437 Forest Av., Locust Valley 11560. (516) 676-7895 ///

OHIO: Edward and Virginia Kluska, New World Center, 3408 Telford, Cincinnati 45220. (513) 961-6400 /// New World Foodshop Restaurant, 347 Ludlow Av., Cincinnati 45220. (513) 861-1101 ///

PENNSYLVANIA: Denny and Judith Waxman, 6 Radcliffe Rd., Bala Cynwyd 19004. (215) 664-1218 ///

TEXAS: Frank and Phyllis Head, 5001 Lynwood, Austin 78756, (512) 459-0670 /// Dr. Norman Ralston, 426 N Buckner, Dallas 75217. (214) 391-3713 ///

WASHINGTON, D.C.: Edward and Wendy Esko, Washington, D.C., Macrobiotic Study Center, 3512 Cummings Lane, Chevy Chase, MD 20015. (301) 657-3329 /// Michael and Jeanne Rossoff, P.O. Box 40012. Zip 20016. (703) 920-2083 ///

WEST VIRGINIA: Jeffrey Esko, Terry Shaffer, Rte. 11, Box 425, Morgantown 26505. (504) 599-3661 ///

International

ARGENTINA: Fundacion Macrobiotica, Perla Jacobovitz, Irene Brocca, Uruguay 1011, Buenos Aires, Argentina ///

AUSTRALIA: Bruce Gyngell, 25 Vaucluse Road, Vaucluse, NSW 2030 /// Daniel Weber, Marcea Newman, Box 496, Double Bay, 2028 ///

BELGIUM: Mark Callebert, Eendracht Straat 37, 9000 Ghent /// Frans Copers, Soven, Hoogpoort 22, Ghent. Phone (091) 23-58-60 /// Boudewijn De Graeve, c/o The Natural Way, Overmeers 40 A, 9821

Afsnee, Ghent /// John-Pierre Dobbelaire, Tennispod 2, 8.300, Knokke /// Pierre Gaevert, Lima Factory, St. Martin, Latem /// Dr. Marc and Suzanne Van Cauwenberghe, Gebroeders Vandeveldestraat 7, Ghent. Phone (091) 23.47.47 /// George Van Wesenbeck, De Brandnetel, Consciense Straat 48, 2000 Antwerp. Phone (050) 60.11.86 ///

BRAZIL: Tomio Kikuchi, Centro Macrobiotico do Brazil, Praca Carlos Gomes, 60-1.0 andar Liberdade, San Paulo. Phone 732-9738 /// Perudah de F. Neves, Associacao Macrobiotica, Rue Marechal Floriano, de Porto Alegre, 72 (terre) (CX.P. 2956), 90.000 Porto Alegre, Rio Grande Do Sul. Phone 25-47-87 ///

CANADA: W. Ray Switzer, 11601-85 St., Edmonton, Alberta. Phone 4776646 /// Duncan and Susan Sim, Box 1620, Fernie, B.C. /// Marjorie Webster, Lower Montague, Prince Edward Island /// Yves Ducharme, 6574 Lebreton St., Montreal PQ, Canada H1M 1L5 /// Claude and Francine Paiement, 6672 St. Denis, Montreal H25 2R9 /// Vert D-Est Restaurant, 969 Rachel St., Montreal /// Stella Belair, 171 Percy St., Ottawa, Ontario. Phone (613) 233-4384 /// Gene and Doris Newman, 10 Brook Av., Toronto, Ontario. Phone (416) 481-5027 /// Verne Verona, Melanie Norman, c/o North American Shiatsu Institute, P.O. Box 1139-A, Vancouver, Canada V6C 2T1. Phone (604) 874-2258 ///

COLOMBIA: Luis Eduardo Molina, Carrera 15 No. 87-94, Apto. 401, Bogota, D. E. ///

COSTA RICA: Julio H. Garcia, Oficina de Planificacion, Nacional Apartado 10127, San Jose, Costa Rica, Central America ///

ENGLAND: Bill Tara, Community Health Foundation, 188 Old St., London EC1 ///

FRANCE: Aux Quatre Oceans, 46 rue des Gravilliers, 75 Paris — 3e. Phone 277-81-08 /// Clim Yoshimi, Mme. Riviere, Institut Tenryu, 8 rue Rochebrune, Paris 75011. Phone 805-91-35 ///

GERMANY: Richard Theobald, An der Kapellenmuhle 6, D-6630 Saarlouis, West Germany. Phone 06831, 40201 /// Richard and Elisabeth Hau, Burgenlandstrasse 104, D. 7000 Stuttgart 30 ///

HOLLAND: Adelbert and Wieke Nelissen, 17-19 Achtergracht, Amsterdam — 1017 WL. Phone 20-24-02-03 ///

INDIA: Dr. Chandrasekkhar G. Thakkur, 375 Kalbadevi, Bombay — 2. Phone 31-59-87, 31-53-52 ///

ITALY: Alois Grassani, Jussi 18, 40068, S. Lazzaro, Savena, Bologna ///

JAPAN: Alcan Yamaguchi, 2 Yamano-Moto-Machi, Kitashirakawa, Sakyo-Ku, Kyoto /// Miles Roberts, Meiji Toyo Igakuin, Kotobuki-Cho 1-20-19, Suita City, Osaka Pref. /// Sekai Seishoku Kyokai — 28,

9-Chome Tani Machi, Tennoji-Ku, Osaka /// Mr. Eiwan Ishida, 7-13 Wadamachi, Takasaki, Phone 0273-33-5484 /// Lima Ohsawa, Masanori Hasimoto, Eiji Kohso, Nippon Centre Ignoramus (also called Nippon C. I. Foundation), 11-5 Ohyamacho, Shibuya-Ku, Tokyo, Japan T 151 ///

PORTUGAL: Jose Gomes Ribeiro and Rosa Maria Calado, c/o Chacra, Rua Augusto Machado, 5—1°—Dt°, Lisboa /// Augusto Leal, Unimave, Centro Macrobiotico Vegetariano, S.C.A.R.L., Rua da Boa Vista 55-2, Lisboa-2 ///

SPAIN: Stephen and Tamra Uprichard left the EWF in Boston in May of 1978 to set up a Center in Spain! The address is Avenida Palma de Mallorca, 43 Torremolinos, Malaga, Spain ///

SWEDEN: SMS (Swedish Macrobiotic Society), c/o Jan Erik Wennerlund, Bergsunds Strand 29 IV, 11738 Stockholm ///

SWITZERLAND: Groupe Macrobiotique, c/o Ted Stadlin, 3 Chemin Francois Lehmann, 1218 Geneva. Phone 98.14.59 /// Wilhelm Keller, Wildbachstrasse 77, CH-8008 Zurich. Phone 01-554826 ///

URUGUAY: Dr. Mateo J. Margarinos de Mello, Echevarriarza 3396, Montevideo, Phone 78-1024 ///

VENEZUELA: Zen-tro Macrobiotico de Venezuela, P.O. Box 51600, Este 105, Caracas, Venezuela ///

Miscellaneous Addresses mentioned in our text:

Michio Kushi stated in his February, 1978, lecture at the United Nations that more than 10,000 food stores in this country are carrying high quality natural foods. But if you're traveling it seems that most of them, as well as most natural food restaurants, are new enough that they're hard to locate. (Often they are too poor to do much advertising, but the *East West Journal* now carries a monthly page for those that can afford it.) In addition to the restaurants and stores among the East West Centers, above, we list a very few others in which we have a personal interest:

Our Daily Bread, 115 E Main St., Atlanta, Indiana 46031. (317) 292-2308 /// Mazda Natural Foods (one of the best-stocked stores in the Midwest), 507 W McGalliard Rd., Muncie, Indiana 47303. (317) 747-9428 /// Eden Foods (store and restaurant), 330 Maynard, Ann Arbor, Michigan 48107. (313) 971-8274. Eden Foods (large-quantity wholesale supplier to businesses and co-ops), 4601 Platt Rd., Ann Arbor 48104. (313) 973-9400 /// Mrs. Gooch's Natural Food Store, 3476 Centinela Av., West Los Angeles, California 90066. (213) 391-5209. Store #2: 526 Pier Av., Hermosa Beach, California. A third was being planned in 1978 /// The *East West Journal* is building up a mail order service to send packages of macrobiotic food. They list their products each month in the *Journal.* (Ask also for a small fine-grater with tray (for ginger, daikon, etc.) 233 Harvard St., Brookline, Massachusetts 02146 ///

Other information related to food: For non-chemicalized cheese made from the milk of organically-fed cows (!): Eilers Cheese Market, Route 2, DePere, Wisconsin 54115. (414) 336-8292. (They don't seem to like to answer mail, so you'd better phone.) /// For many garden seeds needed by macrobiotic people: Johnny's Selected Seeds, Albion, Maine 04910. (207) 437-4303 /// For information on preserving foods by drying: Order flyer from East West Foundation, 359 Boylston St., Boston 02116. Our own summary of the government pamphlets described in Chapter VI is also available from the Foundation.

Alternative cancer-control methods: Kelley Research Foundation, Winthrop, Washington 98862. (509) 997-5405. ("One Answer to Cancer" — see Bibliography) /// Dr. O. Carl Simonton, M.D., D.A.B.R., Oncology Associates, 1413 Eighth Av., Ft. Worth, Texas 76104. (817) 926-7821 /// Ms. Charlotte Gerson Strauss, Mr. Norman Fritz, Gerson Institute, P.O. Box 535, Imperial Beach, California 92032. (714) 575-0967. The Institute is non-profit and educational, teaching doctors and laymen (no chemotherapy patients accepted). A large center, including a hospital with several physicians on the staff and elaborate rehabilitation facilities, is a partially realized goal.

For Massage (EXTREMELY BENEFICIAL!): Dō-In (doe-een) — "the most ancient and effective healing art" — Books I and II, plus supplementary wall-chart and cassette tape if desired, providing a method of self-improvement based on acupressure massage and breathing exercises, utilizing ki energy. Happiness Press, Jacques and Yvette DeLangre, 160 Wycliff Way, Magalia, California 95954. (916) 873-0294 ///

BIBLIOGRAPHY
(with confidential comments)

Literature available from the East West Foundation, 359 Boylston St., Boston, MA 02116. (Phone: (617) 536-3360) (Order a copy of each publication for each room in your house; use these books for Christmas, graduation, wedding, and anniversary gifts! Ask about possible discounts on quantity orders.):

Books

Esko, Edward, ed., *Macrobiotics: Experience the Miracle of Life,* Boston, MA: East West Foundation, 1978. An introduction to basic macrobiotic principles, from lectures of Michio Kushi.

Esko, Wendy, *An Introduction to Macrobiotic Cooking.* Boston, MA: East West Foundation, 1978. Preparation of macrobiotic meals, including special sections on desserts, soups, breads, "extra touches."

Kushi, Aveline, *How to Cook with Miso.* Tokyo, Japan: Japan Publications, Inc., 1978.

Kushi, Michio, *The Book of Dō-In* (pronounced doe-een). Tokyo, Japan: Japan Publications, Inc., 1978.

Kushi, Michio, *The Book of Macrobiotics: The Universal Way of Health and Happiness.* Tokyo, Japan: Japan Publications, Inc., 1977.

Kushi, Michio, *An Introduction to Oriental Diagnosis,* ed. William Tara (see Appendix: ENGLAND). London, England: Sunwheel, Ltd., 1978.

Kushi, Michio, *The Macrobiotic Way of Natural Healing,* ed. Edward Esko, with Marc Van Cauwenberghe, M.D. Boston, MA: East West Foundation, 1978.

Kushi, Michio, *Teachings of Michio Kushi,* Vol. I: *The Spiral of Life.* Boston, MA: East West Foundation, 1977.

Kushi, Michio, *Teachings of Michio Kushi,* Vol. II: *The Origin and Destiny of Man.* Boston, MA: East West Foundation, 1978.

Periodicals

East West Journal, a monthly newspaper. 233 Harvard Street, Brookline, MA 02146. "Explores the dynamic equilibrium that unifies apparently opposite values: Oriental and Occidental, traditional and modern, religious and technological, communal and individual, visionary and practical." Varied, significant material of lasting interest.

Macrobiotic Case Histories, three times per year. Boston, MA: East West Foundation.

The Order of the Universe, quarterly magazine. Boston, MA: East West Foundation. Contains lectures of Michio Kushi and other macrobiotic leaders.

SPECIAL PUBLICATIONS of the East West Foundation, available from the address above:

"A Dietary Approach to Cancer" (according to the Principles of Macrobiotics). Includes "Kass research" on blood pressure and cholesterol mentioned in our Chapters 6 and 8.

"Food Policy Recommendations for the United States." Copies of statements made at the White House on September 21, 1977, by Michio Kushi and macrobiotic associates. This was a two-hour meeting with key government representatives on agriculture, health issues, and food policy.

"A Nutritional Approach to Cancer." A report of the Medical Conference sponsored by the EWF, March 9, 1977, mentioned in our Chapter 6.

Available from Redwing Book Co., 303-B Newbury Street, Boston, MA 02115. (Phone: (617) 267-3338):

DeLangre, Jacques, *Do-In* (doe-een), Books I and II. Magalia, CA: Happiness Press, 1971. (Or, order from DeLangre — discount on quantity orders.)

Illich, Ivan, *Medical Nemesis.* New York, NY: Random House, Inc., 1976, Pantheon Books, 1976.

Muramoto, Naboru, *Healing Ourselves,* ed. Michel Abehsera, from lectures of Muramoto. Binghamton, NY: Swan House Publishing Company; New York, NY: Avon Books, 1973.

Ohsawa, Georges, *Cancer and the Philosophy of the Far East* (Paris, France, 1963), ed. Herman Aihara, trans. Armand la Belle and Ralph Baccash. Binghamton, NY: Swan House Publishing Company, 1971.

Smith, Adam, *Powers of the Mind.* New York, NY: Random House, Inc., 1975.

COOKBOOKS (Redwing Book Co., unless otherwise indicated) Remember to adapt all recipes according to suggestions immediately following the recipe section in our Chapter 13.

Abehsera, Michel, *Cooking for Life.* Binghamton, NY: Swan House Publishing Company, copyright Michel Abehsera 1970, 1972; New York, NY: Avon Books, 1976.

Abehsera, Michel, *Zen Macrobiotic Cooking.* New Hyde Park, NY: University Books, Inc.; New York, NY: Avon Books, First Avon Printing, 1970, Fourth Printing, 1971.

Aihara, Cornelia-San, *Chico-San Cookbook.* See G.O.M.F. Books, below.

Aihara, Cornelia-San, *The Do of Cooking* (pronounced *doe!*). See G.O.M.F., below.

Esko, Wendy, *An Introduction to Macrobiotic Cooking.* See above, East West Foundation BOOKS.

Farmilant, Eunice, *Natural Foods Sweet Tooth Cookbook.* New York, NY: New American Library; Signet Books. (Mostly for parties — use sparingly!)

Ford, Marjorie Winn, Susan Hillyard, and Mary Faulk Koock, *Deaf Smith Country Cookbook,* New York, NY: Collier Books, 1973.

Hurd, Frank J., D.C., and Rosalie Hurd, *Ten Talents.* Chisholm, MN: Dr. and Mrs. Frank J. Hurd, 1968.

Kushi, Aveline, *How to Cook with Miso.* See above, East West Foundation BOOKS.

Ohsawa, Lima, with Nahum Stiskin, *The Art of Just Cooking.* New York; NY: Autumn Press, 1974.

Teeguarden, Iona, *Freedom through Cooking.* See G.O.M.F. Books, below.

Available from the George Ohsawa Macrobiotic Foundation (G.O.M.F.), 1544 Oak St., Oroville, CA 95965. (Phone: (916) 533-7702) See their listing in our Appendix: CALIFORNIA. You may wish to ask for a list of all the books they publish. Two of those below are in our Cancer Victims and Friends section, to help that group; but if you prefer, order from the G.O.M.F., whose goals are also commendable:

Aihara, Cornelia-San, *Chico-San Cookbook.* Held in high regard by Cooks of excellence, this was first published in 1972 by Chico-San, Inc., in Chico, CA. Now by G.O.M.F.

Aihara, Cornelia-San, *The Do of Cooking.* Four books, one for each season of the year — helpful guidance! That word *Do* is pronounced like *doe* (yes, like *dough!),* and translates to something like "natural order."

Morishita, Kieichi, M.D., *The Hidden Truth of Cancer.* See IACVF section below.

Ohsawa, Georges, *Book of Judgment.* Written in 1956. Copyright G.O.M.F. 1966.

Ohsawa, Georges, *Zen Macrobiotics.* See IACVF section, below.

Teeguarden, Iona, *Freedom through Cooking* ("written through Iona Teeguarden"). First published in 1971 by Order of the Universe Publications (East West Foundation), by G.O.M.F. in 1978.

Available from International Association of Cancer Victims and Friends, Inc. (IACVF), 7740 West Manchester Av., Suite 110, Playa del Rey, CA 90291. (Phone: (213) 822-5032 or 822-5132):

Abrahamson, E.M., M.D., and A.W. Pezet, *Body, Mind and Sugar.* New York, NY: Holt, Rinehart, & Winston, Inc., 1951.

Dufty, William, *Sugar Blues,* Radnor, PA: Chilton Book Co., 1975.

Haught, S.J., *Has Dr. Max Gerson a True Cancer Cure?* North Hollywood, CA: London Press, 1962; Twelfth Printing, 1975.

Hunberger, Edyie Mae, and Chris Loeffter, *How I Conquered Cancer Naturally.* San Diego, CA: Production House. (Ann Wigmore's wheat grass, its juice, and other natural foods).

Hutschnecker, Arnold A., M.D., *The Will to Live.* Englewood Cliffs, NJ: Prentice-Hall, Inc., 1961; rev. ed., 1977.

Kelley, William D., D.D.S., *One Answer to Cancer.* Winthrop, Washington: Kelley Research Foundation, Ninth Impression, 1973; rev. ed., 1974.

Kervran, Louis, *Biological Transmutations,* 'rans. M. Abehsera. Paris, France: Maloine, 1962; Binghamton, NY: Swan House Publishing Company, 1972.

Kloss, Jethro, *Back to Eden.* New York, NY: Benedict Lust Publications; Beneficial Books, 1971; Kloss-family ed., 1975.

Livingston, Virginia Wuerthele-Caspe, M.D., *Cancer — a New Breakthrough.* Los Angeles, CA: Nash Publishing Corp., 1972.

Morishita, Kieichi, M.D., *The Hidden Truth of Cancer,* trans. Herman Aihara, Oroville, CA: George Ohsawa Macrobiotic Foundation, 1972.

Morris, Nat, *The Cancer Blackout Amended.* Los Angeles, CA: Regent House, 1976.

Ohsawa, Georges, *Zen Macrobiotics.* Oroville, CA: George Ohsawa Macrobiotic Foundation, 1965.

Available from American Media, P.O. Box 4646, Westlake Village, CA 91359. (Phone: (213) 889-1231):

Corbett, Thomas H., M.D., *Cancer and Chemicals.* Chicago, IL: Nelson-Hall, Inc., 1977.

Davison, Jaquie, *Cancer Winner: How I Purged Myself of Melanoma.* Pierce City, MO: Pacific MO, 1977.

Griffin, Edward G., *World Without Cancer,* Part I and Part II. Thousand Oaks, CA: American Media, Third Printing, 1975.

Heinsohn, Douglas L., *Cancer, Metabolic Therapy, and Laetrile.* Sevierville, TN: Crescent Publishing Company, 1977.

Richardson, John A., M.D., and Patricia Griffin, R.N., *Laetrile Case Histories — the Richardson Cancer Clinic Experience.* Westlake Village, CA: American Media, 1977.

Public Scrutiny (recommended by American Media), published 12 times a year by VOCAL (Victory Over Cancer Action League, a non-profit organization, P.O. Box 4228, Westlake Village, CA 91359. A semi-annual contribution of $3 or $4 is suggested (requested!). We interpret their stated goals as aiming toward complete freedom of choice, for patients and doctors, in the treatment of illness.

Try your favorite bookstore:

Cannon, Walter, *The Wisdom of the Body*. New York, NY: W.W. Norton & Co., Inc., 1963; 2nd ed., Magnolia, MA: Peter Smith, Publisher Inc.

Capra, Fritjof, *The Tao of Physics*. Boulder, CO: Shambhala Publications, Inc., 1975.

Dong, Collin H., M.D., and Jane Banks, *The Arthritic's Cookbook*. New York, NY: Thomas Y. Crowell, 1973. (Not listed with cookbooks because it is unrelated to macrobiotics, and because it seems as much story as cookbook).

Dong, Collin H., M.D., and Jane Banks, *New Hope for the Arthritic*. New York, NY: Thomas Y. Crowell, 1975.

Murphy, Joseph, D.D., D.R.S., Ph.D., LL.D., Fellow of the Andhra Research, University of India, *The Power of Your Subconscious Mind*. Englewood Cliffs, NJ: Prentice-Hall, Inc., 1963; Seventeenth Printing, Reward Books, 1974.

Selye, Hans, M.D., *The Stress of Life*. New York, NY; Toronto, Canada; London, England: McGraw-Hill Book Company, 1956.

Simonton, O. Carl, M.D., and Stephanie Matthews-Simonton, *Getting Well Again*. Los Angeles, CA: J.P. Tarcher, Inc., 1978. (9110 Sunset Blvd., Los Angeles 90069)

Stickle, Robert W., *One Man's Fight to Control Malignancy*. Atlanta, TX: Natural Food Associates, 1976. (NFA Bookstore, P.O. Box 210, Atlanta, TX 75551)

Tompkins, Peter, and Christopher Bird, *The Secret Life of Plants*. New York, NY: Harper & Row Publishers, Inc., 1973; Avon Books, 1974.

For information mentioned in our Chapter 6:

Honorof, Ida, "A Report to the Consumer," P.O. Box 5449, Sherman Oaks, CA 91303.

Honorof, Ida, and Eleanor McBean, *Vaccinations — the Silent Killer*. Lynwood, CA: Honor Publications, 1978. (2901 Los Flores Blvd., Lynwood 90262) An expose of an unsuspected danger.

For valuable breathing exercises mentioned in our Chapter 12 (in addition to those in DeLangre (Redwing, above) and in various yoga methods):

Summit Lighthouse Publications, Institute of Mental Physics, P.O. Box 640, Yucca Valley, CA 92284. For their philosophical information: Summit University, Box A, Malibu, CA 90265.

Available from the U.S. Government:

A Paper presented on July 28, 1976, to the Select Committee on Nutrition and Human Needs, U.S. Congress, by Gio B. Gori, deputy director of the Division of Cancer Cause and Prevention, Department of Health, Education, and Welfare, Public Health Service, National Institutes of Health, Bethesda, MD 20014.

"Dietary Goals for the United States," prepared by the Select Committee on Nutrition and Human Needs, U.S. Congress, Sen. George McGovern, chm., February, 1977. Order from Superintendent of Documents, U.S. Government Printing Office, Washington, D.C. 20402. (95¢ in 1977) Sen. McGovern apparently intended to keep this project alive, as evidenced by such news releases as those in the *Washington Post* and in UPI articles of June 13 and 14, 1978, reporting on U.S. Senate Nutrition Sub-committee hearings. The director of the National Cancer Institute, in response to nutrition deficiencies revealed by the "Dietary Goals," declared that the Institute would be willing to allocate somewhat less money to virus research and more to cancer-and-nutrition relationship if they could find qualified researchers willing to undertake the investigations.

MISCELLANEOUS PERIODICALS:

"The Cures Doctors Can't Explain" was a very enlightening article in McCall's Magazine of April, 1975, which we hope you can locate in your public library. The subject matter was related to books such as *The Power of Your Subconscious Mind,* listed in our "bookstore" section above, and to articles on mental and physical well-being such as appear frequently in *New Realities* (formerly *Psychic Magazine),* a significant bi-monthly magazine to which you may want to subscribe: P.O. Box 26289, San Francisco, CA 94126. Try to get back-issue Vol. II, No. 1, for April, 1978, for a special issue on wholistic health, greater public awareness, and national government stirrings of interest in this awareness. We hope your library will also have a copy of the *Boston Sunday Globe* magazine section *(New England)* for December 4, 1977. Charles Radin's "The Message of Michio Kushi" (p. 67) is an excellent survey of macrobiotics, at once comprehensive and concise.

Index